PRODUCT GUIDE TO
SKIN &
WOUND
CARE

Eighth Edition

Cathy Thomas Hess, RN, BSN, CWCN
Harrisburg, Pennsylvania
2020

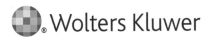 Wolters Kluwer

Philadelphia • Baltimore • New York • London
Buenos Aires • Hong Kong • Sydney • Tokyo

Acquisitions Editor: Nicole Dernoski
Editorial Coordinator: John Larkin
Design Coordinator: Joan Wendt
Manufacturing Coordinator: Kathy Brown
Prepress Vendor: Aptara, Inc.

Eighth edition
Copyright © 2020 Wolters Kluwer.

9 8 7 6 5 4 3 2 1

Printed in Mexico

Library of Congress Cataloging-in-Publication Data

Names: Hess, Cathy Thomas, 1961- author.
Title: Product guide to skin & wound care / Cathy Thomas Hess.
Other titles: Clinical guide to skin & wound care | Product guide to skin and wound care |
    Skin & wound care | Skin and wound care
Description: Eighth edition. | Philadelphia : Wolters Kluwer, [2019] |
    Preceded by Clinical guide to skin & wound care / Cathy Thomas Hess. 7th ed. c2013. |
    Includes bibliographical references and index.
Identifiers: LCCN 2018061424 | ISBN 9781496388094
Subjects: | MESH: Wounds and Injuries–nursing | Bandages | Skin Care–methods |
    Wound Healing | Handbook
Classification: LCC RD95 | NLM WY 49 | DDC 617.1/4–dc23
    LC record available at https://lccn.loc.gov/2018061424

shop.lww.com

Preface

Welcome to the eighth edition of the *Product Guide to Skin & Wound Care!* Your special contribution to wound care is always at the forefront of my efforts each time I revise this worldwide clinical reference and showcase the latest skin and wound care products. I continually strive to bring you the most up-to-date clinical product information and reference materials, and this edition continues with that same tradition—to provide you with relevant information necessary to support the "delicate balance of art and science" in skin and wound care.

We all know that chronic wounds take an emotional toll on patients and their caregivers. As clinicians and physicians, we often feel frustrated and confused when faced with certain skin and wound care options—whether attempting to choose an appropriate product to use on a specific wound type, deciding to change to another dressing to provide the best direction for the wound healing process, determining how to illustrate the wound's progress through appropriate documentation, or providing the best way to benchmark outcomes based on care practices. As dedicated professionals, we find ourselves looking for the best guidance, most reliable tools, and ready answers.

The answers, as it turns out, are commonly found through the delicate balance of art and science: *Art* as it refers to the skill and application techniques utilized when applying the preferred management modality, and *Science* as it refers to the health care team member's knowledge and understanding of the disease process and the preferred modality used in managing the patient. *Art and science*, the fundamental tools of skin and wound healing, directly impact the patient's clinical and financial outcomes.

This edition of the *Product Guide to Skin & Wound Care* focuses solely on the importance of a complete skin and wound care formulary. The section on "Skin Care Products" covers skin cleansers, moisture barriers, antifungal/antimicrobial treatments, therapeutic moisturizers, liquid skin protectants, and other skin care products of interest. Separate sections on "Dressings and Devices" and "Drugs" provide cutting-edge choices for formulary development. Debuting in this edition is "Cellular and Tissue-based Products" as a separate category.

Numerous new products have been introduced within the wound care categories highlighted in these sections. In addition, references for individual products can be found within each product page, if provided by the manufacturer.

Included in this edition are hundreds of individual wound care product profiles and photos. Each profile describes the product in detail, including the product's form, available sizes, actions, indications and contraindications, and application and removal instructions. Photos are displayed on each page, whenever possible. HCPCS codes and sizes are also displayed, when available. Every attempt has been made to accurately detail the product's information. It remains the clinician's responsibility to review each product's insert prior to using the product to ensure accurate and timely information.

Additional dressings and products for effective skin and wound management section details compression bandage systems, as well as various gauze dressings, tapes, wound cleansers, and more. HCPCS codes and sizes are displayed, when available.

The book concludes with a comprehensive list of the manufacturer's websites for your reference.

New products are being introduced to the market all the time. In an effort to have the most up-to-date product information available for you at your fingertips, we have included new products (that were unable to be in the printed book version) within the ebook version only. These can be accessed on the VitalSource ebook and are indicated in the table of contents with an electronic icon ⊙. Instructions for accessing these products can be found on the inside front cover.

Product Guide to Skin & Wound Care, eighth edition, continues to prove to be an essential skin and wound care reference for all team members. Use this book as either a "bedside" or "desk" reference when caring for your patients.

Acknowledgments

"When you learn, teach. When you get, give."

—Maya Angelou

When I began my nursing career, I always sought out mentors. For me, mentors provided guidance and reassurance that I was being the best I could be in my career. Now it is my turn to continue to give back to my wound care community. To that end, my choice was to complete another edition of my book.

The following people graciously helped me achieve this goal while juggling life:

To my husband, Michael: Thank you for your constant love, support, sacrifices, and understanding. You are truly the only person who knows the commitment it takes to complete this "labor of love." Cheers!

To my children, Alex and Max: Thank you for your continuous support and being your unique selves. Keep your tenacity for learning. Nurture your spirituality. And, always, reach for the stars. You both rock! I love you.

To my parents, extended family, and friends: Thank you for your moral support. It is comforting to know you are there for me when I have the chance to come up for air! I am eternally grateful to have all of you in my life.

To my Wolters Kluwer family: Thank you for your guidance, moral support, and leadership. And, especially, your patience. These editions would not have been as successful without all of you.

To all of the manufacturers: A special thank you to all for your contributions; for continuing to work with me to provide your available product information so caregivers can quickly and accurately make determinations for the best course of action for the patients they serve. Your contributions make this edition the valuable resource that it is.

To my readers: Thank you for all of your gracious comments. You inspire me to continue to write.

Contents

Ⓝ *New product*   ◉ *Online product*

Ⓝ *New product*   ⊙ *Online product*

Cellular and Tissue-Based Products (CTPs) — 137

Ⓝ *New product*   ◎ *Online product*

Ⓝ *New product*   ◉ *Online product*

Foams   **226**

Ⓝ *New product*   ⊙ *Online product*

Ⓝ *New product*   ◉ *Online product*

Ⓝ *New product*   Ⓞ *Online product*

Ⓝ *New product*   ⊙ *Online product*

Ⓝ *New product* ◉ *Online product*

Wound Care Products

Overview

The *Product Guide to Skin and Wound Care* can help you, the practitioner, choose the proper skin and wound care products to facilitate skin health and wound healing based on the classification of the wound and skin condition. To use this tool properly, remember that the composition of a product is often key to its success and may be kept a trade secret. However, for fundamental safety reasons, the U.S. Food and Drug Administration requires a basic level of disclosure about the ingredients in products. Some products may contain ingredients that cause an allergic reaction in certain people or ingredients that shouldn't be mixed with certain other ingredients. Labels of most food and household products contain information about their ingredients, which are listed in order of abundance in the mixture. In addition to the label, a Material Safety Data Sheet (MSDS) is available upon request from any manufacturer for any of its products. An MSDS contains health and safety information on the product and its ingredients. Practitioners should be careful when mixing products and should always read the product label and package insert before use.

This resource provides quick-reference descriptions of skin and wound care products grouped under generic categories. Included in Part I, the wound care product section, are alginates, antimicrobials, cellular- and tissue-based products, collagens, composites, contact layers, drugs, foams, hydrocolloids, hydrogels, negative-pressure wound therapy, specialty absorptives, surgical dressings, transparent films, wound fillers, and other devices and products.

The skin care product categories include antifungals and antimicrobials, liquid skin protectants, moisture barriers, skin cleansers, therapeutic moisturizers, and other skin care products. The additional dressings and products are grouped by generic categories and include compression bandage systems, conforming bandages, elastic bandage rolls, gauze impregnated with other than water, gauze impregnated withwater or normal saline, gauze nonimpregnated with adhesive border, gauze nonimpregnated without adhesive border, tapes, and wound cleansers.

For specific product packaging and payment information, contact the manufacturer. (See Manufacturer resource guide, page 485.)

No single skin or wound care product provides an optimum environment for skin health or healing of all wounds. It is your responsibility to understand the characteristics, function, and appropriateness for each patient of the skin care products, dressings, drugs, and devices.

Thank you for your skin and wound caring!

Dressings and Devices

OVERVIEW

With more than 2,000 wound care products on the market, choosing the correct dressing, drug, or device may be difficult. In developing a management pathway and planning wound care, the health care professional must consider:

- Wound- and skin-related factors, such as cause, severity, environment, condition of periwound skin, size and depth, anatomic location, volume of exudate, and the risk or presence of infection.
- Patient-related factors such as vascular, nutritional, and medical status; odor-control requirements; comfort and preferences; and cost-benefit ratio.
- Dressing-related factors, such as availability, durability, adaptability, and uses.

Familiarizing yourself with the major categories of wound care products and their actions, indications, contraindications, advantages, and disadvantages will help you choose the most appropriate dressing. Also consider the product's availability and its application and removal procedures. In many cases, one product can help you meet more than one therapeutic goal.

The wound care products in this section include alginates, antimicrobials, cellular and tissue-based products, collagens, composites, contact layers, drugs, foams, hydrocolloids, hydrogels, specialty absorptives, surgical dressings, transparent films, and more. For each product, you will find the size and configuration of the product, the action, indications, contraindications, and instructions for application and removal, as well as the product's code, as assigned by the Healthcare Common Procedure Coding System (HCPCS), if provided by the manufacturer. Product names may be copyrighted or trademarked even when unaccompanied by copyright or trademark characters.

Alginates

ACTION

Alginates are derived from brown seaweed. The products are composed of soft, nonwoven fibers shaped as ropes (twisted fibers) or pads (fibrous mats). Alginates are absorbent and conform to the shape of a wound. When packed, an alginate interacts with wound exudate to form a soft gel that maintains a moist healing environment. An alginate can absorb up to 20 times its weight.

INDICATIONS

To manage partial- and full-thickness draining wounds; wounds with moderate to heavy exudate; tunneling wounds; infected and noninfected wounds; and "moist" red and yellow wounds.

ADVANTAGES

- Absorb up to 20 times their weight.
- Form a gel within the wound to maintain a moist healing environment.
- Facilitate autolytic debridement.
- Fill in dead space.
- Are easy to apply and remove.

DISADVANTAGES

- Are not recommended for wounds with light exudate or dry eschar.
- Can dehydrate the wound bed.
- Require a secondary dressing.

HCPCS CODE OVERVIEW

The HCPCS codes normally assigned to alginate wound covers or other gelling fiber dressings are:

A6196—pad size <16 in^2.

A6197—pad size >16 in^2 but <48 in^2.

A6198—pad size >48 in^2.

The HCPCS code normally assigned to alginate wound fillers or other gelling fiber dressings is:

A6199—wound filler, per 6 in.

AlgiSite M Calcium Alginate Dressing

Smith & Nephew, Inc.
Wound Management

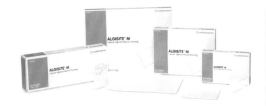

HOW SUPPLIED

Pad	2" × 2"	A6196
Pad	4" × 4"	A6196
Pad	6" × 8"	A6197
Rope	3/4" × 12"	A6199

ACTION

AlgiSite M is a calcium-alginate dressing that forms a soft gel that absorbs wound exudate. AlgiSite M uses the proven benefits of moist wound management. The exudate produces a gel upon contact with the alginate fibers to create a moist wound surface environment. This helps prevent eschar formation and promotes an optimal moist wound environment. The dressing allows wound contraction to occur, which may help reduce scarring, and also allows the gaseous exchange necessary for a healthy wound bed.

INDICATIONS

Under the care of a health care professional, to manage full- and partial-thickness leg ulcers, pressure ulcers, diabetic foot ulcers, and surgical wounds; for over-the-counter applications, to manage lacerations, abrasions, skin tears, and minor burns.

CONTRAINDICATIONS

- Not for use until the packing in cavities and sinuses has been removed.
- Not for use on very lightly exuding wounds.
- Not for use on patients allergic to alginates.

APPLICATION

- Cleanse the wound in accordance with normal procedures.
- Choose a dressing that is slightly larger than the wound and place it in intimate contact with the wound base, making sure that the entire surface is covered. It may be best to use the alginate strip if the wound is deep or undermined. To avoid maceration of the surrounding skin, cut the AlgiSite M to the size of the wound, or fold any dressing material overlying the wound into the wound.
- Apply using an appropriate dressing technique.
- Cover with an appropriate retention dressing. Wound exudate will evaporate from the gel surface; the secondary dressing should not hinder this evaporative process where exudate is heavy.

REMOVAL

- Generally, dressings should be changed daily in heavily draining wounds, reducing to twice weekly (or weekly) as healing proceeds.
- If the dressing is not easily removed, moisten it with saline, then remove.
- To remove AlgiSite M, use tweezers, forceps, or a gloved hand to gently lift the dressing away—the high wet strength generally allows it to remain in one piece. The dressing may adhere if used on a very lightly exuding wound. Removal of the dressing is facilitated by saturating the wound with saline.

AMERX® Calcium Alginate Dressing

AMERX Health Care Corp.

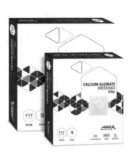

HOW SUPPLIED

Dressing	2″ × 2″	A6196
Dressing	4″ × 4″	A6196

ACTION

AMERX Calcium Alginate highly absorbent dressing quickly forms a hydrophilic gel to create and maintain a moist wound environment for moderate to heavily exudating wounds. The soft, conformable pad enhances patient comfort and can be used on partial- and full-thickness wounds.

INDICATIONS

For use as a primary dressing over moderate to heavily exudating, chronic, and acute wounds.

CONTRAINDICATIONS

- Third-degree burns, dry or low-exudating wounds, or known sensitivities to dressing components.

APPLICATION

- Cleanse the wound with sterile saline solution.
- Remove the dressing from the package and place directly into the wound.
- Any overlap may be folded into the wound or cut away with sterile scissors.

REMOVAL

- If the dressing sticks, moisten with sterile saline solution prior to removal.

New Product: AQUACEL® EXTRA Wound Dressing*

ConvaTec

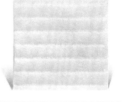

HOW SUPPLIED

Dressing	2″ × 2″	A6196
Dressing	4″ × 4″	A6196
Dressing	6″ × 6″	A6197
Ribbon with Strengthening Fibers	0.39″ × 18″	A6199
Ribbon with Strengthening Fibers	0.75″ × 18″	A6199

ACTION

AQUACEL® EXTRA Wound Dressing is a soft, sterile, nonwoven pad or ribbon dressing made from sodium carboxymethylcellulose fibers. It is composed of two layers of Hydrofiber® stitched together. This conformable and absorbent dressing forms a soft gel that creates a moist wound environment that supports the healing process and autolytic debridement and allows for nontraumatic removal.

INDICATIONS

To manage exuding wounds, pressure ulcers, leg ulcers, abrasions, lacerations, incisions, donor sites, oncology wounds, first- and second-degree burns, and surgical or traumatic wounds that have been left to heal by secondary intent; may be used for wounds that are prone to bleeding, such as mechanically or surgically debrided wounds, donor sites, and traumatic wounds; may also be used to facilitate the control of minor bleeding.

CONTRAINDICATIONS

- Contraindicated for use in patients with sensitivity to this dressing or its components.
- Not intended for use as a surgical sponge.

APPLICATION

- AQUACEL® EXTRA Wound Dressings are sterile and should be handled appropriately.
- If necessary, debride the wound prior to application, then cleanse it with an effective cleansing agent such as SAF-Clens® AF dermal wound cleanser or normal saline solution.
- Apply AQUACEL® EXTRA Wound Dressing to the wound site, and cover with an appropriate secondary dressing, such as a moisture-retentive dressing.
- Change the dressing when it becomes saturated with exudate or when good clinical practice dictates.
- Dressing may remain in place for up to 7 days.

REMOVAL

- Remove the secondary dressing gently, according to the product's package insert.
- Remove the AQUACEL® EXTRA Wound Dressing and discard.
- Without disrupting the delicate granulation tissue, irrigate the wound with SAF-Clens® AF dermal wound cleanser or normal saline solution to remove any residual gel.
- Redress the wound with a new dressing, and cover with a secondary dressing as previously described.

*See package insert for complete instructions for use.

New Product: AQUACEL® Ribbon Hydrofiber® Wound Dressing*

ConvaTec

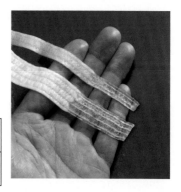

HOW SUPPLIED

Ribbon with Strengthening Fibers	0.39″ × 18″	A6199
Ribbon with Strengthening Fibers	0.75″ × 18″	A6199

ACTION

AQUACEL® Ribbon Hydrofiber® Wound Dressing is a soft, sterile, nonwoven ribbon dressing made from sodium carboxymethylcellulose fibers. This conformable and absorbent dressing forms a soft gel that creates a moist wound environment that supports the healing process and autolytic debridement and allows for nontraumatic removal.

INDICATIONS

Soft, nonwoven ribbon dressing can be used on acute and chronic wounds including leg ulcers, diabetic foot ulcers, pressure injuries, partial-thickness burns, postop wounds or traumatic wounds left to heal by secondary intent, abrasions, lacerations, and donor sites.*

CONTRAINDICATIONS

- Contraindicated for use in patients with sensitivity to this dressing or its components.
- Not intended for use as a surgical sponge.

APPLICATION

- AQUACEL® Ribbon Dressings are sterile and should be handled appropriately.
- If necessary, debride the wound prior to application, then cleanse it with an effective cleansing agent such as SAF-Clens® AF dermal wound cleanser or normal saline solution.
- For deep wounds, loosely pack ribbon or sheet into wound to about 80% of the depth of the wound to accommodate swelling of the dressing, leaving a small overhang (at least 1″ [2.5 cm]) to facilitate removal.
- Change the dressing when it becomes saturated with exudate or when good clinical practice dictates.
- Dressing may remain in place for up to 7 days.

REMOVAL

- Remove the secondary dressing gently, according to the product's package insert.
- Remove the AQUACEL® Ribbon Dressing and discard.
- Without disrupting the delicate granulation tissue, irrigate the wound with SAF-Clens® AF dermal wound cleanser or normal saline solution to remove any residual gel.
- Redress the wound with a new dressing, and cover with a secondary dressing as previously described.

*See package insert for complete instructions for use.

New Product: AquaRite Extra CMC

DermaRite Industries, LLC

Soft, absorbent and resizable when dry

Soothing, clear gel sheet when wet

HOW SUPPLIED

CMC Wound Dressing	0.75″ × 18″	A6199
CMC Wound Dressing	2″ × 2″	A6196
CMC Wound Dressing	4″ × 5″	A6197
CMC Wound Dressing	6″ × 6″	A6197

ACTION

AquaRite™ Extra CMC Wound Dressing is a soft, conformable nonwoven dressing made from sodium carboxymethyl cellulose (CMC) and strengthening cellulose fibers. The dressing forms a soothing gel when saturated with wound exudate or blood, creating a moist wound environment that may support autolytic debridement and the healing process. The gel formation traps debris and bacteria, retaining it inside the fiber dressing. AquaRite Extra CMC's gel fiber retains its structure even when saturated, facilitating removal. The high vertical absorption of exudate into the fiber dressing protects the wound and surrounding skin from maceration.

AquaRite Extra CMC can be cut to fit the wound prior to application.

AquaRite Extra CMC can be used under compression.

INDICATIONS

This product is for single use only.

- Use under the supervision of a qualified health care professional.
- For use in the treatment of moderate to heavily exuding acute or chronic partial or full thickness wounds, including:
  - Pressure ulcers (stages 2, 3, and 4).
  - Leg ulcers.
  - Diabetic ulcers.
  - Surgical wounds.
  - Donor sites.
  - Traumatic wounds (abrasions, lacerations).
  - Exuding oncology wounds.

CONTRAINDICATIONS

- AquaRite Extra CMC should not be used on people who are sensitive or allergic to the dressing and its components. Not intended for use on wounds with severe bleeding, inside internal body cavities, or on closed wounds.
- The treatment should be discontinued after 30 days.

APPLICATION

- Cleanse wound with advised liquid to remove residue according to local infection control protocol. Deep wounds should be well irrigated.
- Skin around wound should be clean and dry. Use protectant shield as needed.
- Remove dressing from package.
- Dressing may be cut to wound size prior to application; avoid overlapping onto skin.

- Apply dressing to moist wound bed. For deep wounds, loosely pack wound with AquaRite Extra CMC Rope wound dressing.
- Cover with appropriate secondary dressing that maintains a moist wound environment.

REMOVAL

- Dressing may be moistened to ease removal.
- Carefully remove adhesive dressings by holding the edge of the dressing and slowly pulling it parallel to the skin.
- Dispose of in accordance with local guidance.

REFERENCES

1. The properties mentioned above refer to the current in vitro data.
2. http://dermarite.com/product/aquarite-extra-cmc/

Biatain® Alginate Dressing and Biatain® Alginate Rope

Coloplast

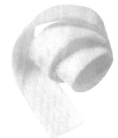

ALGINATES

HOW SUPPLIED

Sheet	2" × 2"	A6196
Sheet	4" × 4"	A6196
Sheet	6" × 6"	A6197
Rope	1" × 17.5"	A6199

ACTION

Biatain® Alginate Dressing and Biatain® Alginate Rope are highly absorbent wound dressings composed of alginate and sodium carboxymethylcellulose. On contact with wound exudate it converts to a soft cohesive gel which provides the optimal moist wound healing environment.

INDICATIONS

Biatain Alginate is indicated for the management of moderately to heavily exuding wounds. Biatain Alginate can be used to facilitate exudate management and local hemostasis during the wound healing process as an external wound dressing in wounds like pressure ulcers, venous leg ulcers, arterial ulcers, diabetic foot ulcers, donor sites, and traumatic wounds. Biatain Alginate can be used for diabetic foot ulcers under the discretion of a physician. Biatain Alginate can be used for sloughy wounds and cavity filling.

CAUTION

Biatain Alginate may be used on infected wounds under the discretion of a health care professional, together with the appropriate therapy and frequent inspections depending on the clinical condition. Biatain Alginate is not intended for controlling heavy or prolonged bleeding which will not stop by physiological means or without surgical intervention. Biatain Alginate is not for use on dry wounds.

APPLICATION

- Rinse the wound with physiological saline or tap water.
- Gently dry the skin around the wound.

Biatain Alginate Dressing

- Cut to fit the wound. If you need to cut the dressing, you are advised to use a sterile pair of scissors.
- Biatain Alginate Dressing should be used with a secondary cover dressing, for example, Comfeel® Plus Transparent Dressing or Biatain® Foam Dressing depending on the clinical condition of the wound.

Biatain Alginate Rope

- Can be cut to fit small or narrow wounds. If you need to cut the dressing, you are advised to use a sterile pair of scissors.
- Biatain Alginate Rope should be applied evenly/loosely into the wound without packing it. This will allow the alginate fiber to form a moist gel and conform to the size of the cavity.
- Biatain Alginate Rope can be soaked in physiological saline prior to application. During absorption the ribbon dressing will not expand from its original size, but adjust to the cavity.
- Biatain Alginate Rope should be used with a secondary cover dressing, for example, Comfeel® Plus Transparent Dressing or Biatain® Foam Dressing depending on the clinical condition of the wound.

REMOVAL

- Should be changed when the secondary wound dressing is changed.
- Should not be left on for more than 7 days.
- Can easily be removed by rinsing with a saline solution. Remove with forceps without causing pain or trauma to the newly formed tissue.
- When exudate levels have decreased and wound healing is progressing, dressing may be discontinued and replaced by another suitable dressing (e.g., Biatain Foam Dressing or Comfeel Plus Ulcer Dressing) to ensure continuation of wound healing.

REFERENCE

1. https://www.coloplast.us/biatain-alginate-en-us.aspx

CalciCare™ Calcium Alginate Dressing*

Hollister Wound Care

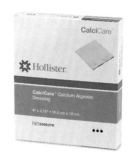

HOW SUPPLIED

Pad	2" × 2"	A6196
Pad	4" × 4"	A6197
Pad	4" × 8"	A6197
Rope	1" × 18"	A6199

ACTION

CalciCare™ calcium alginate dressings are sterile, reinforced nonwoven pads composed of high G (glucuronic acid) calcium/sodium alginate. The dressings are soft and conformable, highly absorbent and fast gelling. As wound fluid is absorbed the alginate forms a gel, which helps support autolytic debridement, while maintaining a moist environment for optimal wound healing. The dressings are reinforced for intact removal.

INDICATIONS

To manage partial- and full-thickness wounds with moderate to heavy exudate, including pressure ulcers, legs ulcers, cavity wounds, lacerations, and postoperative surgical wounds.

CONTRAINDICATIONS

- Contraindicated for direct application on dry to lightly exuding wounds.
- Contraindicated to control heavy bleeding.
- Contraindicated in patients with known sensitivity to calcium alginate, nylon, or with other known allergic conditions.

APPLICATION

- Prepare the wound according to facility policy, or as directed. Make sure the skin is clean and dry.
- Apply the dressing to the wound surface.
- Cover the dressing with a secondary dressing, and secure it.

REMOVAL

- CalciCare calcium alginate dressings can remain in situ for up to 7 days, depending on patient condition and the level of exudate.
- Remove the secondary dressing according to facility policy.
- Remove the CalciCare calcium alginate dressing.
- If necessary, gently rinse away the remaining gel or dressing fibers, using Restore™ wound cleanser or normal saline solution.
- The dressing may adhere if used on dry or very lightly exuding wounds. If the dressing is not easily removed, moisten it with sterile saline solution prior to removal.
- Do not reuse in whole or in part, as it may compromise sterility and/or the performance of the dressing. For external use only.

*See package insert for complete instructions for use.

Calcium Alginate Dressing

Gentell

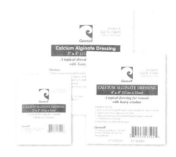

HOW SUPPLIED

Pad	2″ × 2″	A6196
Pad	4″ × 4″	A6196
Pad	5″ × 5″	A6197
Pad	10″ × 10″	A6198
Rope	12″	A6199

ACTION

Gentell Calcium Alginate Dressings are a sterile, comfortable, advanced fiber-structured algi-nate with a highly absorbent capacity. Alginate dressings absorb, collect and contain exudate while providing a moist healing environment. A reaction between the calcium in the dress-ing and the sodium in the wound exudate creates a gel-like substance that promotes moist wound healing.

INDICATIONS

Apply Gentell's Calcium Alginate 2″ × 2″, 4″ × 4″, 5″ × 5″ and 10″ × 10″ pads in dry form on shallow wounds including leg ulcers, pressure ulcers, diabetic foot ulcers, and surgical wounds. May also be used for minor conditions such as lacerations, abrasions, skin tears, and minor burns.

CONTRAINDICATIONS

- Gentell Calcium Alginate Wound Dressings are not indicated for use on third-degree burns or to control heavy bleeding.

APPLICATION

- Irrigate the wound with Gentell Wound Cleanser and gently dry the skin surrounding the wound site.
- Choose appropriate sized dressing based on the dimensions of the wound.
- Cover wound with a secondary dressing such as Gentell Super Absorbent, Gentell Com-fortell™, or Gentell LoProfile Foam Dressing.

REMOVAL

- Change dressing daily or as ordered by a physician.

New Product: CarboFLEX® Odor Control Dressing*

ConvaTec

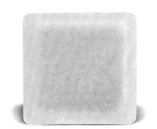

HOW SUPPLIED

Pad	4" × 4"	A6196
Pad	3" × 6"	A6197
Pad	6" × 8"	A6197

ACTION

CarboFLEX® is a sterile nonadhesive dressing with an absorbent wound-contact layer (containing alginate and hydrocolloid), an activated charcoal central pad, and a smooth, water-resistant top layer.

INDICATIONS

To manage acute and chronic wounds; may be used as a primary dressing for shallow wounds or as a secondary dressing over wound fillers for deeper wounds; may also be used on infected malodorous wounds along with appropriate therapy and frequent monitoring of the wound.

CONTRAINDICATIONS

- Contraindicated in patients with a sensitivity to the dressing or its components.

APPLICATION

- If required, debride the wound and remove necrotic tissue. Cleanse the wound site, rinse well, and dry the surrounding skin.
- Do not cut the dressing.
- Choose a dressing that is larger than the wound area to ensure that the dressing overlaps the wound edge by at least 1 1/4" (3 cm). For shallow wounds, the dressing may be placed directly onto the wound as a primary dressing; for cavity wounds, CarboFLEX® can be laid over a wound filler or gel as a secondary dressing.
- Place the fibrous (nonshiny) surface on the wound or cavity filler.
- Secure CarboFLEX® in place with tape or other appropriate material. The wound contact layer absorbs exudate and forms a soft gel.

REMOVAL

- Change the dressing when clinically indicated, when exudate strike-through to the top layer occurs, or when the odor is no longer being absorbed. With noninfected malodorous wounds, CarboFLEX® may be left undisturbed for up to 3 days. If the wound is infected, CarboFLEX® should be changed more frequently.
- Carefully lift the dressing away from the wound by grasping it at one corner.

*See package insert for complete instructions for use.

DermaGinate™

DermaRite Industries, LLC

HOW SUPPLIED

Calcium Alginate Wound Dressing	2″ × 2″	A6196
Calcium Alginate Wound Dressing	4.25″ × 4.25″	A6197
Calcium Alginate Wound Dressing	4″ × 8″	A6197
Calcium Alginate Wound Dressing, Fluffy Rope	12″	A6199
Calcium Alginate Wound Dressing, Rope	12″	

ACTION

DermaGinate™ is a calcium alginate wound dressing for moderate to highly exuding wounds. Forms a soothing, gel-like consistency on contact with moisture, yet maintains integrity for convenient removal. Assists in maintaining a moist wound healing environment.

INDICATIONS

May be used as a primary wound dressing for moderate to highly exuding wounds, such as pressure ulcers, leg ulcers, diabetic ulcers, surgical wounds, donor sites, lacerations, and abrasions. May be used under compression bandages.

CONTRAINDICATIONS

- DermaGinate should not be used on people who are sensitive or allergic to the dressing and its components.
- Not indicated for surgical implantation, dry wounds, or to control heavy bleeding.

APPLICATION

- Cleanse wound with advised liquid to remove residue according to local infection control protocol. Deep wounds should be well irrigated.
- Skin around wound should be clean and dry, use skin barrier prep as needed.
- Remove dressing from package.
- Dressing may be cut to size prior to application.
- Apply dressing to moist wound bed. Loosely pack deep wounds.
- Secure with appropriate cover dressing that manages drainage and maintains a moist wound environment.

REMOVAL

- Carefully remove adhesive dressings by holding the edge of the dressing and slowly pulling it parallel to the skin.
- Dressing may be moistened to ease removal.
- Dispose of in accordance with local guidance.

REFERENCE

1. http://dermarite.com/product/dermaginate/

Drawtex®

Urgo Medical

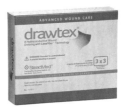

HOW SUPPLIED

Hydroconductive Dressings	2" × 2"	A6196
Hydroconductive Dressings	3" × 3"	A6196
Hydroconductive Dressings	4" × 4"	A6196
Hydroconductive Dressings	6" × 8"	A6197
Hydroconductive Dressings	8" × 8"	A6198
Hydroconductive Rolls	3" × 39"	A6199
Hydroconductive Rolls	4" × 39"	A6199
Hydroconductive Rolls	8" × 39"	A6199
Tracheostomy and Tube Dressing	4" × 4"	
Rope Dressing	3/8" × 18"	
Surgical Dressing	6"	
Surgical Dressing	9.75"	
Surgical Dressing	12"	

ACTION

Drawtex® is a hydroconductive, nonadherent wound dressing with Leva*Fiber* technology. Leva*Fiber* technology is a combination of two types of absorbent, cross-action structures that create the ability to move large volumes of fluid and other debris from the wound through the dressing.

INDICATIONS

Indicated for a variety of wounds, including venous leg ulcers, diabetic foot ulcers, pressure ulcers, burn wounds, dehisced surgical wounds, and difficult-to-heal wounds (mixed etiology leg ulcers, necrotizing fasciitis, chronic wounds with slough, clinically infected wounds, fungating cancer wounds, Buruli ulcers).

CONTRAINDICATIONS

- Cannot be used when arterial bleeding is present.

APPLICATION

- Apply dressing appropriate to the size of the wound bed. Dressing can be cut accordingly. Stack dressing if necessary. Cover with appropriate secondary dressing.

REMOVAL

- Gently lift the dressing away from the wound.
- Clean the wound with saline solution or wound cleanser.

ALGINATES

New Product: Eclypse® Adherent and Eclypse® Adherent Sacral Super Absorbent Dressings

Advancis Medical/DUKAL Corporation

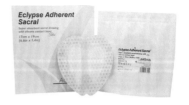

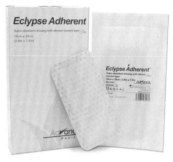

HOW SUPPLIED

Eclypse® Adherent Super Absorbent Dressing	4" × 4"	A6196
Eclypse® Adherent Super Absorbent Dressing	4" × 8"	A6197
Eclypse® Adherent Super Absorbent Dressing	6" × 6"	A6197
Eclypse® Adherent Super Absorbent Dressing	8" × 12"	A6198
Eclypse® Adherent Sacral Super Absorbent Dressing	6.5" × 7.5"	A6197
Eclypse® Adherent Sacral Super Absorbent Dressing	8.5" × 9"	A6198

ACTION

- Super absorbent dressing with self-adhesive soft silicone contact layer.
- Silicone layer does not damage the surrounding skin, periwound area or newly formed tissue and will not adhere to the moist wound bed.
- Can be easily lifted for adjustment without losing its adherent properties and enables single-handed dressing application.
- Features a low profile and rounded edges to prevent dressing lift.
- The Eclypse® Adherent Sacral dressing is anatomically designed to meet the needs of the difficult to dress sacral area, offering a major advancement in the management of sacral pressure ulcers.

INDICATIONS

- Suitable for acute and chronic wounds.
- Cuts and abrasions.
- Superficial burns.
- Surgical wounds.
- Leg ulcers.
- Pressure ulcers.
- Diabetic ulcers.

CONTRAINDICATIONS

- Do not use on arterial bleeds, heavily bleeding wounds.

APPLICATION

- Place face down on wound surface with beige backing uppermost.
- Do not cut Eclypse® Adherent Sacral.

REMOVAL

- Up to 7 days.

REFERENCE

1. http://www.advancis.co.uk/products

ALGINATES

New Product: Eclypse® Boot and Eclypse® Foot Super Absorbent Dressing

Advancis Medical/DUKAL Corporation

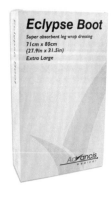

Eclypse Boot
Super absorbent leg wrap dressing
71cm x 80cm
(27.9in x 31.5in)
Extra Large

Advancis
Medical

HOW SUPPLIED

Eclypse® Boot Super Absorbent Dressing, Small	22" × 19"	A6198
Eclypse® Boot Super Absorbent Dressing, Large	24" × 28"	A6198
Eclypse® Boot Super Absorbent Dressing, Large	28" × 32"	A6198
Eclypse® Foot Super Absorbent Dressing	13" × 19"	A6198

ACTION

- Superabsorbent dressing specifically designed to manage high levels of fluid in the lower limb.
- Twelve superabsorbent interconnected compartments to optimize absorbency.
- Significantly improves patient mobility and reduces dressing application time.
- Easy to apply, single dressing design.

INDICATIONS

- Moderate to heavily exuding wounds.
- Leg ulcers.
- Superficial wounds.
- Pressure ulcers.
- Arterial ulcers.
- Leaky legs.
- Diabetic ulcers.
- Lymphedema.

CONTRAINDICATIONS

- Do not use on arterial bleeds and heavily bleeding wounds.
- Do not cut Eclypse® Boot across the absorbent pockets.

APPLICATION

- Open out the dressing fully, white side up placing the heel onto the small triangle, the top of the triangle pointing toward the patient.
- Fold over the foot one at a time the smaller sections to the left and right and secure with tape.
- Fold both the larger sections one at a time around the leg also securing with tape.
- Eclypse® Boot can be used under compression bandaging.

REMOVAL

- Up to 7 days.

REFERENCE

1. http://www.advancis.co.uk/products

New Product: Eclypse® Border and Eclypse® Border Oval Super Absorbent Dressings

Advancis Medical/DUKAL Corporation

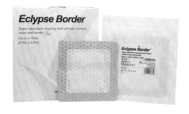

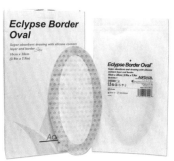

HOW SUPPLIED

Eclypse® Border Super Absorbent Dressing	6" × 6"	A6197
Eclypse® Border Super Absorbent Dressing	8" × 12"	A6198
Eclypse® Border Oval Super Absorbent Dressing	8" × 12"	A6197
Eclypse® Border Oval Super Absorbent Dressing	4" × 8"	A6197
Eclypse® Border Oval Super Absorbent Dressing	6" × 8"	A6197

ACTION

- Superabsorbent dressing with silicone contact layer and border.
- Soft silicone layer provides gentle adherence that facilitates atraumatic removal, does not damage the surrounding skin, periwound area, or newly formed tissue and will not adhere to the wet wound bed.
- Ideal for hard to dress areas.
- Features an enhanced wicking layer, increased absorbency capacity, and breathable, fluid repellent back.

INDICATIONS

- For all exuding wounds.
- Pressure ulcers.
- Leg ulcers.
- Surgical wounds.
- Burns.
- Graft sites.
- Lymphatic legs.
- Fistulas.
- Fungating tumors.

CONTRAINDICATIONS

- Do not use on arterial bleeds or heavily bleeding wounds.

APPLICATION

- Placed face down on wound surface with beige backing uppermost.
- Allow a minimum of a 2-cm border overlap around the wound area.
- Do not cut Eclypse® Border.

REMOVAL

- Up to 7 days.

REFERENCE

1. http://www.advancis.co.uk/products

New Product: Eclypse® Super Absorbent Dressing

Advancis Medical/DUKAL Corporation

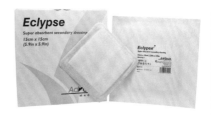

ALGINATES

HOW SUPPLIED

Eclypse® Super Absorbent Dressing	4" × 4"	A6196
Eclypse® Super Absorbent Dressing	6" × 6"	A6197
Eclypse® Super Absorbent Dressing	8" × 12"	A6198
Eclypse® Super Absorbent Dressing	24" × 16"	A6198

ACTION

- High capacity wound dressing designed to absorb and retain fluid, reducing the potential for leaks and minimizing the risk of maceration.
- Rapid wicking face combined with a highly absorbent moisture locking system.
- Absorbent layer provides a large capacity with rapid fluid intake.
- Nonstrikethrough, bacteria-proof backing with a high MVTR rate to prolong wear time.
- Can be used safely under compression without affecting the absorbency.

INDICATIONS

- Moderate to heavily exuding wounds.
- Leg ulcers.
- Pressure ulcers.
- Sloughy or granulating wounds.
- Postoperative or dehisced wounds.
- Fungating wounds.
- Donor site management.

CONTRAINDICATIONS

- Do not use on arterial bleeds or heavily bleeding wounds.

APPLICATION

- Eclypse® is placed white side face down on wound surface with beige backing uppermost.
- For large wounds several dressings can be placed side-by-side and secured with an appropriate tape or bandage.
- Do not cut Eclypse®.

REMOVAL

- Up to 7 days.

REFERENCE

1. http://www.advancis.co.uk/products

ENLUXTRA Smart Self-Adaptive Wound Dressing

OSNovative Systems, Inc.

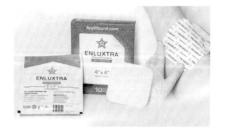

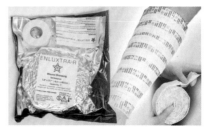

HOW SUPPLIED

ENLUXTRA Wound Dressing—Sterile Pad in a Peelable Foil Pouch	2" × 2" (5 cm × 5 cm)	A6196
ENLUXTRA Wound Dressing—Sterile Pad in a Peelable Foil Pouch	4" × 4" (10 cm × 10 cm)	A6196
ENLUXTRA Wound Dressing—Sterile Pad in a Peelable Foil Pouch	6" × 6" (15 cm × 15 cm)	A6197
ENLUXTRA-R Roll Dressing—A Kit in a Plastic Bag that Contains a Sterile Rolled-Up Strip in a Peelable Foil Pouch, a Roll of Medical Adhesive Tape (Seam Tape), and Instructions for Use	1.5" × 157" (4 cm × 400 cm)	

ACTION

Enluxtra wound dressing belongs to the type of multifunctional wound dressings that perform multiple actions simultaneously.

Enluxtra wound dressings contain smart synthetic superabsorbent and hydrogel polymers sensitive to moisture levels in and around the wound. The polymers adapt to the evolving wound conditions in real time and maintain continuous moist healing environment by automatically controlling on-demand moisture donation or absorption over various wound areas.

Enluxtra dressing material performs the following functions when applied to the wound:

- Superabsorption—Absorbs and retains large amounts of wound exudate, preventing skin maceration.
- Adaptive hydration—Prevents wound desiccation by keeping dry wound parts optimally hydrated and minimizes moisture loss over dry wound areas using embedded hydrogel in combination with adjustable moisture transmission rate membrane.
- Effective continuous wound cleansing—Absorbs and locks in liquefied products of intensive natural autolytic debridement promoted by the stable moist environment.
- Serves as microbial and fluid strikethrough barrier.

INDICATIONS

Enluxtra dressings are suitable for a wide range of wound conditions (acute and chronic) regardless of the wound's etiology and healing stage.

- Enluxtra dressings are indicated for dry and exuding wounds, partial- and full-thickness wounds, such as pressure ulcers (stages II to IV), lower-extremity ulcers (venous or arterial), diabetic foot ulcers, surgical or traumatic wounds, graft and donor sites, burns (thermal, chemical, or radiation).
- Enluxtra dressings can be used on infected and heavy bioburden wounds.

CONTRAINDICATIONS

- Individual sensitivity to the dressing or its components.
- Heavy arterial bleeding.

Precautions

- The following coproducts are not compatible with Enluxtra, may hinder Enluxtra dressing's performance and should not be used under Enluxtra dressings:
  - All petrolatum- or oil-based products.
  - All thick and viscous pastes and ointments.
  - All alginate dressings and fillers.
  - All CMC-based (carboxymethyl cellulose) dressings and fillers.
  - All honey-based products containing thickeners, or honey-impregnated dressings.
  - All creams and ointments containing AHA (alpha-hydroxy acid).

APPLICATION

- *Important:* It is best to avoid using any additional products under Enluxtra dressing. They will prevent full contact of Enluxtra dressing's surface with the wound bed and surrounding skin and may interfere with the vertical draw action.

Instructions for ENLUXTRA dressing

- Cleanse the wound with saline. No need to tap dry.
- Select Enluxtra dressing size large enough to cover all the following areas:
  - Wound bed.
  - Periwound skin.
  - 1″ of healthy skin.
  Important: No need to cut Enluxtra dressings to wound size and shape. Enluxtra can be trimmed or slitted for better fit in difficult areas or around appliances.
- If the wound has depth or conditions such as cavity, tunneling, or undermining, use a nonshrinking wound filler such as AMD gauze or foam strips to fill the wound cavity loosely. Do not use gelling alginates or CMC-based (carboxymethyl cellulose) fiber fillers that are incompatible with Enluxtra.
- Open the peelable foil pouch starting from a corner of chevron shape seal.
- Apply Enluxtra dressing with the white, unprinted fiber side facing down towards the wound.
- Press down on Enluxtra to ensure full contact with:
  - Wound bed and.
  - Wound filler (if any).
- If Enluxtra dressing is tenting over the wound, add folded gauze pads on top of Enluxtra to bend it in toward the wound.
- Secure Enluxtra dressing with a medical tape or wrap or thin film adhesive dressing/drape.

Instructions for ENLUXTRA-R roll dressing

- Cleanse the wound with saline. No need to pat dry.
- If prescribed, apply ointments or wound filler on the wound.
- Open the plastic bag and remove the Enluxtra-R pouch and the seam tape.
- Prepare three to four pieces of the seam tape (about 3″ long each), and keep them conveniently available near the patient.
- Cut open the Enluxtra-R pouch and take out the roll dressing.
- Using a piece of seam tape, secure the end of the roll away from the wound to allow for at least 2″ overlap onto healthy skin. The soft fiber surface must face down towards the skin.
- Wrap the dressing around the body part, making sure the gap between neighboring turns is less than 1/8″ (3 mm). Optionally, use pieces of the seam tape to secure neighboring turns to each other every two to three turns.
- Once the healthy skin at the other end of the wound is overlapped by at least 2″, cut off the excess and secure the roll's end with medical adhesive tape.
  - If one Enluxtra-R strip is not long enough to achieve the 2″ healthy skin overlap at the other end of the wound, use an additional Enluxtra-R strip. Secure the beginning of the second Enluxtra-R strip to the end of the first Enluxtra-R strip with a piece of seam tape.
- Apply the provided seam tape, centering it along the seams of the wrapped roll. Do not stretch the seam tape and avoid creation of any additional compression.
- Optionally, apply a compression wrap.

REMOVAL

- Enluxtra dressing must be removed:
  - Before the exudate reaches the dressing's edge.
  - If the patient is experiencing more pain or discomfort than usual.
- *Important:* Adjust the next Enluxtra dressing's position if the drainage footprint is not centered on the removed dressing.

HOW TO REMOVE

ENLUXTRA dressing

To remove Enluxtra wound dressing, lift one corner of the dressing and slowly peel back until completely removed from the wound.

ENLUXTRA-R roll dressing

Use medical scissors to cut across the wrapped dressing and then slowly and gently peel it away from the wound.

RECOMMENDED ENLUXTRA WEAR TIME

- Copious drainage or very sloughy or infected wounds: 1 to 2 days.
- High drainage or slough presence in the wound bed: 2 to 3 days.
- All other wounds and sites: 3 to 7 days.

New Product: Exufiber®

Mölnlycke Health Care

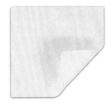

HOW SUPPLIED

Dressing	2″ × 2″	A6196
Dressing	4″ × 4.8″	A6197
Dressing	6″ × 6″	A6197
Dressing	0.8″ × 17.7″	A6199

ACTION

Exufiber® is a sterile nonwoven dressing made from the highly absorbent polyvinyl alcohol fibers. In contact with wound exudate, Exufiber transforms into a gel that facilitates moist wound healing and ease of removal during dressing change. Exufiber absorbs and retains wound exudate. Exufiber is available as sheet and ribbon dressing.

INDICATIONS

Exufiber® wound dressing is intended to be used on a wide range of exuding wounds.
- Leg and foot ulcers.
- Pressure ulcers.
- Partial thickness burns.
- Surgical wounds.
- Donor sites.
- Malignant wounds.

PRECAUTIONS

- Exufiber® is for single use only and should not be reused. Reuse may lead to product deterioration or cross-contamination may occur.
- Sterility is guaranteed unless pouch is opened or damaged prior to use. Do not resterilize.
- All wounds should be inspected frequently. In case of signs of clinical infection, consult a health care professional for adequate infection treatment.
- Exufiber is not intended for dry wounds, full thickness injuries, or surgical implantations.
- If the dressing dries out and is difficult to remove, it should be moistened according to local policies (e.g., sterile saline or sterile water) and allowed to soak until it lifts easily. It may take several minutes for Exufiber to transform into a gel. Remove the dressing by gently cleansing/flushing.

APPLICATION AND REMOVAL

Shallow wounds application

- Cleanse the wound with saline solution or water according to clinical practice.
- Dry the surrounding skin thoroughly.
- Choose the correct size of the dressing to be able to cover the entire wound. For best result, Exufiber should overlap the dry surrounding skin by at least 1 to 2 cm for the smaller sizes (up to 10 × 10 cm) and 5 cm for larger sizes. The dressing will shrink as it absorbs wound fluid and starts gelling.
- Apply a dry Exufiber dressing to the wound.
- Fixate with an appropriate secondary dressing. The choice depends on the exudate level.
- Compression therapy may be used in conjunction with Exufiber.

Dressing change and removal

- Change the Exufiber dressing when saturation is reached. Exufiber can be left in place for up to 7 days depending on wound condition or as indicated by clinical practice.
- Remove the secondary dressing and discard in appropriate ways.
- Remove the Exufiber dressing by gently cleansing/flushing with saline solution or water according to clinical practice. Any nongelled material will moisten in contact with the saline.

Deep wounds and cavities application

- Cleanse the wound with saline solution or water according to clinical practice.
- Dry the surrounding skin thoroughly.
- Loosely packed ribbon or pad into the wound to allow swelling of the dressing. When using the ribbon dressing, cut to appropriate length leaving a small overhang of 2 to 3 cm outside of the wound for easy removal.
- Cover with an appropriate secondary dressing. The choice depends on the exudate level.
- Fixate (or cover) with an adhesive dressing or a bandage as appropriate.

Dressing change and removal

- Change the Exufiber dressing when saturation is reached. Exufiber can be left in place for up to 7 days depending on wound condition or as indicated by clinical practice.
- Remove the secondary dressing and discard in appropriate way.
- Remove the Exufiber dressing by gently cleansing/flushing with saline solution or water according to clinical practice. Any nongelled material will moisten in contact with the saline.

Donor sites application

- Harvest tissue and achieve hemostasis (according to normal routine).
- Choose the correct size of sheet dressing to be able to cover the entire wound. The Exufiber dressing should overlap the dry surrounding skin by at least 5 cm, the dressing will shrink as it absorbs wound fluid and starts gelling.
- Apply a dry Exufiber dressing to the wound.
- Fixate (or cover) with an adhesive dressing or a bandage as appropriate.

Dressing change and removal

- Change the Exufiber dressing when saturation is reached. Exufiber can be left in place for up to 14 days in donor sites depending on wound condition or as indicated by clinical practice.
- Remove the secondary dressing and discard in appropriate way.
- Remove the Exufiber dressing by gently cleansing/flushing with saline solutions or water according to clinical practice. Any nongelled material will moisten in contact with the saline.

New Product: HydraLock™ SA

DermaRite Industries, LLC

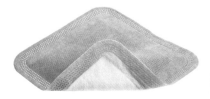

HOW SUPPLIED

Superabsorbent Wound Dressing with Gelling Core and Waterproof Backing	3″ × 3″	A6196
Superabsorbent Wound Dressing with Gelling Core and Waterproof Backing	4″ × 4″	A6196
Superabsorbent Wound Dressing with Gelling Core and Waterproof Backing	6″ × 10″	A6197
Superabsorbent Wound Dressing with Gelling Core and Waterproof Backing	7.87″ × 7.87″	A6197

ACTION

HydraLock™ SA is a superabsorbent primary or secondary wound dressing with a comfortable, nonadherent contact surface and a protective waterproof backing that prevents strikethrough. Rapidly absorbs wound exudate by wicking it into the superabsorbent polymer core which expands as it gels. This locks in the excess moisture, minimizing the risk for maceration while supporting a moist wound environment conducive to autolytic debridement, normalization of wound bed temperature, and the formation of granulation tissue and epithelialization. HydraLock SA must be secured in place with tape or other preferred securement methods. May be used under compression.

INDICATIONS

May be used for the management of moderate to heavily exuding partial- to full-thickness wounds, including pressure ulcers, leg ulcers, diabetic ulcers, surgical wounds, traumatic wounds, graft and donor sites, lacerations, and abrasions.

CONTRAINDICATIONS

- Not for use on people who may be sensitive or allergic to the dressing and its components.

APPLICATION

- Cleanse wound with advised liquid to remove residue according to local infection control protocol. Deep wounds should be well irrigated.
- Skin around wound should be clean and dry, use skin barrier prep as needed.
  Note: When using under compression, select a dressing that is 1″ to 2″ larger than the wound.
- Remove dressing from package.
- Apply white surface of dressing to moist wound bed. Loosely fill empty space in deep wounds with a wound filler dressing.
- Secure with tape or appropriate cover dressing that manages drainage and maintains a moist wound environment.

REMOVAL

- Dressing may be moistened to ease removal.
- Carefully remove adhesive dressings by holding the edge of the dressing and slowly pulling it parallel to the skin.
- Dispose of in accordance with local guidance.

REFERENCE

1. http://dermarite.com/product/hydralock-sa/

KALTOSTAT® Wound Dressing*

ConvaTec

HOW SUPPLIED

Dressing	2″ × 2″	A6196
Dressing	3″ × 4 3/4″	A6196
Dressing	4″ × 4″	A6196
Dressing	4″ × 8″	A6197
Dressing	6″ × 9 1/2″	A6198
Dressing	12″ × 24″	A6198
Rope	2 g	A6199

ACTION

KALTOSTAT® Wound Dressing is a soft, sterile, nonwoven dressing of calcium-sodium alginate fiber. The alginate fibers absorb wound exudate or normal saline solution and form a firm gel-fiber mat. The mat maintains a moist, warm environment at the wound–dressing interface and allows removal of the dressing with little or no damage to newly formed tissue.

INDICATIONS

To manage pressure ulcers, venous stasis ulcers, arterial ulcers, diabetic ulcers, donor sites, abrasions, lacerations, superficial burns, postoperative incisions, and other external wounds inflicted by trauma. Controls minor bleeding. May also be used as a nasal packing for nosebleeds, dental extraction sites, and postoperative wound debridement.

CONTRAINDICATIONS

- Contraindicated for third-degree burns.
- Not intended to control heavy bleeding.
- Not intended for use as a surgical sponge.

APPLICATION

- Debride the wound of excessive necrotic tissue and eschar, and irrigate with an appropriate nontoxic cleansing solution.
- Trim the dressing to the exact size of the wound.
- For heavily exuding wounds, apply the dry dressing to the wound.
- For lightly exuding wounds or nonexuding wounds, place the dressing on the wound, and moisten it with normal saline solution. Reapply normal saline solution, as necessary, to maintain the gel.
- Apply an appropriate secondary dressing to secure the dressing.
- To effect hemostasis on bleeding wounds, apply the dressing to the bleeding area. Remove the dressing after bleeding has stopped, and then apply a new dressing.

REMOVAL

- To remove a dressing from a nonexuding or lightly exuding wound, saturate the dressing with normal saline solution. If the gel has dried, rehydrate it by saturating it with normal saline solution; softening may take several hours if severe drying has occurred.
- Change the dressing on heavily exuding wounds when strike-through to the secondary dressing occurs, or whenever clinical practice dictates. Removal is easy because the dressing forms a gel at the wound–dressing interface.
- Leave the dressing in place for up to 7 days, depending on the wound.
- Cleanse the wound site before applying a new dressing.

*See package insert for complete instructions for use.

New Product: Maxorb II

Medline Industries, Inc.

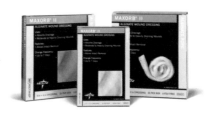

HOW SUPPLIED

Pad	2" × 2"	A6196
Pad	4" × 4"	A6197
Pad	4" × 8"	A6197
Pad	6" × 6"	A6197
Rope	1" × 12" (2 g)	A6199
Rope	1" × 18"	A6199

ACTION

Maxorb II is a 100% calcium alginate dressing designed to deliver superior wet strength and absorbency. Maxorb II is highly conformable and will form a gel as it absorbs wound exudate to provide an optimal moist wound healing environment. Fluid is wicked vertically to prevent potential maceration to periwound tissue.

INDICATIONS

Maxorb II is indicated for all wound depths and moderate to heavily draining pressure injuries, partial- and full-thickness wounds, leg ulcers, diabetic ulcers, surgical wounds, donor sites, lacerations and abrasions, and first- and second-degree burns.

CONTRAINDICATIONS

- Individuals with a known sensitivity to alginates.
- Third-degree burns.
- Not intended for use as a surgical sponge.

APPLICATION

- Cleanse the wound with sterile saline solution or an appropriate wound cleanser, such as Skintegrity Wound Cleanser.
- Apply appropriate skin prep if necessary, such as SurePrep No-Sting.
- Apply the dressing to the wound, covering all areas of the wound with slight overlap to periwound skin. For deep wounds, loosely fill the wound.
- Cover with an appropriate secondary dressing, such as Optifoam Gentle foam.

REMOVAL

- Change when the dressing is saturated or when strike-through to the secondary dressing occurs. Maxorb II may be left in place for up to 7 days.
- Lift one corner of the wound and gently lift the remainder of the dressing.
- If the dressing is dry at the time of removal it may be moistened with sterile saline or wound cleanser to ease removal.
- Rinse the wound with sterile saline solution or an appropriate wound cleanser.

REFERENCE

1. https://www.medline.com/product/Maxorb-II-Alginate-Dressings/Alginate-Dressings/Z05-PF43435?question=maxorb±&=2&=2

ALGINATES

Maxorb Extra CMC/Alginate Dressing

Medline Industries, Inc.

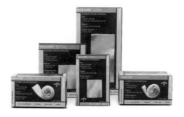

HOW SUPPLIED

Pad	1″ × 12″	A6196
Pad	2″ × 2″	A6196
Pad	4″ × 4″	A6196
Pad	4″ × 8″	A6197
Rope	12″ (2 g)	A6199

Dressings are supplied in sterile form in single pouches or a lidded tray. The lidded tray package on the rope is important because it keeps the fibers from compressing. As a result, fluid-handling capacity is increased.

ACTION

Maxorb Extra CMC/Alginate Dressing's nonwoven alginate and carboxymethylcellulose fiber combination reacts with wound exudate to form a gel, providing a moist healing environment. The added presence of carboxymethylcellulose in Maxorb improves the wicking and fluid-handling ability of this dressing and increases wet strength. Because the product does not wick exudate laterally, it reduces the potential for damage to delicate periwound tissue.

INDICATIONS

To manage partial- and full-thickness wounds with moderate to heavy exudate, including venous stasis ulcers, pressure ulcers (stages 2, 3, and 4), arterial ulcers, diabetic ulcers, donor sites, lacerations, abrasions, postsurgical incisions, and second-degree burns; may also be used for infected and noninfected wounds, tunneling wounds, and wounds with serosanguineous or purulent drainage.

CONTRAINDICATIONS

- Contraindicated for third-degree burns.
- Not intended for use as a surgical sponge.

APPLICATION

- Clean the wound with normal saline solution or an appropriate wound cleanser, such as Skintegrity Wound Cleanser.
- Apply the dressing to a moist wound bed. The dressing can be cut to fit if necessary. Loosely pack deep or tunneling wounds.
- Cover the dressing with an appropriate secondary dressing, such as Optifoam Gentle silicone-faced foam.

REMOVAL

- Change the dressing when strike-through to the secondary dressing occurs, as directed by the physician or up to 7 days.
- The gelatinous pad may be easily lifted away in one piece from the wound bed, making dressing changes easier.
- Remove the secondary dressing as well as gelled and nongelled Maxorb dressing.
- Irrigate the wound with normal saline solution or another appropriate solution, such as Skintegrity Wound Cleanser, to remove any remaining gel.
- If the dressing is dry at the time of removal, moisten it with saline or wound cleanser before removing it. This may indicate the need to consider replacing this type of dressing with a moistening, hydrogel product instead.

REFERENCE

1. https://www.medline.com/product/Maxorb-Extra-CMC/Alginate-Dressings/Alginate-Dressings/Z05-PF00125?question=maxorb±extra&index=P2&indexCount=2

ALGINATES

Melgisorb® Plus Alginate Dressing

Mölnlycke Health Care

Melgisorb® Plus

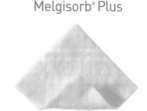

HOW SUPPLIED

Pad	2″ × 2″	A6196
Pad	4″ × 4″	A6196
Pad	4″ × 8″	A6197
Rope	12.5″	A6199

ACTION

Melgisorb® Plus is a hydrophilic calcium alginate dressing that absorbs wound exudate. As the alginate fibers absorb exudate, they become gel-like providing a moist environment conducive to wound healing.

INDICATIONS

To manage infected and noninfected wounds with moderate to heavy exudate, such as pressure ulcers, venous ulcers, arterial ulcers, diabetic ulcers, donor sites, postoperative wounds, and dermal lesions.

CONTRAINDICATIONS

- Contraindicated for dry wounds.
- Contraindicated on third-degree burns.
- Not recommended for surgical implantation.

APPLICATION

- Clean and flush the wound with normal saline solution, then dry the healthy surrounding skin.
- Apply Melgisorb Plus dry to a moist wound bed. For shallow wounds, choose the correct size of the flat dressing to cover the entire wound. For deep or tunneling wounds, choose and cut an appropriate length and pack loosely.
- Cover the dressing with an appropriate secondary dressing.

REMOVAL

- Gently flush the wound with normal saline solution or another appropriate solution. Any nongelled Melgisorb Plus can be moistened with saline and removed.

New Product: Mextra® Superabsorbent

Mölnlycke Health Care

HOW SUPPLIED

Dressing	5″ × 5″	A6196
Dressing	5″ × 7″	A6197
Dressing	5″ × 9″	A6197
Dressing	7″ × 9″	A6197
Dressing	9″ × 11″	A6198
Dressing	9″ × 13″	A6198

ACTION

Mextra® Superabsorbent is a superabsorbent dressing with a fluid-repellent nonwoven backing, a core consisting of superabsorbent particles and a nonwoven contact layer. Mextra® Superabsorbent absorbs wound exudate through the wound contact layer, retains the exudate within the core, and minimizes the risk for maceration. The fluid-repellent nonwoven backing acts as a barrier and prevents exudate strike-through.

INDICATIONS

Mextra® Superabsorbent is intended for use on moderately to heavily exuding wounds.

CONTRAINDICATIONS

* Do not use Mextra® Superabsorbent in cavities.

APPLICATION

* Cleanse the wound in accordance with normal procedures.
* Apply Mextra® Superabsorbent directly on the wound area with the white side of the dressing onto the wound. For the best result, the pad should overlap the dry surrounding skin by at least 2 cm.
* Secure the dressing, for example, with a suitable bandage or tape.
* Mextra® Superabsorbent can be used in conjunction with compression therapy for venous leg ulcers.

REMOVAL

* The wound and Mextra® Superabsorbent should be inspected regularly. The dressing should be changed based on the condition of the wound or before the dressing has become saturated. Mextra® Superabsorbent may be left on the wound for a maximum of 7 days.

New Product: Opticell

Medline Industries, Inc.

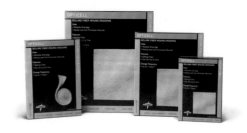

HOW SUPPLIED

Pad	2″ × 2″	A6196
Pad	4″ × 4″	A6197
Pad	6″ × 6″	A6197
Pad	8″ × 12″	A6198
Rope	0.75″ × 18″	A6199

ACTION

Opticell is a chitosan-based gelling fiber made with Chytoform technology that brings the benefits of chitosan to a conformable and highly absorbent wound dressing. Opticell controls minor bleeding and is designed to minimize pain upon removal. As it absorbs wound exudate, Opticell will not shrink and will maintain its size using surface area memory. Lateral wicking limits the risk of maceration to periwound skin.

INDICATIONS

Opticell is indicated for partial- and full-thickness wounds, venous stasis ulcers, pressure injuries, first- and second-degree burns, diabetic foot ulcers, surgical wounds, trauma wounds, donor sites, arterial ulcers and leg ulcers of mixed etiology, and oncology wounds.

CONTRAINDICATIONS

- Individuals with a known sensitivity to chitosan, which is derived from shellfish.
- Third-degree burns.

APPLICATION

- Cleanse the wound with sterile saline solution or an appropriate wound cleanser, such as Skintegrity Wound Cleanser.
- Apply appropriate skin prep if necessary, such as SurePrep No-Sting.
- Apply the dressing to the wound, covering all areas of the wound with slight overlap to periwound skin. For deep wounds, loosely fill the wound.
- Cover with an appropriate secondary dressing, such as Optifoam Gentle foam.

REMOVAL

- Opticell may be left in place for up to 7 days depending on wound exudate.
- Lift one corner of the dressing and gently lift the remainder of the dressing.
- If the dressing is dry at the time of removal it may be moistened with sterile saline or wound cleanser to ease removal.
- Rinse the wound with sterile saline solution or an appropriate wound cleanser.

REFERENCE

1. https://www.medline.com/product/Opticell-Gelling-Fiber-Wound-Dressing/Gelling-Fiber-Dressings/Z05-PF50473?question=opticell&index=P6&indexCount=6

New Product: Optilock

Medline Industries, Inc.

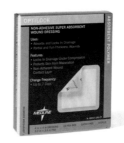

HOW SUPPLIED

Nonadhesive Superabsorbent Wound Dressing	3″ × 3″	A6196
Nonadhesive Superabsorbent Wound Dressing	4″ × 4″	A6196
Nonadhesive Superabsorbent Wound Dressing	5″ × 5.5″	A6197
Nonadhesive Superabsorbent Wound Dressing	6.5″ × 10″	A6198
Nonadhesive Superabsorbent Wound Dressing	8″ × 12″	A6198

ACTION

OptiLock is a superabsorbent polymer core dressing. It takes in a remarkable amount of wound fluid—even under compression—and locks it away to help prevent maceration. Even more, this wound dressing is nonadhesive, meaning minimal disruption to the wound and gentle, pain-free removal. OptiLock can be used as a primary dressing on partial-thickness and full-thickness wounds, such as pressure, venous or neuropathic ulcers; postoperative wounds; superficial or partial-thickness burns (first- or second-degree); lacerations; abrasions. OptiLock can also be used as a secondary dressing on full-thickness wounds.

INDICATIONS

Partial-thickness and full-thickness wounds, such as pressure, venous or neuropathic ulcers; postoperative wounds; superficial or partial-thickness burns (first- or second-degree); lacerations; abrasions. OptiLock can also be used as a secondary dressing on full-thickness wounds.

CONTRAINDICATIONS

- Third-degree burns. Do not use on nonexudating or minimally exudating wounds.

APPLICATION

- Clean the wound using Skintegrity Wound Cleanser or an appropriate solution. Dry the surrounding skin.
- Select the appropriate size dressing to allow the dressing to cover all breached or compromised skin. DO NOT cut Optilock.
- Apply the dressing blue side facing away from the wound, and secure with appropriate cover dressing.

REMOVAL

- The dressing may be left in place for up to 7 days. Dressing change frequency will depend on amount of drainage.
- Clean the wound again before applying a new dressing.

New Product: Qwick

Medline Industries, Inc.

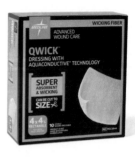

HOW SUPPLIED

Nonadhesive Wicking Fiber Dressing with Aquaconductive Technology	2" × 2"	A6196
Nonadhesive Wicking Fiber Dressing with Aquaconductive Technology	4.25" × 4"	A6197
Nonadhesive Wicking Fiber Dressing with Aquaconductive Technology	6.125" × 8"	A6198

ACTION

Qwick wound dressing is intended for use on moderate to heavily draining wounds. The dressing's fast wicking and super absorbent layers absorb and retain wound exudate that contains harmful Matrix metalloproteinase (MMPs), bacteria, and necrotic debris. Its flexible material makes it versatile for use on any wound with exudate. Aquaconductive Technology is the mechanism by which the three layers of Qwick wound dressing pull exudate away or out of the wound to help create an optimal, moist wound healing environment.

INDICATIONS

Pressure injuries, partial- and full-thickness wounds, and diabetic foot ulcers.

CONTRAINDICATIONS

- Third-degree burns and lesions with active vasculitis.

APPLICATION

- Clean the wound using Skintegrity Wound Cleanser or an appropriate solution. Dry the surrounding skin.
- Select the appropriate size dressing to allow the dressing to cover all breached or compromised skin.
- Apply the dressing blue side facing away from the wound, and secure with appropriate cover dressing.

REMOVAL

- The dressing may be left in place for up to 7 days or until exudate is visible and nears the edge of the dressing.
- Clean the wound again before applying a new dressing.

3M™ Tegaderm™ High Integrity and High Gelling Alginate Dressing

3M™ Health Care

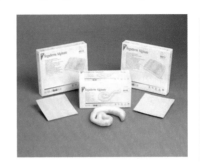

HOW SUPPLIED

High integrity

Pad	4″ × 4″	A6196
Rope	1″ × 12″	A6199

High gelling

Pad	4″ × 4″	A6196
Rope	12″	A6199

ACTION

3M™ Tegaderm™ Alginate Dressings are gel-forming, absorbent, versatile alginates, which provide for optimum wound healing. 3M™ Tegaderm™ High Integrity Dressing offers high integrity for quick dressing changes. 3M™ Tegaderm™ High Gelling Alginate Dressing offers high-gelling properties, which may be preferable for gentle removal of the dressing from fragile tissue.

INDICATIONS

3M™ Tegaderm™ Alginate Dressings are primary dressings intended for use on partial and full thickness wounds with moderate to heavy exudate. The dressings may be used for pressure injuries, arterial ulcers, venous ulcers, diabetic ulcers, superficial wounds such as cuts and abrasions, donor sites, postoperative wounds, trauma wounds, and other dermal lesions. They are also intended to help control minor bleeding. Use of any dressing, including 3M™ Tegaderm™ Alginate dressings, should be part of a well-defined protocol for dermal wound management.

CONTRAINDICATIONS

- Contraindicated for surgical implantation.
- Contraindicated for third-degree burns.

APPLICATION

Pad

- Moisten the wound site with normal saline solution or other sterile irrigation solution, according to facility policy. Dry the periwound skin.
- If the patient's skin is fragile or wound drainage may contact the periwound skin, apply barrier film around the wound.
- Select the appropriate dressing size for the wound. 3M™ Tegaderm™ High Integrity and High Gelling Alginate dressings may be trimmed to fit the wound site.
- Apply the dressing to the wound bed with minimal overlap to the periwound skin.
- Loosely pack deep wounds.
- Cover the dressing with an appropriate secondary dressing.

Rope

- Fluff the rope dressing as needed for light packing.
- Make sure the dressing lightly contacts all wound surfaces, including areas of undermining.
- Loosely pack deep wounds by fluffing and layering the dressing back and forth into the wound.
- Cover the rope dressing with an appropriate secondary dressing.
- Extend the cover dressing at least 1″ (2.5 cm) beyond the edge of the wound.

REMOVAL

- Remove secondary dressing and nongelling alginate dressing. Rinse away remaining gel with gentle irrigation.
- If the dressing appears dry, saturate it with sterile saline solution to help remove it.
- Dressing may be removed using sterile forceps or gentle irrigation.

REFERENCE

1. https://www.3m.com/3M/en_US/company-us/all-3m-products/~/3M-Tegaderm-Alginate-Dressing?N=5002385±3293321971&rt=rud

Antimicrobials

ACTION

Antimicrobial dressings are topical wound care products derived from agents such as silver, iodine, and polyhexethylene biguanide. These products combine active ingredients with a dressing to deliver an antimicrobial or antibacterial action to the wound. Silver dressings come in various delivery systems as well as shapes and sizes. The silver is activated from the dressing to the wound's surface based on the amount of exudate and bacteria in the wound. Silver dressings are available in foams, hydrocolloids, alginates, barrier layers, charcoal cloth dressings, or a combination of different forms. Silver dressings may be used with select topical and adjunctive therapies to, among other things, decrease the bacterial load and manage exudate, and as a result, optimize the appearance of the wound's granulation tissue.

Gauze products containing antibacterial properties have been designed to provide a barrier to specific organisms but also inhibit the growth of bacteria within the dressing, thus protecting the wound and potential spread of bacteria from the dressed site.

INDICATIONS

Antimicrobial dressings are intended for use in draining, exuding, and nonhealing wounds where protection from bacterial contamination is desired. These dressings may be used as primary or secondary dressings to manage various amounts of exudate (minimal, moderate, or heavy) for both acute and chronic wounds, including burns, surgical wounds, diabetic foot ulcers, pressure ulcers, and leg ulcers. Select dressings may also be used under compression.

ADVANTAGES

- Provides a broad range of antimicrobial or antibacterial activity.
- Reduces infection.
- Prevents infection.
- May alter metalloproteinases within wounds with select dressings.

DISADVANTAGES

- May cause staining on wound and intact skin with silver dressings.
- May cause stinging or sensitization.
- Development of resistant organisms not yet known.

HCPCS CODE OVERVIEW

Each product under this category description has been assigned a different code based on its physical size and characteristics; or the manufacturer hasn't yet received or applied for a code. Please refer to individual product listings for further information about each product.

New Product: ACTISORB™ Silver 220 Antimicrobial Binding Dressing

Systagenix, An ACELITY™ Company

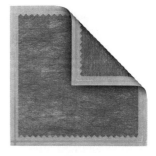

HOW SUPPLIED

ACTISORB™ Silver 220 Antimicrobial Binding Dressing	2 1/2" × 3 3/4"	A6206
ACTISORB™ Silver 220 Antimicrobial Binding Dressing	4 1/8" × 4 1/8"	A6207
ACTISORB™ Silver 220 Antimicrobial Binding Dressing	4 1/8" × 7 1/2"	A6207

ACTION

ACTISORB™ Silver 220 Antimicrobial Binding Dressing is a sterile primary dressing, comprised of activated charcoal cloth, impregnated with silver, within a spun bonded nylon envelope. Within the dressing, there is 220 mg of silver per 100 g activated charcoal cloth equating to 33 g of silver per square centimeter of cloth.

INDICATIONS

ACTISORB™ Silver 220 Dressing provides an effective barrier to bacterial penetration and for absorbing offending odor resulting from wounds; the binding properties of the dressing trap bacteria, bacterial toxins, and odor. ACTISORB™ Silver 220 Dressing may help reduce infection in partial- and full-thickness wounds, including:

- Pressure ulcers.
- Venous ulcers.
- Diabetic ulcers.
- First- and second-degree burns.
- Donor sites.
- Surgical wounds.
  ACTISORB™ Silver 220 Dressing is suitable for use under compression bandaging.

CONTRAINDICATIONS

- ACTISORB™ Silver 220 Dressing should not be used on third-degree burns or used on patients with a known sensitivity to silver.

APPLICATION

- This product should not be cut, otherwise particles of activated charcoal may get into the wound and cause discoloration.
- The dressing performance may be impaired by excess use of petrolatum-based ointments.
- Clinicians/Health care Professionals should be aware that there are very limited data on prolonged and repeated use of silver containing dressings, particularly in children and neonates.
- Prepare wound bed according to wound management protocol, ensuring removal of necrotic tissue.

- The properties of the dressing are most fully utilized when ACTISORB™ Silver 220 Antimicrobial Binding Dressing makes direct contact with the wound.
- Either side of ACTISORB™ Silver 220 dressing can be applied to the wound bed.
- Do not cut the dressing. Fold or pack as necessary.
- ACTISORB™ Silver 220 Dressing can be easily packed into deep wounds.
- The outer nylon envelope enables removal from the majority of wounds with minimal adherence or trauma.
- For lightly exuding wounds, ACTISORB™ Silver 220 Dressing can be used in combination with a nonadherent wound contact layer.
- Depending on the level of exudate, an absorbent secondary dressing may be placed on top of ACTISORB™ Silver 220 Dressing.
- Secure the dressing in a manner appropriate for the indication.

REMOVAL

- ACTISORB™ Silver 220 Antimicrobial Binding Dressing can remain in situ up to 7 days, dependent on the level of exudate, while the secondary absorbent dressing is changed as required. Initially it may be necessary to change ACTISORB™ Silver 220 Dressing every 24 hours to ensure optimal dressing performance.

REFERENCES

1. Jackson L. Use of a charcoal dressing with silver on a MRSA-infected wound. *British J Community Nurs.* 2001;6(Suppl3):19–26.
2. Hampton S. Actisorb Silver 220: a unique antibacterial dressing. *British J Nurs.* 2001;10 (Suppl4): 17–19.
3. Stadler R, Wallenfang K. Survey of 12444 patients with chronic wounds treated with charcoal dressing (Actisorb). *Aktuelle Dermatologie.* 2002;28(10):351–354.

ANTIMICROBIALS

Algidex Ag

DeRoyal

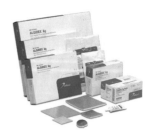

HOW SUPPLIED

Foam Back	2" × 2"	A6209
Foam Back	4" × 4"	A6209
Foam Back	4" × 5"	A6210
Foam Back	6" × 6"	A6210
Foam Back	8" × 8"	A6211
Thin Sheet	2" × 2"	A6196
Thin Sheet	4" × 4"	A6196
Thin Sheet	4" × 8"	A6197
Thin Sheet	6" × 6"	A6197
Thin Sheet	8" × 8"	A6198
Thin Sheet	8" × 16"	A6198
Thin Sheet	16" × 16"	A6198
Paste	10 cc	A6261

ACTION

Algidex Ag provides slow, extended release of active ionic silver for broad antimicrobial effectiveness. The unique matrix formulation of silver, alginate, and maltodextrin allows Algidex Ag to absorb wound exudates, decrease surface wound contaminates, decrease wound odor, and create a moist environment conducive to healing.

INDICATIONS

For use in infected and noninfected wounds of all types; dermal ulcers (leg ulcers, pressure ulcers); diabetic ulcers; abdominal wounds; superficial wounds; lacerations, cuts, and abrasions; donor sites; second-degree burns; and dry, moist, or wet wounds.

CONTRAINDICATIONS

- Not for use on third-degree burns.
- Not for use on ulcers resulting from infections.
- Contraindicated for lesions associated with active vasculitis.
- Contraindicated for patients with sensitivity to alginates.

APPLICATION

For Algidex Ag Foam

- Thoroughly cleanse wound with normal saline.
- Apply Algidex Ag with silver matrix touching the wound.
- Secure dressing in place with retention dressing such as gauze, transparent film, or tape.
- Algidex Ag is antimicrobial for up to 7 days and may be worn until dressing has reached saturation.

ANTIMICROBIALS

For Algidex Ag Thin Sheet

- Thoroughly cleanse wound with normal saline.
- Remove backing from Algidex Ag Thin Sheet.
- Place Algidex Ag Thin Sheet over shallow wounds, or pack into deep wounds.
- Cover with appropriate secondary dressing based on wound drainage.
- Algidex Ag Thin Sheet is antimicrobial for up to 7 days and may be worn until secondary dressing requires changing.

For Algidex Ag Paste

- Thoroughly cleanse wound with normal saline.
- Apply 1/4" thickness of paste to shallow wounds, or completely fill deep wounds.
- Cover with appropriate secondary dressing based on wound drainage.
- Algidex Ag Paste is antimicrobial for up to 7 days and may be worn until secondary dressing requires changing.

REMOVAL

For Algidex Ag Foam

- Remove retention dressing, if applicable.
- Gently lift Algidex Ag from the wound. If dressing adheres to wound, gently irrigate with saline to help loosen dressing.
- Discard according to institutional policy.
- Once dressing is removed, thoroughly cleanse wound with normal saline to remove any residue or debris from the wound.

For Algidex Ag Thin Sheet or Paste

- Remove secondary dressing.
- Gently irrigate wound with saline to help loosen Algidex Ag.
- Continue to thoroughly cleanse wound to remove wound drainage or any residue left from Algidex Ag.

ANTIMICROBIALS

Algidex Ag I.V. Patch

DeRoyal

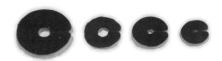

HOW SUPPLIED

I.V. Patch	3/4" disc w/2 mm opening	A6209
I.V. Patch	1" disc w/4 mm opening	A6209
I.V. Patch	1" disc w/7 mm opening	A6209
I.V. Patch	1" disc w/4 mm opening (with insert)	A6209
I.V. Patch	1 1/2" disc w/7 mm opening	A6209

ACTION

Algidex Ag I.V. patch is an effective bacterial barrier that helps to prevent catheter-related infections. It is an ideal dressing for intravenous catheters, tube sites, or external fixator pin sites. With a unique combination of silver, alginate, and maltodextrin, Algidex Ag I.V. patch provides a sustained antimicrobial activity against a broad spectrum of pathogens without inducing bacterial resistance. The antimicrobial activity remains effective for up to 7 days.

INDICATIONS

Algidex Ag I.V. patch is indicated for dialysis catheters, central venous lines, arterial catheters, external fixator pins, epidural catheters, peripheral I.V. catheters, gastrostomy feeding tubes, and nonvascular percutaneous devices.

CONTRAINDICATIONS

- Not for use on third-degree burns.
- Contraindicated for patients with sensitivity to alginates.

APPLICATION

- May be applied immediately following initial catheter placement or during routine catheter dressing change.
- Apply Algidex Ag I.V. Patch with dark side touching the catheter and skin.
- Secure patch in place with retention dressing such as gauze, transparent film, or tape.
- Patch may be worn up to 7 days.

REMOVAL

- Remove retention dressing, if applicable.
- Lift Algidex Ag I.V. patch from the catheter and gently wipe any Algidex matrix residue during routine dressing change, using saline or antiseptic skin prep as stated in the institutional procedural guidelines.
- Discard according to institutional policy.

ANTIMICROBIALS

Algidex Ag Packing Gauze

DeRoyal

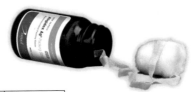

HOW SUPPLIED

Algidex Ag Packing Gauze	1/2″ × 5 yd	A6407
Algidex Ag Packing Gauze	1/4″ × 5 yd	A6407

ACTION

Algidex Ag provides slow, extended release of active ionic silver for broad antimicrobial effectiveness. The unique matrix formulation of silver, alginate, and maltodextrin allows Algidex Ag to absorb wound exudates, decrease surface wound contaminates, decrease wound odor, and create a moist environment conducive to healing.

INDICATIONS

Algidex Ag Packing Gauze is used for the management of "deeper" wounds that require packing such as tunneling or undermining wounds (pressure ulcers, venous ulcers, diabetic ulcers, and surgical wounds).

CONTRAINDICATIONS

- None provided by the manufacturer.

APPLICATION

- Thoroughly cleanse wound with normal saline.
- Remove appropriate amount of packing gauze from bottle.
- Completely fill wound with packing gauze (lightly packing).
- Cover with appropriate secondary dressing such as gauze, hydrocolloid, foam, or film dressing. Secondary dressing selection should be based on the amount of wound drainage.
- Dressing may be worn up to 5 days or until cover dressing reaches saturation.

REMOVAL

- Remove secondary dressing.
- Gently remove packing gauze.
- Thoroughly cleanse wound to remove wound drainage or residue from Algidex Ag.
- Reapply as necessary following directions above.

New Product: Algidex Ag Tracheostomy Dressing

DeRoyal

HOW SUPPLIED

Dressing	2″ × 2″, precut	A6209
Dressing	4″ × 4″, precut	A6209

ACTION

Algidex Ag provides slow, extended release of active ionic silver for broad antimicrobial effectiveness. The unique matrix formulation of silver, alginate, and maltodextrin allows Algidex Ag to absorb wound exudates, decrease surface wound contaminants, decrease wound odor, and create a moist environment conducive to healing. The maltodextrin creates an environment that helps the body's own cells to carry out the task of granulation tissue formation while eliminating wound odor. Algidex Ag is not absorbed systemically.

INDICATIONS

Algidex Ag Tracheostomy Dressings are for use in the treatment of wounds associated with tracheostomy, other intubation, and cannula sites. Additional uses may include nonvascular percutaneous devices such as external fixator pins, peritoneal dialysis catheters, and other tube sites.

CONTRAINDICATIONS

- Not for use on third-degree burns.
- Contraindicated for patients with sensitivity to alginates.

APPLICATION

- Clean the site according to institutional policy and procedures. Prepare and clean the skin surrounding the tracheostomy tube to remove excess moisture.
- Remove the Algidex Ag Tracheostomy Dressing, locate the precut opening and position it around the stoma or tracheostomy tube. Apply with the silver side (dark side) toward the patient.
- If needed, the dressing may be cut to shape or size.
- If additional fixation is required, transparent film dressings or tape may be used to help secure the dressing.
- The tracheostomy site should be inspected frequently during the early stages of treatment to ensure skin integrity and clear airway. The dressing can be left in place undisturbed for up to 7 days, or until the foam pad becomes saturated with exudates.

REMOVAL

- Remove retention dressing, if applicable.
- Lift the Algidex Ag Tracheostomy Dressing from around the tube and discard according to institutional policy.

ANTIMICROBIALS

New Product: AQUACEL® Ag EXTRA™ Wound Dressing*

ConvaTec

HOW SUPPLIED

Dressing	2″ × 2″	A6196
Dressing	4″ × 5″	A6197
Dressing	6″ × 6″	A6197
Dressing	8″ × 12″	A6198

ACTION

AQUACEL® Ag EXTRA™ Wound Dressing is an advanced technology, sterile, single use wound dressing comprised of sodium carboxymethylcellulose and ionic silver. It is composed of two layers of Hydrofiber® Technology stitched together. It is a soft and conformable dressing that remains integral when wet or dry. This highly absorbent dressing interacts with wound exudate and forms a soft gel that maintains a moist environment for optimal wound healing and easy removal with little or no damage to healing wounds. The ionic silver gives AQUACEL® Ag EXTRA™ dressing its silver-gray appearance and broad-spectrum antimicrobial properties.

INDICATIONS

To manage wounds at risk of infection; partial-thickness (second-degree) burns; diabetic foot ulcers; venous stasis ulcers, arterial ulcers, and other leg ulcers; pressure ulcers (partial- and full-thickness); surgical wounds left to heal by secondary intent; traumatic wounds prone to bleeding, such as those that have been mechanically or surgically debrided; oncology wounds with exudate, such as fungoides-cutaneous tumors, fungating carcinoma, cutaneous metastasis, Kaposi's sarcoma, and angiosarcoma.

CONTRAINDICATIONS

- Not for use on patients who are sensitive to or who have had an allergic reaction to the dressing or its components.

APPLICATION

- Clean the wound with water or saline. Apply the dressing to shallow wounds with an adequate overlap (at least 3/8″ [1 cm]) of the wound edges. For deep wounds, loosely pack ribbon or sheet into wound to about 80% of the depth of the wound to accommodate swelling of the dressing, leaving a small overhang (at least 1″ [2.5 cm]) to facilitate removal.
- For dry wounds, place the AQUACEL® Ag EXTRA™ dressing in the wound and then wet with sterile saline over the wound area only. The vertical absorption properties of the dressing will help to maintain the moist area over the wound only and reduce the risk of maceration. Cover the dressing with a moisture-retentive dressing to avoid drying out the dressing and subsequent dressing adherence to the wound.
- Cover and secure with an appropriate dressing.

REMOVAL

- AQUACEL® Ag EXTRA™ dressing is designed to be easy to remove without leaving residue or causing trauma to the wound bed. In the unlikely event of adhesion to the wound bed, the dressing can be easily removed by soaking.

*See package insert for complete instructions for use.

ANTIMICROBIALS

New Product: AQUACEL™ Ag Foam Wound Dressing*

ConvaTec

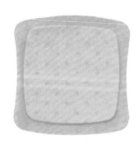

HOW SUPPLIED

Dressing, Adhesive	3.2" × 3.2"
Dressing, Adhesive	4" × 4"
Dressing, Adhesive	5" × 5"
Dressing, Adhesive	7" × 7"
Dressing, Adhesive	10" × 12"
Dressing, Heel	8" × 5(1/2)"
Dressing, Sacral	8" × 7"
Dressing, Sacral	9.4" × 8.4"
Dressing, Nonadhesive	2" × 2"
Dressing, Nonadhesive	4" × 4"
Dressing, Nonadhesive	6" × 6"
Dressing, Nonadhesive	6" × 8"
Dressing, Nonadhesive	8" × 8"

ACTION

AQUACEL™ Ag Foam dressing offers the healing benefits of a Hydrofiber™ interface layer, the comfort of foam, and the bacteria-killing power of ionic silver.

INDICATIONS

AQUACEL™ Ag Foam may be used for the management of both chronic and acute wounds, such as: leg ulcers, pressure ulcers (stage 2 to 4) and diabetic ulcers; surgical wounds (post-operative, donor sites, dermatologic); partial thickness (second-degree) burns; traumatic or surgical wounds left to heal by secondary intention such as dehisced surgical incisions; surgical wounds that heal by primary intent, such as dermatologic and surgical incisions (e.g., orthopedic and vascular); local management of wounds that are prone to bleeding, such as wounds that have been mechanically or surgically debrided and donor sites; painful wounds; abrasions; lacerations; minor cuts; minor scalds and burns.

CONTRAINDICATIONS

- AQUACEL™ Ag Foam dressings should not be used on individuals who are sensitive to or who have had an allergic reaction to the dressing or its components.

APPLICATION

- If the immediate sterile product pouch is damaged, do not use.

Wound site preparation and cleansing

- Before applying the dressing, cleanse the wound area with an appropriate wound cleanser and dry the surrounding skin.

Dressing preparation and application

- Choose a dressing size and shape to ensure that the central absorbent pad (area within the adhesive window) is 1 cm larger than the wound area. Remove the dressing from the sterile pack, minimizing finger contact with the wound contact surface and the adhesive surface where applicable. Remove the release liner if using the adhesive dressing.
- The dressing can be cut to shape for convenience. Hold the dressing over the wound and line up the center of the dressing with the center of the wound. Place the pad directly over the wound. For adhesive dressing, smooth down the adhesive border. An appropriate retention bandage or tape should be used to secure the dressing in place if the dressing does not have an adhesive border or if the adhesive dressing has been cut. For difficult to dress anatomical locations, such as the heel or the sacrum, the specially shaped adhesive dressings may be used. Discard any unused portion of the product after dressing the wound.

REMOVAL

- The dressing should be changed when clinically indicated (i.e., leakage, bleeding, increased pain, suspicion of infection). Maximum recommended wear time is up to 7 days. The wound should be cleansed at appropriate intervals. To remove the dressing, press down gently on the skin and carefully lift one corner of the dressing. Continue until all edges are free. Carefully lift away the dressing and discard according to local clinical protocols.

*See package insert for complete instructions for use.

ANTIMICROBIALS

New Product: AQUACEL® Ag Ribbon Dressing*

ConvaTec

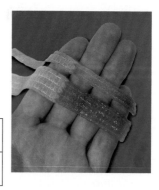

HOW SUPPLIED

Ribbon with Strengthening Fibers	0.39" × 18"	A6199
Ribbon with Strengthening Fibers	0.75" × 18"	A6199

ACTION

AQUACEL® Ag Ribbon dressing is an advanced technology, sterile, single use wound dressing comprised of sodium carboxymethylcellulose and ionic silver. It is a soft and conformable dressing that remains integral when wet or dry. This highly absorbent dressing interacts with wound exudate and forms a soft gel that maintains a moist environment for optimal wound healing and easy removal with little or no damage to healing wounds. The ionic silver gives AQUACEL® Ag Ribbon dressing its silver-gray appearance and broad-spectrum antimicrobial properties.

INDICATIONS

To manage wounds at risk of infection; partial-thickness (second-degree) burns; diabetic foot ulcers; venous stasis ulcers, arterial ulcers, and other leg ulcers; pressure ulcers (partial- and full-thickness); surgical wounds left to heal by secondary intent; traumatic wounds prone to bleeding, such as those that have been mechanically or surgically debrided; oncology wounds with exudate, such as fungoides-cutaneous tumors, fungating carcinoma, cutaneous metastasis, Kaposi's sarcoma, and angiosarcoma.

CONTRAINDICATIONS

- Not for use on patients who are sensitive to or who have had an allergic reaction to the dressing or its components.

APPLICATION

- Clean the wound with water or saline. Apply the dressing to shallow wounds with an adequate overlap (at least 3/8" [1 cm]) of the wound edges. For deep wounds, loosely pack ribbon into wound to about 80% of the depth of the wound to accommodate swelling of the dressing, leaving a small overhang (at least 1" [2.5 cm]) to facilitate removal.
- For dry wounds, place the AQUACEL® Ag Ribbon dressing in the wound and then wet with sterile saline over the wound area only. The vertical absorption properties of the dressing will help to maintain the moist area over the wound only and reduce the risk of maceration. Cover the dressing with a moisture-retentive dressing to avoid drying out the dressing and subsequent dressing adherence to the wound.
- Cover and secure with an appropriate dressing.

REMOVAL

- AQUACEL® Ag Ribbon dressing is designed to be easy to remove without leaving residue or causing trauma to the wound bed. In the unlikely event of adhesion to the wound bed, the dressing can be easily removed by soaking.

*See package insert for complete instructions for use.

New Product: AQUACEL® Ag Surgical Slim Profile (SP) Wound Dressing*

ConvaTec

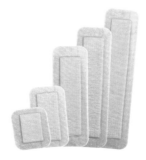

HOW SUPPLIED

Dressing	3(1/2)" × 4"
Dressing	3(1/2)" × 6"
Dressing	3(1/2)" × 10"
Dressing	3(1/2)" × 12"
Dressing	3(1/2)" × 14"

ACTION

AQUACEL® Ag Surgical SP dressing is a sterile postoperative dressing comprising of an inner nonwoven pad composed of Hydrofiber® technology and ionic silver. The pad is composed of a hydrocolloid adhesive (top layer) bound to an outer polyurethane film and a windowed polyurethane film skin contact layer, sandwiched between one layer of acrylic and one layer of hydrocolloid contacting the skin.

INDICATIONS

AQUACEL® Ag Surgical SP may be used for the management of wounds healing by primary intent and as an effective barrier to bacterial penetration to help reduce infection.

CONTRAINDICATIONS

- AQUACEL® Ag Surgical SP Dressing should not be used on individuals who are sensitive to the dressing or its components or have had an allergic reaction to the dressing or its components.

APPLICATION

- Before applying the dressing, cleanse the wound/incision site, rinse well with sterile saline and dry the surrounding skin. Choose a dressing size and shape to ensure direct contact between the wound/incision area and the Hydrofiber® pad. Remove the dressing from the sterile pack. Initially remove 3/4 of the backing paper along the length of the dressing minimizing finger contact with the central pad and the adhesive surface. Place at one side of the wound/incision line. Gently roll the dressing over the wound/incision line and mold into place. Remove the remaining 1/4 backing paper and gently mold the dressing in place with hand for a secure adhesion. Do not stretch. The translucent hydrocolloid backing allows the clinician to monitor the central Hydrofiber® pad and assess when the dressing needs to be changed.
- The dressing can be left in place for up to 7 days subject to regular clinical assessment and local dressing protocol. All wounds/incisions should be monitored frequently. Remove AQUACEL® Ag Surgical SP Dressing when clinically indicated (i.e., leakage, excessive bleeding, suspicion of infection, or at 7 days).
- To dress knee incisions.
- Knee should be approximately at a 30-degree angle for optimal dressing application.

REMOVAL

- To remove dressing, press down on the skin with one hand and carefully lift an edge of the dressing with the other hand. Stretch the dressing to break the adhesive seal and remove. TIP: For ease of removal, use Sensi-Care® Sting Free Adhesive Remover spray or Sensi-Care® Sting Free Adhesive Remover wipes.

*See package insert for complete instructions for use.

ANTIMICROBIALS

ANTIMICROBIALS

New Product: AQUACEL® Ag Surgical Wound Dressing*

ConvaTec

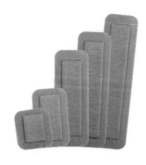

HOW SUPPLIED

Dressing	3(1/2)" × 4"
Dressing	3(1/2)" × 6"
Dressing	3(1/2)" × 10"
Dressing	3(1/2)" × 12"
Dressing	3(1/2)" × 14"

ACTION

AQUACEL® Ag Surgical dressing is a sterile postoperative dressing comprising of an inner nonwoven pad composed of Hydrofiber® Technology and ionic silver. The pad is composed of a hydrocolloid adhesive (top layer) bound to an outer polyurethane film and a windowed polyurethane film skin contact layer, sandwiched between one layer of acrylic and one layer of hydrocolloid contacting the skin.

INDICATIONS

AQUACEL® Ag Surgical dressing may be used for the management of wounds healing by primary intent and as an effective barrier to bacterial penetration to help reduce infection.

CONTRAINDICATIONS

- AQUACEL® Ag Surgical dressing should not be used on individuals who are sensitive to the dressing or its components or have had an allergic reaction to the dressing or its components.

APPLICATION

- Before applying the dressing, cleanse the wound/incision site, rinse well with sterile saline and dry the surrounding skin. Choose a dressing size and shape to ensure direct contact between the wound/incision area and the Hydrofiber® pad. Remove the dressing from the sterile pack. Initially remove 3/4 of the backing paper along the length of the dressing minimizing finger contact with the central pad and the adhesive surface. Place at one side of the wound/incision line. Gently roll the dressing over the wound/incision line and mold into place. Remove the remaining 1/4 backing paper and gently mold the dressing in place with hand for a secure adhesion. Do not stretch. The translucent hydrocolloid backing allows the clinician to monitor the central Hydrofiber® pad and assess when the dressing needs to be changed.
- The dressing can be left in place for up to 7 days subject to regular clinical assessment and local dressing protocol. All wounds/incisions should be monitored frequently. Remove AQUACEL® Ag Surgical dressing when clinically indicated (i.e., leakage, excessive bleeding, suspicion of infection, or at 7 days).
- To dress knee incisions.
- Knee should be approximately at a 30-degree angle for optimal dressing application.

REMOVAL

- To remove dressing, press down on the skin with one hand and carefully lift an edge of the dressing with the other hand. Stretch the dressing to break the adhesive seal and remove. TIP: For ease of removal, use Sensi-Care® Sting Free Adhesive Remover spray or Sensi-Care® Sting Free Adhesive Remover wipes.

*See package insert for complete instructions for use.

Biatain® Ag Non-Adhesive Foam Dressing; Biatain® Ag Adhesive Foam Dressing

Coloplast

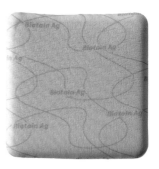

HOW SUPPLIED

Biatain Ag Non-Adhesive Foam Dressing

Square	4″ × 4″	A6209
Square	6″ × 6″	A6210

Biatain Ag Adhesive Foam Dressing

Square	5″ × 5″	A6212
Square	7″ × 7″	A6213
Heel	7.5″ × 8″	A6212
Sacral	9″ × 9″	A6213

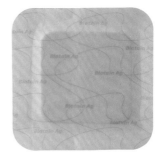

ACTION

Biatain® Ag Foam Dressings are sterile, single use, soft, highly absorbent, and conformable antibacterial polyurethane foam dressings with ionic silver as the active component. Biatain Ag Foam Dressings provide an optimal moist wound environment and effective exudate management. Biatain Ag Foam Dressings contain an antibacterial silver complex homogeneously dispersed throughout the foam. In the presence of exudate the release of ionic silver will continue for up to 7 days.

INDICATIONS

Biatain Ag Foam Dressings are indicated for wounds with moderate to high amounts of exudate, including leg ulcers and Category II–IV pressure ulcers with delayed wound healing due to bacteria, or where there is a risk of infection. They may be used for second-degree burns, donor sites, postoperative wounds, and skin abrasions with delayed wound healing due to bacteria, or where there is a risk of infection. In addition, Biatain Ag Non-Adhesive Foam Dressing is indicated for diabetic foot ulcers.

CAUTION

- A health care professional should frequently inspect and manage diabetic wounds and wound which are solely or partially caused by arterial insufficiency, in accordance with local standards.
- Should not be used in patients with a known sensitivity to silver.
- Do not use with oxidizing solutions (e.g., hypochlorite and hydrogen peroxide solutions). Ensure that any other evaporating solution is completely dried off before dressing application.
- May cause a transient discoloration of the wound bed, which can be removed by gentle washing.
- Must be removed prior to radiation treatment or examinations that include x-rays, ultrasonic treatment, diathermy, or microwaves. However, it is MR safe and compatible up to 3 Tesla and can therefore be left in place during an MR scan.
- Use during pregnancy, lactation, and on children has not been demonstrated.
- Application with enzymatic debriding agents has not been demonstrated.

ANTIMICROBIALS

APPLICATION

- Rinse the wound with lukewarm water or physiological saline. Gently dry the skin around the wounds. The safe use of other cleansing agents, in combination with Biatain Ag Foam Dressings has not been demonstrated.
- If any film, cream, ointment or similar product is used, allow the skin to dry before applying the dressing.
- Remove the dressing aseptically from the packaging. Do not touch the plain (nonprinted) side of the foam.
- Select a dressing where the foam pad overlaps the wound edge by at least 2 cm. For small size dressings an overlap of only 1 cm is necessary.

Biatain Ag Non-Adhesive Foam Dressing

- Must be applied with the plain (nonprinted) side toward the wound.
- Must be secured with a secondary bandage or compression.

Biatain Ag Adhesive Foam Dressing

- Use the handles to prevent touching the dressing and to ensure aseptic application. Remove the protective film first and place the foam part of the dressing over the wound. Then remove the release films on the sides as part of the dressing application.

Biatain Ag Sacral Foam Dressing

- Use the handles to ensure aseptic application. Remove the central protective film. Place the narrow end of the dressing as far down over the wound as possible and fix the dressing working up and outwards. Remove the handles.

Biatain Ag Heel Foam Dressing

- Use the handles to ensure aseptic application. Remove the central protective film. The dressing is shaped like an "arrow." Fold the dressing at a 90-degree angle between the "arrow head" and "arrow tail." Let the "arrow" point away from the heel tip and fix the "arrow tail" first. Secondly, fix the "arrow head." Remove the handles one by one and fix the sides carefully, in order that the foam parts touch or overlap.

REMOVAL

- Dressing should be changed when clinically indicated or when visible signs of exudate approach the edge of the dressing.
- Dressing may be left in place for up to 7 days, depending on the amount of exudate, dressing condition, and type of wound.
- To remove the dressing, gently lift the corners of the dressing away from the wound.
- To remove the adhesive dressings, loosen the adhesive border before lifting the dressing away from the wound.
- Biatain Ag Sacral Foam Dressing should be removed from the top edge and down toward the anus to minimize the risk of transmitting infection.

REFERENCES

Biatain Ag Non-Adhesive Foam Dressing

1. https://www.coloplast.us/wound/wound-/solutions/#section=Effective-management-of-wounds-at-risk-of-infection_82172

Biatain Ag Adhesive Foam Dressing

2. https://www.coloplast.us/wound/wound-/solutions/#section=Effective-management-of-wounds-at-risk-of-infection_82172

Biatain® Alginate Ag Dressing and Biatain® Alginate Ag Rope

Coloplast

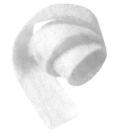

HOW SUPPLIED

Sheet	2″ × 2″	A6196
Sheet	4″ × 4″	A6196
Rope	6″ × 6″	A6197

ACTION

Biatain® Alginate Ag Dressing and Biatain® Alginate Ag Rope are a unique mix of calcium alginate and highly absorbent carboxymethyl-cellulose with the addition of an ionic silver complex, which releases silver ions in the presence of wound exudate. As exudate is absorbed, the dressing forms a soft, cohesive gel that intimately conforms to the wound surface. Silver ions protect the dressing from a broad spectrum of microorganisms over a period of up to 14 days.

INDICATIONS

To manage moderate to heavily exuding wounds such as pressure ulcers, leg ulcers, diabetic ulcers, second-degree burns, grafts, donor sites, trauma wounds, as well as cavity wounds; may be used on infected wounds under the discretion of a health care professional.

CAUTIONS

The dressing may adhere if used on dry or very lightly exuding wounds. If the dressing is not easily removed, moisten it with sterile saline prior to removing. The dressing performance may be impaired by excess use of petrolatum-based ointments. The dressing must be removed prior to undergoing MRI examinations. Systemic antimicrobial therapy should be considered when wound infection is evident. Biatain Alginate Ag may be used, under medical supervision, in conjunction with systemic antibiotics. In the event of clinical infection, topical silver does not replace the need for systemic therapy or other adequate infection treatment.

APPLICATION

- Debride when necessary, and irrigate the wound site in accordance with standard protocols.
- Remove excess solution from surrounding skin.
- Select a size of Biatain Alginate Ag that is slightly larger than the wound.
- Cut or fold the dressing to fit the wound.
- Apply to wound bed directly.
- Cover and secure with a nonocclusive secondary dressing, such as Comfeel® Plus Transparent Dressing or Biatain® Foam Dressing.

REMOVAL

- Dressing change frequency will depend on wound condition and the level of exudate. Initially, it may be necessary to change the dressing every 24 hours.

REFERENCE

1. https://www.coloplast.us/wound/wound-/solutions/#section=Effective-management-of-wounds-atrisk-of-infection_82172

Bordered Foam with Silver

Gentell

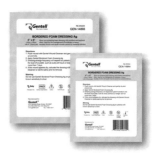

HOW SUPPLIED

Pad	4″ × 4″	A6212
Pad	6″ × 6″	A6212

ACTION

Gentell Bordered Foam Ag is a silver ion-containing foam dressing with excellent antibacterial effects.

INDICATIONS

It is ideal for the treatment of moderate or heavy exudate chronic and acute wounds caused by bacterial infections, including leg ulcers, pressure injuries, diabetic foot ulcers, second degree burns, donor sites, postoperative wounds, and skin abrasions.

CONTRAINDICATIONS

- Do not use Gentell Bordered Foam Dressing Ag on patients with known sensitivity to silver.

APPLICATION

- Irrigate the wound with Gentell Wound Cleanser and gently dry the skin surrounding the wound site.
- Choose the appropriate sized dressing based on the dimensions of the wound.
- Apply Gentell Bordered Foam Ag directly to the wound bed.

REMOVAL

- If the wound appears dry, saturate the dressing with Gentell Wound Cleanser or sterile saline prior to removal. Change daily or as ordered by a physician.

ANTIMICROBIALS

CalciCare™ Calcium Alginate, Silver*

Hollister Wound Care

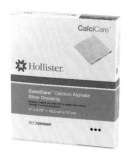

HOW SUPPLIED

Dressing	2″ × 2″	A6196
Dressing	4″ × 4.75″	A6197
Rope	1″ × 18″	A6199

ACTION

CalciCare™ calcium alginate dressing, silver is a sterile, reinforced nonwoven pad composed of high G (glucuronic acid) and calcium alginate, carboxymethylcellulose (CMC), and ionic silver complex (Silver Sodium Hydrogen Zirconium Phosphate) which releases silver ions in the presence of wound fluid. As wound fluid is absorbed the alginate forms a gel, which assists in maintaining a moist environment for optimal wound healing. The dressings are reinforced for intact removal. The silver ions protect the dressing from a broad spectrum of microorganisms over a period of up to 14 days, based on *in vitro* testing. Odor reduction results from the antibacterial effect of the dressing. CalciCare calcium alginate dressing, silver is an effective barrier to bacterial penetration.

CalciCare calcium alginate dressing, silver protects the wound and aids autolytic debridement, therefore facilitating wound healing.

INDICATIONS

Indicated for moderate to heavily exuding partial- to full-thickness wounds, such as postoperative wounds, trauma wounds, leg ulcers, pressure ulcers, diabetic ulcers, graft and donor sites, first- and second-degree burns.

CONTRAINDICATIONS

- Not for use on individuals with a known sensitivity to alginates or silver.
- Not for use to control heavy bleeding.
- Not for direct application on dry or lightly exuding wounds.

APPLICATION

- Debride when necessary and irrigate the wound site in accordance with standard protocols.
- Remove excess solution from surrounding skin.
- Select a size of CalciCare calcium alginate dressing, silver that is slightly larger than the wound.
- Cut (using sterile scissors) or fold the dressing to fit the wound. Loosely fill deep wounds, ensuring the dressing does not overlap the wound margins.
- Apply to wound bed directly.
- Cover and secure CalciCare calcium alginate dressing, silver with a nonocclusive secondary dressing.
- The dressing performance may be impaired by excess use of petroleum-based ointments.
- The dressing must be removed prior to patients undergoing Magnetic Resonance Imaging (MRI) examinations.

ANTIMICROBIALS

- Avoid contact with electrodes or conductive gels during electronic measurements, for example, electrocardiograms (ECG) and electroencephalograms (EEG).
- In the event of clinical infection, topical silver does not replace the need for systemic therapy or other adequate infection treatment.

REMOVAL

- Dressing change frequency will depend on wound condition and the level of exudate. Initially it may be necessary to change the dressing every 24 hours.
- Reapply CalciCare calcium alginate dressing, silver when the secondary dressing has reached its absorbent capacity or whenever good wound care practice dictates that the dressing should be changed.
- Gently remove the secondary dressing.
- If the wound appears dry, saturate the dressing with sterile saline solution prior to removal.
- Gently remove the dressing from the wound bed and discard.
- Irrigate the wound site in accordance with standard protocols prior to application of a new dressing.

*See package insert for complete instructions for use.

ANTIMICROBIALS

Calcium Alginate with Silver

Gentell

HOW SUPPLIED

Pad	2" × 2"	A6196
Pad	4.5" × 4.5"	A6197
Rope	12"	A6199

ACTION

Gentell's Calcium Alginate Rope Dressing with Silver is a sterile, antimicrobial, comfortable, fiber-structured alginate with high absorbency. This advanced alginate dressing with silver fights bacteria and a broad spectrum of microorganisms while absorbing and containing exudate in a moist healing environment. A reaction between the calcium in the dressing and the sodium in the wound exudate creates a gel-like substance that promotes moist wound healing.

INDICATIONS

Gentell's Calcium Alginate with Silver Dressings should be applied in dry form on infected shallow wounds including leg ulcers, pressure ulcers, diabetic foot ulcers, and surgical wounds. May also be used for minor conditions such as lacerations, abrasions, skin tears, and minor burns.

CONTRAINDICATIONS

- Gentell Calcium Alginate with Silver should not be used on third-degree burns or to control heavy bleeding.

APPLICATION

- Irrigate the wound with Gentell Wound Cleanser and gently dry the skin surrounding the wound site.
- Choose the appropriate sized dressing based on the dimensions of the wound.
- Cover wound with a secondary dressing such as Gentell Super Absorbent, Gentell Comfortell™, or Gentell LoProfile Bordered Foam.

REMOVAL

- Change daily or as ordered by a physician.

ANTIMICROBIALS

New Product: ComfortFoam/Ag

DermaRite Industries, LLC

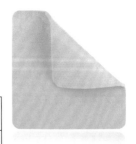

HOW SUPPLIED

Foam Wound Dressing with Soft Silicone Adhesive and Silver	2″ × 2″	A6209
Foam Wound Dressing with Soft Silicone Adhesive and Silver	4″ × 5″	A6210
Foam Wound Dressing with Soft Silicone Adhesive and Silver	6″ × 6″	A6210

ACTION

ComfortFoam/Ag® absorbs exudate, maintains a moist wound healing environment and has good antibacterial preservative properties. ComfortFoam/Ag foam dressing consists of 0.25–0.35 mg/cm^2 of silver ions that demonstrate in vitro antibacterial preservative effectiveness within the dressing for up to 7 days.

ComfortFoam/Ag consists of a vapor permeable waterproof polyurethane top film, an absorbent polyurethane foam pad containing polyvinyl alcohol, silver sulfate, and silver chloride with a soft silicone wound contact surface.

INDICATIONS

ComfortFoam/Ag is indicated for the management of exuding wounds, such as leg and foot ulcers, pressure ulcers, traumatic and surgical wounds, superficial and partial thickness burns. Silver compounds present in the dressing help reduce bacterial colonization in the dressing.

CONTRAINDICATIONS

- ComfortFoam/Ag should not be used on patients with a known sensitivity to silver or any other contents of the dressing.

APPLICATION

- Cleanse wound with sterile saline or sterile water to remove residue according to local infection control protocol. Deep wounds should be well irrigated.
- Skin around wound should be clean and dry, use skin barrier prep as needed.
- Remove dressing from package.
- Dressing may be cut to size prior to application.
- Remove backing paper from dressing.
- Apply sticky side of dressing to moist wound bed overlapping 1 to 2 inches of dry skin; gently smooth into place.
- Secure edges with tape if desired.

REMOVAL

- Dressing may be moistened to ease removal.
- Carefully remove adhesive dressings by holding the edge of the dressing and slowly pulling it parallel to the skin.
- Dispose of in accordance with local guidance.

REFERENCE

1. http://dermarite.com/product/comfortfoamag/

New Product: ComfortFoam/Ag Border

DermaRite Industries, LLC

HOW SUPPLIED

Bordered Foam Wound Dressing with Soft Silicone Adhesive and Silver	2″ × 2″	A6212
Bordered Foam Wound Dressing with Soft Silicone Adhesive and Silver	4″ × 4″	A6212
Bordered Foam Wound Dressing with Soft Silicone Adhesive and Silver	6″ × 6″	A6212

ACTION

ComfortFoam/Ag® Border absorbs exudate, maintains a moist wound healing environment and has good antibacterial preservative properties. ComfortFoam/Ag Border contains 0.25–0.35 mg/cm² of silver ions that demonstrate in vitro antibacterial preservative effectiveness within the dressing for up to 7 days.

ComfortFoam/Ag Border consists of a vapor permeable waterproof polyurethane top film, a nonwoven fabric layer, and an absorbent polyurethane foam pad containing polyvinyl alcohol, silver sulfate, and silver chloride, with a soft silicone wound contact surface.

INDICATIONS

ComfortFoam/Ag Border is indicated for the management of exuding wounds, such as leg and foot ulcers, pressure ulcers, traumatic and surgical wounds, superficial and partial-thickness burns. Silver compounds present in the dressing help reduce bacterial colonization in the dressing.

CONTRAINDICATIONS

- ComfortFoam/Ag Border should not be used on patients with a known sensitivity to silver or any other contents of the dressing.

APPLICATION

- Cleanse wound with sterile saline or sterile water to remove residue according to local infection control protocol. Deep wounds should be well irrigated.
- Skin around wound should be clean and dry, use skin barrier prep as needed.
- Remove dressing from package.
- Remove backing paper from dressing.
- Apply sticky side of dressing to moist wound bed overlapping 1″ to 2″ of dry skin; gently smooth into place.

REMOVAL

- Dressing may be moistened to ease removal.
- Carefully remove adhesive dressings by holding the edge of the dressing and slowly pulling it parallel to the skin.
- Dispose of in accordance with local guidance.

REFERENCE

1. http://dermarite.com/product/comfortfoamag-border/

ANTIMICROBIALS

DermaCol/Ag

DermaRite Industries, LLC

HOW SUPPLIED

| Collagen Matrix Dressing with Silver | 2" × 2" | A6021 |
| Collagen Matrix Dressing with Silver | 4" × 4" | A6021 |

ACTION

DermaCol/Ag™ Collagen Matrix Dressing with Silver is an advanced wound care dressing made of collagen, sodium alginate, carboxyl methylcellulose, ethylenediaminetetraacetic acid (EDTA), and silver chloride. The topically applied wound dressing will transform into a soft gel sheet when in contact with wound exudates. The dressing maintains a moist wound environment at the wound surface that aids in the formation of granulation tissue and epithelialization. The EDTA in the dressing removes zinc to inhibit the activity of matrix metalloproteinases (MMP), thus creating a suitable environment for wound healing. The silver chloride in the dressing is an effective antimicrobial intended to prevent colonization of the dressing. The dressings may be trimmed and layered for the management of deep wounds.

INDICATIONS

DermaCol/Ag is indicated for management of full and partial thickness wounds including pressure ulcers, diabetic ulcers, ulcers caused by mixed vascular etiologies, venous ulcers, donor and graft sites, abrasions, traumatic wounds healing by secondary intention, dehisced surgical wounds, first- and second-degree burns.

CONTRAINDICATIONS

- DermaCol/Ag dressing should not be used on third-degree burns or on patients with a known allergy or sensitivity to collagen, silver, or any other ingredient.
- If sensitivity to DermaCol/Ag develops, discontinue use.
- DermaCol/Ag may be used under compression therapy under the supervision of a health care professional.

APPLICATION

- Debride and irrigate the wound bed with an appropriate wound cleanser or distilled water before application. The use of saline may affect the efficacy of the silver.
- Cut the dressing to fit the exact wound size. For heavily exuding wounds, apply the dressing directly to the wound bed. For dry wounds with very little exudate, moisten the wound bed with distilled water to begin the gelling process.
- Cover with an appropriate secondary dressing.
- Change dressings daily or as good nursing practice dictates.

REMOVAL

- Remove the secondary dressing with care. Gently remove DermaCol/Ag dressing ensuring that the dressing removal does not damage any newly formed tissues.
- Use an appropriate wound cleanser or distilled water to cleanse the wound site prior to applying a new DermaCol/Ag dressing as per application instructions.

REFERENCE

1. http://dermarite.com/product/dermacolag/

ANTIMICROBIALS

DermaGinate/Ag

DermaRite Industries, LLC

HOW SUPPLIED

Calcium Alginate Wound Dressing with Antibacterial Silver, Rope	2″ × 2″	A6196
Calcium Alginate Wound Dressing with Antibacterial Silver, Rope	4″ × 5″	A6197
Calcium Alginate Wound Dressing with Antibacterial Silver, Rope	4″ × 8″	A6197
Calcium Alginate Wound Dressing with Antibacterial Silver, Rope	12″	A6199

ACTION

DermaGinate/Ag™ is a calcium alginate wound dressing with antibacterial silver composed of calcium alginate, sodium alginate, and silver particles. DermaGinate/Ag is made of natural fibers derived from seaweed, and is designed to be highly absorbent. The dressing absorbs exudate and forms a gel-like surface over the wound that supports a moist wound healing environment and keeps the dressing from adhering to the wound. DermaGinate/Ag Silver Alginate Dressing can restrain bacterial growth within the dressing for 24 hours. DermaGinate/Ag Silver Alginate Dressing has been tested in vitro and found to be effective against bacteria such as *Staphylococcus aureus, Streptococcus pyogenes, Escherichia coli, Pseudomonas aeruginosa, Klebsiella pneumoniae,* and *Staphylococcus epidermis.*

INDICATIONS

- OTC: May be used as first aid to help in minor abrasions, minor cuts, lacerations, scrapes, minor scalds, and burns.
- PRESCRIPTION: May be used as a primary wound dressing for moderate to heavily exuding partial- to full-thickness wounds, including postoperative wounds, trauma wounds, leg ulcers, pressure ulcers, diabetic ulcers, and graft and donor sites.

CONTRAINDICATIONS

- DermaGinate/Ag should not be used on patients with a known sensitivity to silver. Not intended for use on third-degree burns.

APPLICATION

- Cleanse wound with advised liquid to remove residue according to local infection control protocol. Deep wounds should be well irrigated.
- Skin around wound should be clean and dry, use skin barrier prep as needed.
- Choose a dressing size that can cover the wound bed. Remove from package. May be cut to size prior to application to fit wound bed.
- Apply dressing to moist wound bed. Loosely pack deep wounds.
- Secure with appropriate cover dressing that manages drainage and maintains a moist wound environment.

REMOVAL

- Gently remove the secondary dressing. Carefully remove adhesive dressings by holding the edge of the dressing and slowly pulling it parallel to the skin.
- If the wound appears dry, saturate the dressing with sterile saline or sterile water prior to removal.
- Dispose of in accordance with local guidance.

REFERENCE

1. http://dermarite.com/product/dermaginate-ag/

Dermanet Ag⁺

DeRoyal

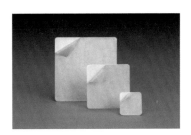

HOW SUPPLIED

Dressing	2″ × 2″	A6206
Dressing	4″ × 4″	A6206
Dressing	4″× 8″	A6207
Dressing	6″ × 6″	A6207
Dressing	8″ × 8″	A6208
Dressing	8″ × 16″	A6208

ANTIMICROBIALS

ACTION

Dermanet Ag⁺ is a combination of Dermanet wound contact layer and Algidex Ag Silver Technology. Dermanet is an inert, nonadherent material that helps to shield and protect fragile granulation tissue. It helps to reduce trauma and pain that can be caused during dressing changes. Algidex Ag technology is a unique formulation of ionic silver combined in an alginate and maltodextrin matrix. Algidex Ag provides an extended release of active ionic silver for broad antimicrobial effectiveness and helps to prevent contamination from external bacteria.

INDICATIONS

Dermanet Ag⁺ can be used on infected and noninfected wounds, including dermal ulcers (e.g., leg ulcers, pressure ulcers), diabetic ulcers, abdominal wounds, superficial wounds, lacerations, cuts, abrasions, donor sites, and burn wounds. The unique formulation can be used on dry, moist, or wet wounds.

CONTRAINDICATIONS

- Not for use on third-degree burns.
- Not for use on ulcers resulting from infections.
- Contraindicated for lesions associated with active vasculitis.
- Contraindicated for patients with sensitivity to alginates.

APPLICATION

- Thoroughly cleanse wound.
- Remove Dermanet Ag⁺ from the backing material.
- Place Dermanet Ag⁺ over shallow wounds or pack into deep wounds.
- Cover with appropriate secondary dressing based on wound drainage.
- Dermanet Ag⁺ can be worn up to 5 days or until the secondary dressing is saturated and requires changing.

REMOVAL

- Remove secondary cover dressing.
- Gently remove Dermanet Ag⁺ from wound.
- Irrigate wound with saline as needed to help loosen dressing.
- Continue to thoroughly cleanse wound to remove wound drainage or any residue left by the Dermanet Ag⁺.

ANTIMICROBIALS

Dermanet Ag⁺ Border

DeRoyal

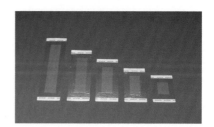

HOW SUPPLIED

Dressing	4″ × 4″
Dressing	4″ × 6″
Dressing	4″ × 8″
Dressing	4″ × 10″
Dressing	4″ × 14″

ACTION

Dermanet Ag⁺ Border is a combination of Dermanet Ag and Transeal polyurethane dressing. The Dermanet Ag⁺ is "Island Placed" in the center of Transeal and is the perfect dressing for surgical incisions, lacerations, and vascular access sites. The Dermanet Ag⁺ "Island" creates an antimicrobial, nonadherent surface that will not adhere to sutures or staples while the Transeal holds the dressing securely in place and provides a breathable barrier to external contaminants. In addition, the dressing is transparent, which provides for easy inspection of the wound, surgical site, or vascular access site.

INDICATIONS

For the management of surgical site incisions, lacerations, and vascular access sites.

CONTRAINDICATIONS

- Not for use on third-degree burns.
- Not for use on ulcers resulting from infections.
- Contraindicated for lesions associated with active vasculitis.
- Contraindicated for patients with sensitivity to alginates.

APPLICATION

- Thoroughly cleanse wound.
- Peel release liner from center of dressing while aligning the Dermanet Ag⁺ center over the site.
- Press dressing into place.
- Remove the "Top Clear Carrier Film" by lifting away at the tab.

REMOVAL

- Gently grasp a corner on the edge of the dressing and slowly pull the dressing from the skin in the direction of hair growth.

DermaSyn/Ag

DermaRite Industries, LLC

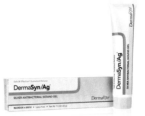

HOW SUPPLIED

Silver Antibacterial Wound Gel	1.5 oz	A6248

ACTION

DermaSyn/Ag® is a water-based amorphous hydrogel dressing with antibacterial silver.

INDICATIONS

DermaSyn/Ag Silver Antibacterial Wound Gel is indicated for the management of:

- First- and second-degree burns.
- Stasis ulcers.
- Pressure ulcers.
- Diabetic ulcers.
- Lacerations.
- Abrasions.
- Skin tears.
- Graft sites.
- Donor sites.
- Surgical incision sites.
- Device insertion sites.

CONTRAINDICATIONS

- There are no known or reasonably suspected adverse reactions associated with the use of DermaSyn/Ag.

APPLICATION

- Cleanse wound.
- Apply directly to wound area and cover with appropriate dressing.
- Reapply every 24 to 72 hours based on condition of wound, surrounding skin and dressing, or as directed by a qualified health professional.

REFERENCE

1. http://dermarite.com/product/dermasyn-ag/

New Poduct: Exufiber® Ag⁺

Mölnlycke Health Care

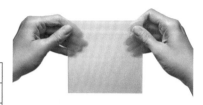

Exufiber® Ag+

HOW SUPPLIED

Dressing	2″ × 2″	A6196
Dressing	4″ × 4.8″	A6197
Dressing	6″ × 6″	A6197
Dressing	8″ × 12″	A6198
Dressing	0.8″ × 17.7″	A6199

ACTION

Exufiber® Ag⁺ wound dressing is a sterile, soft, nonwoven pad or ribbon. Exufiber Ag⁺ consists of highly absorbents and gel forming polyvinyl alcohol (PVA) nonwoven fibers. The nonwoven pad or ribbon is coated with silver sulfate on both sides. The silver is released within the dressing in contact with fluid, and acts as a preservative in the dressing to inhibit or reduce microbial growth in the dressing.

In vitro testing demonstrates that the Exufiber Ag⁺ kills a wide range of wound pathogens and creates an antimicrobial environment within the dressing. Exufiber Ag⁺ gives a ≥4 log reduction, in the dressing, of the following Gram-positive bacteria, Gram-negative bacteria, and fungi through seven (7) days in *in vitro* studies. By reducing the number of microorganisms, Exufiber Ag⁺ may also reduce dressing odor.

Exufiber® Ag⁺ has shown to have an unchanged microbial reduction through seven (7) days when tested *in vitro* with a secondary dressing.

Exufiber® Ag⁺ maintains a moist wound environment in combination with a secondary dressing.

Exufiber® Ag⁺ can be used under compression bandaging.

INDICATIONS

Exufiber® Ag⁺ is intended to be used on the following medium to high exuding wounds.

- Leg ulcers (venous stasis ulcers, arterials ulcers, and ulcers of mixed etiology) and diabetic foot ulcers.
- Pressure ulcers (partial and full thickness).
- Partial-thickness burns (second degree).
- Donor sites and other wounds that are prone to bleeding, such as debrided wounds (mechanically and surgically).
- Traumatic wounds.
- Surgical wounds that heal by primary intention, such as dermatological and surgical incisions (e.g., orthopedic and vascular), and surgical wounds left to heal by secondary intention, such as dehisced surgical incisions.
- Oncology wounds with exudate, such as fungoides-cutaneous tumors, fungating carcinoma, cutaneous metastasis, Kaposi's sarcoma, and angiosarcoma.
- Exufiber Ag⁺ may be used for management of wounds as an effective barrier to bacterial penetration of the dressing, as this may help to reduce the risk of infection.
- Indicated wear time: Up to seven (7) days.

CONTRAINDICATIONS

- Exufiber Ag⁺ is not intended for dry wounds or full-thickness injuries.
- For external use only.
- Do not use on patients with known sensitivity to silver or any other contents of the dressing.

APPLICATION AND REMOVAL

Shallow wounds application

- Cleanse the wound with saline solution or water according to clinical practice.
- Dry the surrounding skin thoroughly.
- Choose the correct size of the dressing to be able to cover the entire wound. For best result, Exufiber Ag⁺ should overlap the dry surrounding skin by at least 1 to 2 cm for the smaller sizes (up to 10×10 cm) and 5 cm for larger sizes. The dressing will swell, causing contraction of the dressing edges, as it absorbs wound fluid and starts gelling.
- Apply a dry Exufiber Ag⁺ dressing to the wound.
- Fixate with an appropriate secondary dressing. The choice depends on the exudate level.
- Compression therapy may be used in conjunction with Exufiber Ag⁺.

Deep wounds and cavities

- Cleanse the wound with saline solution or water according to clinical practice.
- Dry the surrounding skin thoroughly.
- Loosely pack the ribbon or pad into the wound to allow room for swelling of the dressing. When using the ribbon dressing, cut to appropriate length leaving a small overhang of 2 to 3 cm outside of the wound for easy retrieval.
- Cover with an appropriate secondary dressing. The choice depends on the exudate level.
- Fixate (or cover) with an adhesive dressing or a bandage as appropriate.

Donor sites application

- Harvest tissue and achieve hemostasis (according to normal routine).
- Choose the correct size of sheet dressing to be able to cover the entire wound. The Exufiber Ag⁺ dressing should overlap the dry surrounding skin by at least 5 cm, the dressing will swell, causing contraction of the dressing edges, as it absorbs wound fluid and starts gelling.
- Apply a dry Exufiber Ag⁺ dressing to the wound.
- Cover with an appropriate secondary dressing. The choice depends on the exudate level.
- Fixate (or cover) with an adhesive dressing or a bandage as appropriate.

Dressing change and removal

- Change the Exufiber Ag⁺ dressing when saturation is reached. Exufiber Ag⁺ can be left in place for up to 7 days depending on wound condition or as indicated by clinical practice.
- Remove the secondary dressing and discard in appropriate way.
- Remove the Exufiber Ag⁺ dressing by gently cleansing/flushing with saline solution or water according to clinical practice. Any nongelled material will moisten in contact with the saline.
- If this dressing dries out and is difficult to remove, it should be moistened with saline solution or water according to local policies and allowed to soak until it lifts easily. It may take several minutes for Exufiber® Ag⁺ to transform into a gel. Remove the dressing by gently cleansing/flushing.

ANTIMICROBIALS

KALGINATE Thin Calcium Alginate Wound Dressing

DeRoyal

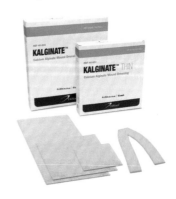

HOW SUPPLIED

Pad	2″ × 2″	A6196
Pad	4″ × 4″	A6196
Pad	4″ × 8″	A6197

ACTION

KALGINATE Thin is a sterile, nonwoven, calcium alginate dressing of heavy fiber. Thick and substantial, it provides maximum absorption of exudate with minimal dressing changes. It allows for gaseous exchange, can be layered or packed for absorbency, and maintains its shape and integrity during removal.

INDICATIONS

To manage pressure ulcers (stages 3 and 4); full-thickness wounds; tunneling, infected, and draining wounds; and wounds with moderate to heavy exudate.

CONTRAINDICATIONS

- Contraindicated for third-degree burns.

APPLICATION

- Clean the wound area with normal saline solution.
- Place KALGINATE Thin pad or rope into the wound, packing deep wounds loosely.
- Cover the dressing with an absorptive cover dressing, and secure in place.

REMOVAL

- Change the dressing when the outer dressing is saturated with drainage.
- Remove the outer dressing.
- Irrigate the wound with normal saline solution, and lift the dressing from the wound bed.

Maxorb Extra Ag Antimicrobial Silver CMC/Alginate Dressing

Medline Industries, Inc.

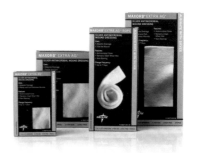

HOW SUPPLIED

Pad	2″ × 2″	A6196
Pad	4″ × 8″	A6197
Pad	4″ × 4.75″	A6197
Pad	6″ × 6″	A6197
Pad	8″ × 12″	A6198
Rope	1″ × 12″ (2 g)	A6199

ACTION

Maxorb Extra Ag CMC/Alginate Dressing's nonwoven alginate and carboxymethylcellulose fiber combination reacts with wound exudate to form a gel, providing a moist healing environment. The added presence of carboxymethylcellulose in Maxorb improves the wicking and fluid-handling ability of this dressing and increases wet strength. Because the product does not wick exudate laterally, it reduces the potential for damage to delicate periwound tissue. Maxorb Extra Ag is biocompatible, nonirritating, nonsensitizing, nonstaining, and will not harm new granulation tissue.

INDICATIONS

To manage partial- and full-thickness wounds with moderate to heavy exudate, including venous stasis ulcers, pressure ulcers (stages), arterial ulcers, diabetic ulcers, donor sites, lacerations, abrasions, postsurgical incisions, and second-degree burns; may also be used for infected and noninfected wounds, tunneling wounds, and wounds with serosanguineous or purulent drainage.

CONTRAINDICATIONS

- Contraindicated for third-degree burns.
- Not intended for use as a surgical sponge.

APPLICATION

- Clean the wound with normal saline solution or an appropriate wound cleanser, such as Skintegrity Wound Cleanser.
- Apply the dressing to a moist wound bed. The dressing may be cut to fit if necessary. Loosely fill deep or tunneling wounds.
- Cover the dressing with an appropriate secondary dressing, such as Optifoam Gentle silicone faced foam.

REMOVAL

- Change the dressing when strike-through to the secondary dressing occurs. Maxorb Extra Ag$^+$ may be left in place up to 21 days.
- The gelatinous pad may be easily lifted away in one piece from the wound bed, making dressing changes easier.

ANTIMICROBIALS

- Remove the secondary dressing as well as gelled and nongelled Maxorb dressing.
- Irrigate the wound with normal saline solution or another appropriate solution, such as Skintegrity Wound Cleanser, to remove any remaining gel.
- If the dressing is dry at the time of removal, moisten it with saline or wound cleanser before removing it.

REFERENCE

1. https://www.medline.com/product/Maxorb-Extra-Ag-CMC/Alginate-Dressings/Alginate-Dressings/ Z05-PF00123?question=maxorb±extra&index=P1&indexCount=1

Melgisorb® Ag Antimicrobial Alginate Dressing

Mölnlycke Health Care

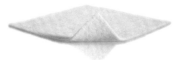

Melgisorb® Ag

HOW SUPPLIED

Pad	2″ × 2″	A6196
Pad	4″ × 4″	A6196
Pad	6″ × 6″	A6197
Pad	8″ × 12″	A6198
Rope	1.2″ × 18″	A6199

ACTION

Melgisorb® Ag is a highly absorbent antimicrobial alginate dressing containing an ionic silver complex that releases silver ions in the presence of wound fluid. As wound fluid is absorbed, the alginate forms a gel, which assists in maintaining a moist environment for optimal wound healing. The silver ions protect the dressing from a broad spectrum of microorganisms over a period of up to 14 days.

INDICATIONS

To manage wounds with moderate to heavy exudate, surgical wounds, trauma injuries, leg ulcers, pressure ulcers, diabetic and neuropathic ulcers, graft and donor sites, critically colonized wounds, and partial-thickness burns. Melgisorb Ag may also be used under compression bandages.

CONTRAINDICATIONS

- Contraindicated for dry wounds.
- Do not use on individuals known to have sensitivity to silver or alginates.
- Not recommended for surgical implantation.

APPLICATION

- Debride when necessary and irrigate the wound site in accordance with standard protocols. Dry the surrounding skin.
- Apply Melgisorb Ag dry to a moist wound bed. For shallow wounds, choose the correct size of the flat dressing to cover the entire wound. For deep or tunneling wounds, choose and cut an appropriate length and pack loosely.
- Cover and secure Melgisorb Ag with a nonocclusive secondary dressing.

REMOVAL

- Gently flush the wound with normal saline solution or another appropriate solution. Any nongelled Melgisorb Ag can be moistened with saline and removed.

Mepilex® Ag Antimicrobial Foam Dressing

Mölnlycke Health Care

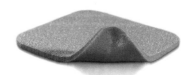

HOW SUPPLIED

Dressing	4″ × 4″	A6209
Dressing	4″ × 5″	A6210
Dressing	4″ × 8″	A6210
Dressing	6″ × 6″	A6210
Dressing	8″ × 8″	A6211
Dressing	8″ × 20″	A6211

ACTION

Mepilex® Ag consists of a Safetac® (soft silicone) technology wound layer, a grey absorbent polyurethane foam pad containing a silver compound, activated carbon, and a vapor permeable and waterproof film. It effectively absorbs wound exudate, maintains a moist wound healing environment, and releases silver ions to inactivate a wide range of wound-related pathogens within 30 minutes. The Safetac technology layer minimizes the risk of periwound maceration and allows for atraumatic dressing changes. Mepilex Ag may be used under compression bandages and may also be cut to size.

INDICATIONS

For the management of moderately exuding wounds such as leg and foot ulcers, pressure ulcers, partial-thickness burns, and graft and donor sites. The silver sulfate in the dressing helps reduce microbial colonization on the dressing.

CONTRAINDICATIONS

- Not for use on patients with known sensitivity to silver.
- Not for use during radiation treatments or examinations.
- Avoid contact with electrodes or conductive gels during electronic measurements.
- Do not use with oxidizing agents such as hydrogen peroxide.

APPLICATION

- Cleanse or flush the wound with normal saline solution or water, then dry the surrounding skin thoroughly.
- Remove the release films and apply the adherent side to the wound. Do not stretch.
- For best results, Mepilex Ag should overlap dry surrounding skin by at least 2 cm.
- Secure Mepilex Ag with a bandage or other fixation, as needed.

REMOVAL

- Leave Mepilex Ag in place for several days, depending on the condition of the wound and the surrounding skin or facility policy.

ANTIMICROBIALS

Mepilex® Border Ag Antimicrobial Bordered Foam Dressing

Mölnlycke Health Care

Mepilex® Border Ag

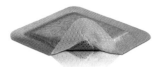

HOW SUPPLIED

Dressing	3" × 3"	A6212
Dressing	4" × 4"	A6212
Dressing	4" × 10"	A6212
Dressing	6" × 6"	A6213
Dressing	6" × 8"	A6213
Dressing	4" × 8"	A6213
Dressing	4" × 12"	A6213
Sacrum	7.2" × 7.2"	A6213
Sacrum	9.2" × 9.2"	A6213

Mepilex® Border Sacrum Ag

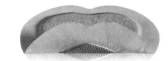

ANTIMICROBIALS

ACTION

Mepilex® Border Ag is a self-adhesive antimicrobial foam dressing consisting of a Safetac (soft silicone) technology wound contact layer, an absorbent polyurethane foam pad containing a silver compound and activated carbon, a layer with superabsorbent polyacrylate fibers, and a nonwoven and vapor permeable waterproof film. It effectively absorbs wound exudate, maintains a moist wound healing environment, and has antimicrobial properties known to inactivate wound related pathogens for up to 7 days. The Safetac technology layer minimizes the risk of periwound maceration and allows for pain- and trauma-free dressing changes. Mepilex Border Ag may also be used under compression.

INDICATIONS

For the management of exuding wounds such as leg and foot ulcers, pressure ulcers, traumatic and surgical wounds, and superficial and partial-thickness burns. The silver sulfate in the dressing helps reduce microbial colonization on the dressing.

CONTRAINDICATIONS

- Not for use on patients with known sensitivity to silver.
- Not for use during radiation treatments or examinations.
- Avoid contact with electrodes or conductive gels during electronic measurements.
- Not for use with oxidizing agents such as hydrogen peroxide.

APPLICATION

- Cleanse or flush the wound with normal saline solution or water, then dry the surrounding skin thoroughly.
- Remove the release films and apply the adherent side to the wound. Do not stretch.
- For best results, Mepilex Border Ag's wound pad should overlap the wound edges by at least 2 cm.

REMOVAL

- Leave Mepilex Border Ag in place for several days, depending on the condition of the wound and the surrounding skin, or facility policy.

New Product: Mepilex® Border Post-Op Ag with Safetac Technology

Mölnlycke Health Care

Mepilex® Border Post-Op Ag

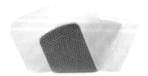

HOW SUPPLIED

Dressing	4″ × 6″	A6212
Dressing	4″ × 8″	A6212
Dressing	4″ × 10″	A6212
Dressing	4″ × 12″	A6213
Dressing	4″ × 14″	A6213

ACTION

Mepilex® Border Post-Op Ag consists of a Safetac® soft silicone wound contact layer, an absorbent polyurethane foam pad containing a silver compound and activated carbon, a layer with superabsorbent polyacrylate fibers, a nonwoven and a vapor permeable waterproof film.

Mepilex® Border Post-Op is a soft silicone foam dressing that absorbs exudates, maintains a moist wound healing environment, and has antimicrobial properties.

Mepilex® Border Post-Op Ag has been shown to inactivate wound related pathogens up to 7 days in vitro.

INDICATIONS

Mepilex® Border Post-Op Ag is indicated for the management of exudating wounds such as surgical and traumatic wounds. It can also be used under compression bandaging. Silver sulfate present in the dressing helps reduce microbial colonization in the dressing.

PRECAUTIONS

- Do not use on patients with a known sensitivity to silver or any contents of this dressing.
- Mepilex® Border Post-Op Ag may cause transient discoloration of the wound bed and surrounding skin. Frequent or prolonged use of the product may result in permanent discoloration of skin.
- In the event of clinical infection, Mepilex® Border Post-Op Ag does not replace the need for systematic therapy or other adequate infection treatment.
- Prior to commencing radiation therapy remove the Mepilex® Border Post-Op Ag if product is present in the treatment area. A new dressing can be applied following the treatment.
- Avoid contact with electrodes or conductive gels during the electronic measurements, for example, electrocardiograms (ECG) and electroencephalograms (EEG).
- Do not use Mepilex® Border Post-Op Ag together with oxidizing agents such as hypochlorite solution or hydrogen peroxide.
- Carbon black contained in the device may cause mild irritation and redness. Discontinue if any symptoms develop.
- Other saline solution or water, the interaction of cleansing agents in combination with Mepilex® Border Post-Op Ag has not been demonstrated.
- The interaction of Mepilex® Border Post-Op Ag with other topical treatments had not been demonstrated.

ANTIMICROBIALS

- For external use only. Sterile. Do not use if inner package is damaged or opened prior to use. Do not re-sterilize.
- Do not use after expiration date. If the product is used after the expiration date product properties cannot be ensured.

APPLICATION

- Note that local hygiene procedures should be followed prior to and following the dress change.
    - Cleanse the wound with saline solution or water according to standard clinical practice.
    - Dry the surrounding skin thoroughly.
    - Remove the middle release film and apply the adherent side to the wound, allowing initial fixation of the dressing. One at a time, gently remove the remaining release films while gradually adhering the dress toward the skin, avoiding wrinkles in the dressing border. Do not stretch the product.
    - Secure that the nonholed area, of the wound contact layer, is placed on intact skin.
- Mepilex® Border Post-Op Ag is intended for short-term use up to 4 weeks. For long-term use, a clinical assessment by physician is recommended.

REMOVAL

- Mepilex® Border Post-Op Ag may be left in place for up to 7 days, depending on the patient, the condition of the wound, and surrounding skin, or as indicated by accepted clinical practice. Initially, it might be required to change Mepilex® Border Post-Op Ag more frequently due to the change in treatment regime may result in an initial increase in exudation.

ANTIMICROBIALS

New Product: Mepilex® Transfer Ag with Safetac® Technology

Mölnlycke Health Care

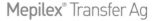

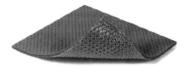

HOW SUPPLIED

Dressing	4″ × 5″	A6210
Dressing	6″ × 8″	A6210
Dressing	8″ × 20″	A6211
Dressing	4″ × 47″	A6211

ACTION

Mepilex® Transfer Ag is a soft silicone wound contact layer that absorbs and transfers exudate, maintains a moist wound environment and has antimicrobial properties. A moist wound environment is shown to be beneficial for wound healing.

Mepilex® Transfer Ag contains silver sulfate which acts as a preservative to reduce or minimize growth of microorganisms within the dressing.

Mepilex® Transfer Ag has been shown to inactivate the microorganism for up to 14 days *in vitro*.

Mepilex® Transfer Ag consists of:

- A Safetac adhesive layer.
- A compressed polyurethane foam containing silver sulfate and activated carbon.
  Safetac is a unique and a patented adhesive technology.
  The wound pad is Mepilex® Transfer Ag contains 1.2 mg/cm² silver.

INDICATIONS

Mepilex® Transfer Ag is indicated for the management of a wide range of exuding wounds such as leg and foot ulcers, pressure ulcers, partial-thickness burns, and traumatic and surgical wounds. Mepilex® Transfer Ag can also be used under compression bandaging.

PRECAUTIONS

- Mepilex® Transfer Ag should be used under the supervision of a qualified health care professional.
- Do not use on patients with a known sensitivity to silver or any other contents of the dressing. Mepilex® Transfer Ag may cause transient discoloration of the wound bed and surrounding skin. Frequent or prolonged use of this product may result in permanent discoloration of skin.
- In the event of clinical infection Mepilex® Transfer Ag does not replace the need for systemic therapy or other adequate infection treatment.
- Do not use Mepilex® Transfer Ag during radiation treatment or examinations (e.g., x-ray, ultrasound, or diathermy).
- Avoid contact with electrodes or conductive gels during electronic measurements, for example, electrocardiograms (ECG) and electroencephalograms (EEG).
- Do not use Mepilex® Transfer Ag together with oxidizing agents such as hypochlorite solutions or hydrogen peroxide.

- Other than saline solution or water, the interaction of cleansing agents in combination with Mepilex® Transfer Ag has not been demonstrated.
- The interaction of Mepilex® Transfer Ag with topical treatments has not been demonstrated.

APPLICATION

- Note that local hygiene procedures should be followed prior to and following the dressing change.
  - Cleanse the wound with saline solution or water according to standard clinical practice.
  - Dry the surrounding skin thoroughly.
  - Cut to appropriate size (if needed), remove the release films, and apply the adherent side to the wound. Do not stretch.
- For the best results, cut Mepilex® Transfer Ag to a size that overlaps the dry surrounding skin by approximately 2 cm for the smaller product sizes and 5 cm for the larger product sizes.
  - Apply the appropriate secondary dressing that overlaps the edges of Mepilex® Transfer Ag. Fixate if required.

REMOVAL

- Mepilex® Transfer Ag is intended for short-term use for up to 4 weeks. For continued use, a re-assessment by a physician is recommended.

ANTIMICROBIALS

ANTIMICROBIALS

New Product: Mepitel® Ag with Safetac® Technology

Mölnlycke Health Care

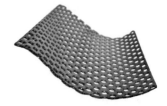

Mepitel® Ag

HOW SUPPLIED

Dressing	2″ × 3″	A6206
Dressing	3″ × 4″	A6206
Dressing	4″ × 5″	A6207
Dressing	4″ × 7″	A6207
Dressing	8″ × 12″	A6208
Dressing	8″ × 20″	A6208

ACTION

Mepitel® Ag is a soft silicone wound contact layer that allows exudate to pass vertically into a secondary dressing.

Mepitel® Ag makes it possible to change only the secondary absorbent dressing. It maintains its structural integrity and can be left in place for up to eight (8) days depending on the wound condition and surrounding skin (or as indicated by accepted clinical practice). *In vitro* testing demonstrates the Mepitel® Ag gives a ≥4 log, on the dressing of the following Gram-positive bacteria, Gram-negative bacteria and yeast; *Enterococcus faecalis* (VRE), *Staphylococcus aureus* (MRSA), *Staphylococcus epidermidis*, *Acinetobacter baumannii*, *Enterobacter cloacae*, *Pseudomonas aeruginosa*, *Candida albicans*, *Candida guilliermondii*, *Candida lusitaniae*. The dressing sustains antimicrobial activity for up to eight (8) days *in vitro* studies. By reducing the number of micro-organisms, Mepitel® Ag may also reduce odor.

Mepitel® Ag has shown to have a 4 log microbial reduction up to eight (8) days when tested with *in vitro* with a secondary dressing. Mepitel® Ag maintains a moist wound environment in combination with a secondary dressing. Mepitel® Ag can be used under compression bandaging.

Mepitel® Ag consists of:

- A Safetac adhesive layer containing silver sulfate and cellulose compound. Safetac is a unique and a patented adhesive technology.
- A polyamide net.

Contents of the dressing: Polydimethylsiloxane, Polyamide, Silver sulfate, Sodium carboxymethylcellulose.

The product and its packaging are not made with natural rubber latex.

INDICATIONS

Mepitel® Ag is intended for the management of a wide range of exuding wounds such as skin tears, skin abrasions, sutured/surgical wounds, partial-thickness burns, partial- and full-thickness grafts, lacerations, diabetic ulcers, venous ulcers, and arterial ulcers. Silver sulfate is added to the dressing as a preservative to inhibit or reduce microbial growth on the dressing.

- Mepitel® Ag contains 1.8 to 3.0 mg/cm^2 silver.

PRECAUTIONS

- Mepitel® Ag may cause transient discoloration of the wound bed and surrounding skin. Frequent or prolonged use of this product may result in permanent discoloration of skin.
- The silver sulfate component in Mepitel® Ag is intended to act as a preservative for the dressing materials. It is not intended to treat infection. In the event of clinical infection Mepitel® Ag does not replace the need for systemic therapy or other adequate infection treatment.
- Prior to commencing radiation therapy remove Mepitel® Ag if product is present in the treatment area. A new dressing can be applied following treatment.
- If present during conventional X-ray imaging Mepitel® Ag will appear as a grid-like pattern artifact.
- Avoid contact with electrodes or conductive gels during electronic measurements, for example, electrocardiograms (ECG) and electroencephalograms (EEG).
- Other than saline solution or water, the interaction of cleansing agents in combination with Mepitel® Ag has not been demonstrated.
- The interaction of Mepitel® Ag with topical treatments has not been demonstrated.
- When used on bleeding wounds or wounds with high viscosity exudate, Mepitel® Ag should be covered with a moist absorbent dressing.
- When Mepitel® Ag is used for the fixation of skin grafts, the dressing should not be changed before the fifth day of post application.

APPLICATION

- Note that local hygiene procedures should be followed prior to and following the dressing change.
  - Cleanse the wound in accordance with normal procedures and dry the surrounding skin thoroughly.
  - Choose the size of Mepitel® Ag that covers the wound and the surrounding skin by at least 2 cm. Mepitel® Ag can be cut to size to suit various wound shapes and locations.
  - While holding the larger protective film, remove the smaller one. If needed, moisten gloves to avoid adherence to Mepitel® Ag.
  - Apply Mepitel® Ag over the wound and remove the remaining protective film. Smooth Mepitel® Ag in place onto the surrounding skin, ensuring a good seal. If more than one piece of Mepitel Ag is required, overlap the dressing, ensuring that the holes are not blocked.
  - Apply a secondary dressing on top of Mepitel® Ag. In contoured or jointed areas (e.g., under arm, under breast, inner elbow, groin, deep wounds), ensure sufficient padding is applied to keep the Mepitel Ag held flat against the surface of the wound.
  - Apply a suitable fixation.

REMOVAL

- Duration of treatment is determined by the physician and depends on the wound type and healing conditions. One product of Mepitel® Ag may be left in place for up to eight (8) days depending on the patient, condition of the wound and surrounding skin, or as indicated by accepted clinical practice (exudates should pass freely through the dressing and these holes should not be blocked).
- If saturated, the secondary absorbent dressing could be changed with the Mepitel® Ag left in place.
- In the condition where the wound deteriorates unexpectedly, consult a health care professional for the appropriate medical treatment.

ANTIMICROBIALS

New Product: Opticell Ag Gelling Fiber with Silver

Medline Industries, Inc.

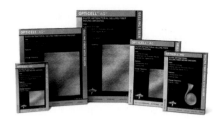

HOW SUPPLIED

Pad	2″ × 2″	A6196
Pad	4″ × 4″	A6197
Pad	6″ × 6″	A6197
Pad	8″ × 12″	A6198
Rope	0.75″ × 18″	A6199

ACTION

Opticell Ag$^+$ is a chitosan-based gelling fiber made with Chytoform technology that brings the benefits of chitosan to a conformable and highly absorbent wound dressing. Opticell Ag$^+$ offers broad spectrum antibacterial ionic silver to protect the wound from bacterial burden. Opticell controls minor bleeding and is designed to minimize pain upon removal. As it absorbs wound exudate, Opticell Ag$^+$ will not shrink and will maintain its size using surface area memory. Lateral wicking limits the risk of maceration to periwound skin.

INDICATIONS

Opticell Ag$^+$ is indicated for partial- and full-thickness wounds, venous stasis ulcers, pressure injuries, first- and second-degree burns, diabetic foot ulcers, surgical wounds, trauma wounds, donor sites, arterial ulcers and leg ulcers of mixed etiology, and oncology wounds.

CONTRAINDICATIONS

- Individuals with a known sensitivity to silver or chitosan, which is derived from shellfish.
- Third-degree burns.

APPLICATION

- Cleanse the wound with sterile saline solution or an appropriate wound cleanser, such as Skintegrity Wound Cleanser.
- Apply appropriate skin prep if necessary, such as SurePrep No-Sting.
- Apply the dressing to the wound, covering all areas of the wound with slight overlap to periwound skin. For deep wounds, loosely fill the wound.
- Cover with an appropriate secondary dressing, such as Optifoam Gentle foam.

REMOVAL

- Opticell may be left in place for up to 7 days depending on wound exudate.
- Lift one corner of the dressing and gently lift the remainder of the dressing.
- If the dressing is dry at the time of removal it may be moistened with sterile saline or wound cleanser to ease removal.
- Rinse the wound with sterile saline solution or an appropriate wound cleanser.

REFERENCE

1. http://www.medline.com/product/Opticell-Ag-Gelling-Fiber-with-Silver/Z05-PF50474

ANTIMICROBIALS

New Product: Optifoam Ag⁺ Post-Op

Medline Industries, Inc.

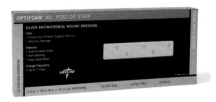

HOW SUPPLIED

Antimicrobial Silver Foam Post-Op Dressing	3.5" × 6"	A6212
Antimicrobial Silver Foam Post-Op Dressing	3.5" × 10"	A6212
Antimicrobial Silver Foam Post-Op Dressing	3.5" × 14"	A6213

ACTION

Optifoam Ag⁺ postop strips use a thin and conformable adhesive border that is waterproof, flexible, and breathable. This dressing provides a powerful antimicrobial protection from a comfortable foam dressing. Optifoam Ag⁺ eliminates 99.99% of bacteria within 2 hours and remains effective for up to 7 days. The ionic silver in Optifoam Ag⁺ provides an effective barrier for managing repeated bacterial introduction.

INDICATIONS

Postoperative wounds, donor sites, skin tears, and lesions.

CONTRAINDICATIONS

- Third-degree burns, lesions with active vasculitis, individuals with a known sensitivity to silver.

APPLICATION

- Clean the wound using SurePrep or an appropriate cleansing solution. Dry the surrounding skin.
- Remove one release liner and apply dressing to one side of wound.
- Gentle rub the dressing border until it sticks to the skin. Try to avoid wrinkling.
- Carefully remove the other release liner. Gently rub the dressing border against the skin.

REMOVAL

- The dressing may be left in place for up to 7 days. Dressing change frequency will depend on amount of drainage.
- To remove, lift up an edge of the dressing while pressing down on the skin.
- Carefully stretch the dressing in the direction of the skin, relax the dressing, and then repeat the process in a new area until the dressing has been removed.
- Clean the wound again before applying a new dressing.

ANTIMICROBIALS

New Product: Optifoam Gentle Ag⁺ Non-Bordered

Medline Industries, Inc.

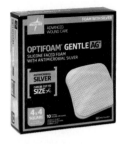

HOW SUPPLIED

Antimicrobial Nonbordered Silicone Faced Foam Dressing	4" × 4"	A6209
Antimicrobial Nonbordered Silicone Faced Foam Dressing	6" × 6"	A6210
Antimicrobial Nonbordered Silicone Faced Foam Dressing	8" × 8"	

ACTION

Optifoam Gentle Ag⁺ Nonbordered dressings have a silicone face that is soft and conformable. This conformable nonbordered foam can be cut to size. The ionic silver provides an antimicrobial barrier and continuous antimicrobial protection while helping create an ideal healing environment. The outer layer helps provide low friction and shear.

INDICATIONS

Pressure injuries, partial- and full-thickness wounds, lower-extremity ulcers, donor sites, lesions with active vasculitis.

CONTRAINDICATIONS

- Third-degree burns.

APPLICATION

- Clean the wound using SurePrep or an appropriate cleansing solution. Dry the surrounding skin.
- Remove one release liner and apply dressing to one side of wound.
- Carefully remove the other release liner.
- Secure in place using tape or a secondary dressing such as an elastic net.

REMOVAL

- The dressing may be left in place for up to 7 days. Dressing change frequency will depend on amount of drainage.
- To remove, lift up gently while pressing down on the skin.
- Clean the wound again before applying a new dressing.

ANTIMICROBIALS

New Product: Optifoam Gentle Ag⁺ Post-Op

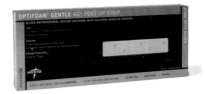

Medline Industries, Inc.

HOW SUPPLIED

Antimicrobial Silicone Bordered Postoperative Foam Dressing	3.5″ × 6″	A6212
Antimicrobial Silicone Bordered Postoperative Foam Dressing	3.5″ × 10″	A6212
Antimicrobial Silicone Bordered Postoperative Foam Dressing	3.5″ × 14″	A6213

ACTION

Optifoam Gentle postop strips use a thin and conformable adhesive border that is waterproof, flexible, and breathable. The new silicone adhesive is designed for a gentler feel and allows for the dressing to be repositioned. Optifoam Gentle Ag⁺ eliminates 99.99% of bacteria within 2 hours and remains effective for up to 7 days. The ionic silver in Optifoam Gentle Ag⁺ provides an effective barrier for managing repeated bacterial introduction.

INDICATIONS

Postoperative wounds, donor sites, skin tears, and lesions.

CONTRAINDICATIONS

- Third-degree burns, lesions with active vasculitis, individuals with a known sensitivity to silver.

APPLICATION

- Clean the wound using SurePrep or an appropriate cleansing solution. Dry the surrounding skin.
- Remove one release liner and apply dressing to one side of wound.
- Gentle rub the dressing border until it sticks to the skin. Try to avoid wrinkling.
- Carefully remove the other release liner. Gently rub the dressing border against the skin.

REMOVAL

- The dressing may be left in place for up to 7 days. Dressing change frequency will depend on amount of drainage.
- To remove, lift up an edge of the dressing while pressing down on the skin.
- Carefully stretch the dressing in the direction of the skin, relax the dressing, and then repeat the process in a new area until the dressing has been removed.
- Clean the wound again before applying a new dressing.

ANTIMICROBIALS

New Product: Optifoam Gentle Ag⁺ Superabsorbent Post-Op

Medline Industries, Inc.

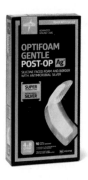

HOW SUPPLIED

Antimicrobial Silicone Bordered and Face Postoperative Foam Dressing with Superabsorbent Core and Flexible Design	4" × 6"	A6254
Antimicrobial Silicone Bordered and Face Postoperative Foam Dressing with Superabsorbent Core and Flexible Design	4" × 8"	A6212
Antimicrobial Silicone Bordered and Face Postoperative Foam Dressing with Superabsorbent Core and Flexible Design	4" × 10"	A6212
Antimicrobial Silicone Bordered and Face Postoperative Foam Dressing with Superabsorbent Core and Flexible Design	4" × 12"	A6213
Antimicrobial Silicone Bordered and Face Postoperative Foam Dressing with Superabsorbent Core and Flexible Design	4" × 14"	A6255

ACTION

Optifoam Gentle Ag⁺ Superabsorbent postop dressings use a gentle and conformable silicone border that is waterproof, flexible, and breathable. This dressing has a new silicone adhesive face and border that is designed for a gentler feel and allows for the dressing to be repositioned. Optifoam Gentle Ag⁺ eliminates 99.99% of bacteria within 2 hours and remains effective for up to 7 days. The ionic silver in Optifoam Gentle Ag⁺ provides an effective barrier for managing repeated bacterial introduction.

INDICATIONS

Postoperative wounds, donor sites, skin tears, and lesions.

CONTRAINDICATIONS

- Third-degree burns, lesions with active vasculitis, individuals with a known sensitivity to silver.

APPLICATION

- Clean the wound using SurePrep or an appropriate cleansing solution. Dry the surrounding skin.
- Remove one release liner and apply dressing to one side of wound.
- Gentle rub the dressing border until it sticks to the skin. Try to avoid wrinkling.
- Carefully remove the other release liner. Gently rub the dressing border against the skin.

REMOVAL

- The dressing may be left in place for up to 7 days. Dressing change frequency will depend on amount of drainage.
- To remove, lift up an edge of the dressing while pressing down on the skin.
- Carefully stretch the dressing in the direction of the skin, relax the dressing and then repeat the process in a new area until the dressing has been removed.
- Clean the wound again before applying a new dressing.

ANTIMICROBIALS

PolyMem® MAX® Silver™ Dressing

Ferris Mfg. Corp.

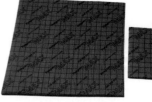

HOW SUPPLIED

Extra-absorbent Nonadhesive PMD Pad with Silver	4" × 4"	A6209
Extra-absorbent Nonadhesive PMD Pad with Silver	8" × 8"	A6211

ACTION

PolyMem MAX Silver is an extra-absorbent multifunctional,[1–4] interactive[5] polymeric membrane dressing (PMD) with silver added. PolyMem Silver dressings contain small particle silver.[6] All PolyMem dressings pull exudate, drainage, dirt, slough, and fibrin into the dressing matrix[7–9]; PolyMem Silver dressings also help manage bioburden by killing microbes as they come in contact with the dressing.[1,10–12] Rather than placing silver directly into the wound bed, the silver in PolyMem Silver is built into the dressing to help eliminate the bioburden and microbes in the dressing, doing potentially less damage to the healing wound.[1,10,13–16]

PolyMem MAX Silver is designed for handling exudate[3,9,17–19] while providing protection from contamination,[3,9] continuously cleansing,[9,20] balancing moisture,[3,5,17,21,22] helping to subdue and focus inflammation,[1,23–25] and reducing odor[3,5,9,26] and wound pain.[4,9,27–29] Many new wound products are being developed to include small aspects of PolyMem dressings' many benefits, but none are able to furnish the integrated solutions PolyMem products have reliably provided for nearly three decades.[9]

Activated by moisture, PolyMem products gradually release a nontoxic surfactant cleanser and glycerin to loosen bonds between the wound bed and adherent substances that may impair healing.[1,5,30–32] Glycerin pulls nutrient-filled, enzyme-rich fluid from the body into the wound bed, enhancing healing and autolytic debridement while floating the contaminants.[3,5,17,33,34] The PolyMem membrane pulls in the undesirable substances along with the fluid, which are locked into the porous superabsorbent structure.[1,7–9] The wound contaminants are atraumatically removed and discarded when the PolyMem dressing is changed, eliminating the need for routine rinsing at dressing changes.[7,8,22,31]

The glycerin and surfactant in PolyMem products help moisturize dry areas of wounds while pulling fluid from the body into the wound bed and redistributing it.[3,5,17,21,22] Simultaneously, excess fluid from overly wet areas is absorbed into the dressing and is locked into a gel.[3,5,7,35] The "intelligent" backing allows excess fluid to evaporate while retaining the fluid needed to keep dry wounds moist.[36] Other available dressings have only portions of this complete moisture balancing system.[9]

All occlusive dressings provide some pain relief. However, PolyMem products are the only drug-free dressings with evidence showing that they also relieve pain by altering the response of the pain-sensing nerves (nociceptors).[21,23–25,32,37,38] PolyMem products' alteration of the nociceptor response occurs even on intact skin, and has been shown in clinical studies to decrease the excess inflammation that leads to excess swelling and often slows healing.[9,21,23–25,38]

PolyMem dressings are nonadherent while conforming to the wound bed.[5,7,17,22,33,37,39,40] They are flexible and comfortable to wear.[1,9,33,39–41]

INDICATIONS

Indicated for virtually all wounds at every stage of healing,[1,3,7,17,31] including closed tissue injuries,[24,38,42,43] multifunctional PolyMem dressings meet or exceed every criterion wound experts identify for an *Ideal Dressing*.[8,44,45] PolyMem dressings are safe for use over structures like tendon, bone, and exposed vessels because they can donate moisture.[1,5,17,33,34] PolyMem is suitable for use even when wounds are infected, provided that the infection is otherwise appropriately addressed.[1,5,9,46,47] PolyMem is especially suitable for chronic, trauma, and burn wounds because it helps subdue excess inflammation and is a pain relieving dressing.[2,9,19,21,23,27,35,47,48]

- PolyMem MAX Silver is especially suited for moderately to heavily exudating wounds when the wound displays signs of delayed healing or the patients is immune compromised.[45,49,50] It is 60% more absorbent and has a higher MVTR than standard thickness PolyMem Dressings.

CONTRAINDICATIONS

- None.

APPLICATION

- Initially, irrigate or debride the wound bed as indicated or prescribed. Rinse with water or saline. Additional topical products are not necessary or recommended for use with PolyMem. Simply pat the periwound dry, leaving the wound bed slightly moist.
- Select a PolyMem MAX Silver dressing with a membrane pad that is large enough to cover the open wound **AND** all of the surrounding inflamed (reddened, raw, tender, warm, itchy, or swollen) skin. Fill any deep cavities lightly with PolyMem WIC Silver or WIC Silver Rope, allowing for about 30% expansion. Apply the PolyMem dressing with the moisture-barrier film (printed side) out.
- Secure PolyMem appropriately. Apply adhesives without tension.

How to know when to change PolyMem dressings

- Do NOT change PolyMem on a calendar schedule, especially in the first week of use; anticipate changes in exudate levels, which may dramatically increase initially.
- PolyMem is an indicator dressing: The backing will become a darker color when the membrane becomes saturated. Change the dressing when the darker color reaches any of the wound edges.

REMOVAL

- Simply, gently remove the PolyMem Silver MAX dressing and replace it with an appropriate new PolyMem configuration. In most cases, when using PolyMem, there is no need to rinse the wound.
- PolyMem is designed to continuously cleanse the wound and does not leave residue that needs to be removed. Excessive cleaning may injure regenerating tissue and delay wound healing.

Guidelines for optimal use

(See *Instructions for Use* provided in each box and **PolyMem.com for detailed information.**)

Independent wound experts have created a robust evidence base for PolyMem dressings by documenting their success in using PolyMem over the past 25+ years. Ferris has developed these guidelines, which are based upon their documented experiences.

- Using PolyMem is simple. However, using PolyMem optimally (knowing which dressing configuration to use, and how) is an art.[9,51] PolyMem use saves time, giving wound specialists more time to address the whole patient, improving healing by optimizing offloading, compression, circulation, nutrition, medications, and so forth.[4,21,27,33,35,37,43,51–53]

ANTIMICROBIALS

ANTIMICROBIALS

- PolyMem dressings should be changed when indicated, rather than on a schedule. Changing PolyMem more frequently than necessary on a healthy, granulating wound bed may slow healing. Tracing the approximate wound borders on the outer film of the PolyMem dressing makes it easy to see when a change is needed without "peeking" at the wound.[44]
- PolyMem is an interactive dressing. PolyMem often recruits LARGE amounts of wound fluid, containing debris and metabolic wastes, for the first few days of use, which may prompt frequent dressing changes.[1,31,52] When the wound is clean and granulating, reduced exudate may allow PolyMem to be left in place for up to 7 days.[9]
- On first application, irrigate or debride the wound to remove causes of delayed healing that are easy to address; then allow PolyMem to remove the remainder of the contaminants atraumatically. The PolyMem membrane may become discolored or malodorous, but the wound bed itself will become cleaner and healthier.
- Experienced users gain the confidence to avoid routine rinsing at dressing changes.[3,4,9,53,54] Simply applying a PolyMem dressing **IS** wound cleansing.[9,51] Because rinsing cools the wound bed, washes away valuable nutrients, and can damage fragile new tissue, it is best to rinse only if loose contaminants are visible or the dressing has become dislodged prior to the dressing change, allowing the wound to become dirty and dry.[55]
- Patients with large surface area third-degree burns must be carefully supervised by a burn specialist, especially when any absorptive dressing is used, including PolyMem.
- Healing wounds quickly is the most cost-saving choice. PolyMem is proven to help close wounds quickly.

*See package insert for complete information.

REFERENCES

PDFs of many of the footnoted references are available at www.polymem.com/clinicalguide/

1. Benskin LL. PolyMem Wic Silver Rope: a multifunctional dressing for decreasing pain, swelling, and inflammation. *Adv Wound Care (New Rochelle)*. 2012;1(1):44–47.
2. Dawson, Lewis C, Boch R. Total Joint Replacement Surgical Site Infections Eliminated by Using Multifunctional Dressing. 900 Cases Report over 4 years. May 2010.
3. Cutting KF, Vowden P, Wiegand C. Wound inflammation and the role of a multifunctional polymeric dressing. *Int Wound J*. 2015;6(2):41–46.
4. White L. Optimal Management for Upper Extremity Wounds with a Multifunctional Polymeric Membrane Dressing. September 2015.
5. Denyer J, White R, Ousey K, Agathangelou C, HariKrishna R. PolyMem dressings Made Easy. *Wounds International*. May 2015. http://www.woundsinternational.com/made-easys/view/polymem-dressings-made-easy. Accessed May 7, 2016.
6. Wilson D. Stalled diabetic ulcer closed in six weeks using PolyMem Silver dressings. June 2007.
7. Fowler E, Papen JC. Clinical evaluation of a polymeric membrane dressing in the treatment of dermal ulcers. *Ostomy Wound Manage*. 1991;35:35–38, 40–44.
8. Yastrub DJ. Relationship between type of treatment and degree of wound healing among institutionalized geriatric patients with stage II pressure ulcers. *Care Manag J*. 2004;5(4):213–218.
9. Benskin LL. Polymeric Membrane Dressings for topical wound management of patients with infected wounds in a challenging environment: A protocol with 3 case examples. *Ostomy Wound Manage*. 2016;62(6):42–50. (OWM website adds evidence summaries, Tables 1 & 2)
10. Benskin LL. Limitations of in vitro antimicrobial dressings study. *Burns*. 2016;42(5):1147–1148. doi:10.1016/j.burns.2016.01.034.
11. Larkö E, Blom K. Assessment of a Multifunctional Wound Dressing Using an Ex Vivo Wound Infection Healing Model. May 2012.
12. Boonkaew B, Barber PM, Rengpipat S, et al. Development and characterization of a novel, antimicrobial, sterile hydrogel dressing for burn wounds: single-step production with gamma irradiation creates silver nanoparticles and radical polymerization. *J Pharm Sci*. 2014;103(10):3244–3253.
13. Burd A, Kwok CH, Hung SC, et al. A comparative study of the cytotoxicity of silver-based dressings in monolayer cell, tissue explant, and animal models. *Wound Repair Regen*. 2007;15(1):94–104.

14. Tamir J. Mesh reinforced silver rope dressing for acute infected cavity wounds. April 2010.
15. Yeo ED, Yoon SA, Oh SR, Choi YS, Lee YK. Degree of the hazards of silver- containing dressings on MRSAInfected wounds in Sprague-Dawley and streptozotocin-induced diabetic rats. *Wounds.* 2015;27(4):95–102.
16. Benskin L. Letter to the Editor: Degree of the hazards of silver-containing dressings on MRSA-infected wounds in Sprague-Dawley and streptozotocin-induced diabetic rats. *Wounds.* 2015;27(7):A10.
17. Dabiri G, Damstetter E, Phillips T. Choosing a wound dressing based on common wound characteristics. *Adv Wound Care (New Rochelle).* 2016;5(1):32–41.
18. Langemo DK, Black J; National Pressure Ulcer Advisory Panel. Pressure ulcers in individuals receiving palliative care: a National Pressure Ulcer Advisory Panel white paper. *Adv Skin Wound Care.* 2010;23(2):59–72.
19. Edwards J, Mason S. An evaluation of the use of PolyMem Silver in burn management. *Journal of Community Nursing.* 2010;24(6):16–19.
20. Blackman JD, Senseng D, Quinn L, Mazzone T. Clinical evaluation of a semipermeable polymeric membrane dressing for the treatment of chronic diabetic foot ulcers. *Diabetes Care.* 1994;17(4):322–325.
21. Weissman O, Hundeshagen G, Harats M, et al. Custom-fit polymeric membrane dressing masks in the treatment of second degree facial burns. *Burns.* 2013;39(6):1316–1320.
22. Scott A. Polymeric membrane dressings for radiotherapy-induced skin damage. *Br J Nurs.* 2014; 23(10):S24, S26–S31. doi:10.12968/bjon.2014.23.Sup10.S24.
23. Kim YJ, Lee SW, Hong SH, Lee HK, Kim EK. The effects of PolyMem(R) on the wound healing. *J Korean Soc Plast Reconstr Surg.* 1999;26(6):1165–1172.
24. Hayden JK, Cole BJ. The effectiveness of a pain wrap compared to a standard dressing on the reduction of postoperative morbidity following routine knee arthroscopy: a prospective randomized single-blind study. *Orthopedics.* 2003;26(1):59–63; discussion 63.
25. Beitz AJ, Newman A, Kahn AR, Ruggles T, Eikmeier L. A polymeric membrane dressing with antinociceptive properties: analysis with a rodent model of stab wound secondary hyperalgesia. *J Pain.* 2004;5(1):38–47.
26. Agathangelou C. Treating Fungating Breast Cancer Wounds with Polymeric Membrane Dressings, an Innovation in Fungating Wound Management. May 2015.
27. Haik J, Weissman O, Demetrius S, Tamir J. Polymeric Membrane Dressings* for Skin Graft Donor Sites: 6 Years Experience on 1200 Cases. April 2011.
28. Man D, Aleksinko P. Use of Polymeric Membrane Dressings After Occlusive Deep Facial and Neck Chemical Peel Improves Outcomes. April 2010.
29. Man D, Aleksinko P. Intra-Operative Use Followed with Post-Op Application of Polymeric Membrane Dressings Reduces Post-Op Pain, Edema and Bruising After Full Face Lift Surgery. April 2010.
30. Rodeheaver GT, Kurtz L, Kircher BJ, Edlich RF. Pluronic F-68: a promising new skin wound cleanser. *Ann Emerg Med.* 1980;9(11):572–576.
31. Denyer JE, Pillay E. Best practice guidelines for skin and wound care in epidermolysis bullosa—International Consensus. 2012. http://www.woundsinternational.com/other-resources/view/best-practice-guidelines-for-skin-and-wound-care-in-epidermolysis-bullosa. Accessed March 30, 2015.
32. Davies SL, White RJ. Defining a holistic pain-relieving approach to wound care via a drug free polymeric membrane dressing. *J Wound Care.* 2011;20(5):250, 252, 254 passim.
33. Rafter L, Oforka E. Standard versus polymeric membrane finger dressing and outcomes following pain diaries. *Wounds UK.* 2014;10(2):40–49.
34. Cahn A, Kleinman Y. A novel approach to the treatment of diabetic foot abscesses—a case series. *J Wound Care.* 2014;23(8):394, 396–399. doi:10.12968/jowc.2014.23.8.394.
35. Stoddart J. Circumferential Wrap Technique with Polymeric Membrane Dressings after Arthroscopic ACL Reconstruction Reduces Blistering, Inflammation and Bruising; Rapid Recovery and Improved Patient Satisfaction: 80 Prospective Patient Series. May 2013.
36. Fulton JA, Blasiole KN, Cottingham T, Tornero M, Graves M, Smith LG, Mirza S, Mostow EN. Wound dressing absorption: a comparative study. *Adv Skin Wound Care.* 2012;25(7):315–320.
37. Bolhuis J. Evidence-based skin tear protocol. *Long-Term Living: For the Continuing Care Professional.* 2008;57(6):48–52.
38. Kahn AR, Sessions RW, Apasova EV. A superficial cutaneous dressing inhibits pain, inflammation and swelling in deep tissues. *Pain Medicine.* 2000;1(2):187.
39. Bauer J, Diem A, Ploder M. Efficiency and Safety of Using a Polymeric Membrane Wound Dressing in Patients with Epidermolysis Bullosa after a Release Operation. May 2013.

ANTIMICROBIALS

40. Bauer J, Brandtner G. Chirurgische Korrektur der Handfehlbildungen bei Epidermolysis bullosa dystrophicans. *Arzt+Kind*. 2013.

41. Rafter L, Oforka E. Trauma-free fingertip dressing changes. *Wounds UK*. 2013;9(1):96–100.

42. Hegarty F, Wong M. Polymeric membrane dressing for radiotherapy-induced skin reactions. *Br J Nurs*. 2014;23 Suppl 20:S38–S46.

43. Wilson D. Application of Polymeric Membrane Dressings to Stage I Pressure Ulcers Speeds Resolution, Reduces Ulcer Site Discomfort and Reduces Staff Time Devoted to Management of Ulcers. April 2010.

44. Carr RD, Lalagos DE. Clinical evaluation of a polymeric membrane dressing in the treatment of pressure ulcers. *Decubitus*. 1990;3(3):38–42.

45. Benskin L. PolyMem The Ideal Dressing. August 2015.

46. Denyer JE. Wound management for children with epidermolysis bullosa. *Dermatol Clin*. 2010;28(2):257–264.

47. Aaltonen M. Developing a Protocol For Burns in a Private Out-Patient Wound Clinic. May 2015.

48. Rahman S, Shokri A. Total Knee Arthroplasty (TKA) Infections Eliminated and Rehabilitation Improved Using Polymeric Membrane Dressing Circumferential Wrap Technique: 120 Patients at 12-month Follow-up. May 2013.

49. Agathangelou C. Huge sacral pressure ulcer closed in four months using silver polymeric membrane cavity filler and dressings. February 2009.

50. Benskin L. Combining Email Wound Consulting and Polymeric Membrane Dressings to Dramatically Improve Quality of Life. April 2009.

51. Denyer J. Six Years' Experience Of PolyMem Dressings Used On Children With Epidermolysis Bullosa (EB). September 2015.

52. Denyer J. Managing pain in children with epidermolysis bullosa. *Nurs Times*. 2012;108(29):21–23.

53. Vanwalleghem G. A New Protocol for the Treatment of Pilonidal Cysts. May 2011.

54. Agathangelou C. Patients with Chronic Wound Pain Stop Hurting, Why? May 2011.

55. McGuiness W, Vella E, Harrison D. Influence of dressing changes on wound temperature. *J Wound Care*. 2004;13(9):383–385.

ANTIMICROBIALS

PolyMem® Silver™ Cloth Adhesive Dressing

Ferris Mfg. Corp.

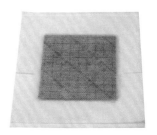

HOW SUPPLIED

Silver Cloth Adhesive PMD Island	3.5" × 3.5" pad with 6" × 6" adhesive	A6212

ACTION

PolyMem Silver with Cloth Adhesive Border is an antimicrobial,[1] multifunctional,[2–5] interactive[6] polymeric membrane dressing (PMD) with a comfortable cloth border.[1] These polymeric membrane dressings are designed to control inflammation,[2,7–9] pain[5,10–13] and odor,[4,6,13,14] and to protect wounds[4,13] while partnering with the body to promote quick healing.[10,15–21] All PolyMem dressings pull exudate, drainage, dirt, slough, and fibrin into the dressing matrix[13,22,23]; PolyMem Silver dressings also help manage bioburden by killing microbes as they come in contact with the dressing.[2,24–26] Rather than placing silver directly into the wound bed, the silver in PolyMem Silver is built into the dressing to help eliminate the bioburden and microbes in the dressing, doing potentially less damage to the healing wound.[2,24,27–30] Many new wound products are being developed to include small aspects of PolyMem dressings' many benefits, but none are able to furnish the integrated solutions PolyMem products have reliably provided for nearly three decades.[13]

Activated by moisture, PolyMem products gradually release a nontoxic surfactant cleanser and glycerin to loosen bonds between the wound bed and adherent substances that may impair healing.[2,6,31–33] Glycerin pulls nutrient-filled, enzyme-rich fluid from the body into the wound bed, enhancing healing and autolytic debridement while floating the contaminants.[4,6,21,34,35] The PolyMem membrane pulls in the undesirable substances along with the fluid, which are locked into the porous superabsorbent structure.[2,13,22,23] The wound contaminants are atraumatically removed and discarded when the PolyMem dressing is changed, eliminating the need for routine rinsing at dressing changes.[18,22,23,32]

The glycerin and surfactant in PolyMem products help moisturize dry areas of wounds while pulling fluid from the body into the wound bed and redistributing it.[4,6,15,18,21] Simultaneously, excess fluid from overly wet areas is absorbed into the dressing and is locked into a gel.[4,6,22,36] The "intelligent" backing allows excess fluid to evaporate while retaining the fluid needed to keep dry wounds moist.[37] Other available dressings have only portions of this complete moisture balancing system.[13]

All occlusive dressings provide some pain relief. However, PolyMem products are the only drug-free dressings with evidence showing that they also relieve pain by altering the response of the pain-sensing nerves (nociceptors).[7–9,15,33,38,39] PolyMem products' alteration of the nociceptor response occurs even on intact skin, and has been shown in clinical studies to decrease the excess inflammation that leads to excess swelling and often slows healing.[7–9,13,15,35,39]

PolyMem dressings are nonadherent while conforming to the wound bed.[6,18,21,22,34,38,40,41] They are flexible and comfortable to wear.[2,13,34,40–42]

INDICATIONS

Indicated for virtually all wounds at every stage of healing,[2,4,21,22,32] including closed tissue injuries,[8,39,43,44] multifunctional PolyMem dressings meet or exceed every criterion wound experts identify for an *Ideal Dressing*.[1,23,45] PolyMem dressings are safe for use over structures like tendon, bone, and exposed vessels because they can donate moisture.[2,6,21,34,35] PolyMem is suitable for use even when wounds are infected, provided that the infection is otherwise appropriately addressed.[2,6,13,19,46] PolyMem is especially suitable for chronic, trauma, and burn wounds because it helps subdue excess inflammation and is a pain relieving dressing.[3,7,10,13,15,19,36,47,48]

- PolyMem Silver with Cloth Adhesive Border is especially suited for low to moderately exudating wounds when a wound displays signs of delayed healing or the patient is immune compromised. The breathable, adhesive-coated cloth backing provides exceptional comfort for patients.[1,13]

CONTRAINDICATIONS

- None.

APPLICATION

- Initially, irrigate or debride the wound bed as indicated or prescribed. Rinse with water or saline. Additional topical products are not necessary or recommended for use with PolyMem. Simply pat the periwound dry, leaving the wound bed slightly moist.
- Fill any deep cavities lightly with PolyMem WIC silver or WIC Silver Rope, allowing for about 30% expansion. Apply the PolyMem Silver with Cloth Adhesive dressing with the membrane pad covering the open wound **AND** all of the surrounding inflamed (reddened, raw, tender, warm, itchy, or swollen) skin.
- Apply the adhesive borders without tension. Smooth into place. See Instructions for Use for details.

How to know when to change PolyMem dressings

- Do NOT change PolyMem on a calendar schedule, especially in the first week of use; anticipate changes in exudate levels, which may dramatically increase initially.
- PolyMem is an indicator dressing: The backing will become a darker color when the membrane becomes saturated. Change the dressing when the darker color reaches any of the wound edges.

REMOVAL

- Simply, gently remove the PolyMem Silver with Cloth Adhesive dressing and replace it with an appropriate new PolyMem configuration. In most cases, when using PolyMem, there is no need to rinse the wound.
- PolyMem is designed to continuously cleanse the wound and does not leave residue that needs to be removed. Excessive cleaning may injure regenerating tissue and delay wound healing.

Guidelines for optimal use

(See *Instructions for Use* provided in each box and **PolyMemzz.com for detailed information.**)

Independent wound experts have created a robust evidence base for PolyMem dressings by documenting their success in using PolyMem over the past 25+ years. Ferris has developed these guidelines based upon their documented experiences.

- Using PolyMem is simple. However, using PolyMem optimally (knowing which dressing configuration to use, and how) is an art.[13,16] PolyMem use saves time, giving wound specialists more time to address the whole patient, improving healing by optimizing offloading, compression, circulation, nutrition, medications, and so forth.[5,10,15,16,34,36,38,44,49,50]
- PolyMem dressings should be changed when indicated, rather than on a schedule. Changing PolyMem more frequently than necessary on a healthy, granulating wound bed may slow healing. Tracing the approximate wound borders on the outer film of the PolyMem dressing makes it easy to see when a change is needed without "peeking" at the wound.[45]

- PolyMem is an interactive dressing. PolyMem often recruits LARGE amounts of wound fluid, containing debris and metabolic wastes, for the first few days of use, which may prompt frequent dressing changes.[2,32,49] When the wound is clean and granulating, reduced exudate may allow PolyMem to be left in place for up to 7 days.[13]
- On first application, irrigate or debride the wound to remove causes of delayed healing that are easy to address; then allow PolyMem to remove the remainder of the contaminants atraumatically. The PolyMem membrane may become discolored or malodorous, but the wound bed itself will become cleaner and healthier.
- Experienced users gain the confidence to avoid routine rinsing at dressing changes.[4,5,13,50,51] Simply applying a PolyMem dressing **IS** wound cleansing.[13,16] Because rinsing cools the wound bed, washes away valuable nutrients, and can damage fragile new tissue, it is best to rinse only if loose contaminants are visible or the dressing has become dislodged prior to the dressing change, allowing the wound to become dirty and dry.[52]
- Patients with large surface area third-degree burns must be carefully supervised by a burn specialist, especially when any absorptive dressing is used, including PolyMem.
- Healing wounds quickly is the most cost-saving choice. PolyMem is proven to help close wounds quickly.

*See package insert for complete information.

REFERENCES

PDFs of many of the footnoted references are available at www.polymem.com/clinicalguide/

1. Benskin L. PolyMem The Ideal Dressing. August 2015.
2. Benskin LL. PolyMem Wic Silver Rope: a multifunctional dressing for decreasing pain, swelling, and inflammation. *Adv Wound Care (New Rochelle).* 2012;1(1):44–47.
3. Dawson, Lewis C, Boch R. Total Joint Replacement Surgical Site Infections Eliminated by Using Multifunctional Dressing. 900 Cases Report over 4 years. May 2010.
4. Cutting KF, Vowden P, Wiegand C. Wound inflammation and the role of a multifunctional polymeric dressing. *Inter Wound J.* 2015;6(2):41–46.
5. White L. Optimal Management for Upper Extremity Wounds with a Multifunctional Polymeric Membrane Dressing. September 2015.
6. Denyer J, White R, Ousey K, Agathangelou C, HariKrishna R. PolyMem dressings Made Easy. *Wounds International.* May 2015. http://www.woundsinternational.com/made-easys/view/polymem-dressings-made-easy. Accessed May 7, 2016.
7. Kim YJ, Lee SW, Hong SH, Lee HK, Kim EK. The effects of PolyMem(R) on the wound healing. J Korean Soc Plast Reconstr Surg. 1999;26(6):1165–1172.
8. Hayden JK, Cole BJ. The effectiveness of a pain wrap compared to a standard dressing on the reduction of postoperative morbidity following routine knee arthroscopy: a prospective randomized single-blind study. *Orthopedics.* 2003;26(1):59–63; discussion 63.
9. Beitz AJ, Newman A, Kahn AR, Ruggles T, Eikmeier L. A polymeric membrane dressing with anti-nociceptive properties: analysis with a rodent model of stab wound secondary hyperalgesia. *J Pain.* 2004;5(1):38–47.
10. Haik J, Weissman O, Demetrius S, Tamir J. Polymeric Membrane Dressings* for Skin Graft Donor Sites: 6 Years Experience on 1200 Cases. April 2011.
11. Man D, Aleksinko P. Use of Polymeric Membrane Dressings After Occlusive Deep Facial and Neck Chemical Peel Improves Outcomes. April 2010.
12. Man D, Aleksinko P. Intra-Operative Use Followed with Post-Op Application of Polymeric Membrane Dressings Reduces Post-Op Pain, Edema and Bruising After Full Face Lift Surgery. April 2010.
13. Benskin LL. Polymeric Membrane Dressings for topical wound management of patients with infected wounds in a challenging environment: A protocol with 3 case examples. *Ostomy Wound Manage.* 2016;62(6):42–50. (OWM website adds evidence summaries, Tables 1 & 2)
14. Agathangelou C. Treating Fungating Breast Cancer Wounds with Polymeric Membrane Dressings, an Innovation in Fungating Wound Management. May 2015.
15. Weissman O, Hundeshagen G, Harats M, et al. Custom-fit polymeric membrane dressing masks in the treatment of second degree facial burns. *Burns.* 2013;39(6):1316–1320.

ANTIMICROBIALS

16. Denyer J. Six Years' Experience Of PolyMem Dressings Used On Children With Epidermolysis Bullosa (EB). September 2015.

17. Scott A. Involving patients in the monitoring of radiotherapy-induced skin reactions. *J Community Nurs.* 2013;27(5):16–22.

18. Scott A. Polymeric membrane dressings for radiotherapy-induced skin damage. *Br J Nurs.* 2014;23(10):S24, S26–31. doi:10.12968/bjon.2014.23.Sup10.S24.

19. Aaltonen M. Developing a Protocol For Burns in a Private Out-Patient Wound Clinic. May 2015.

20. Curtin C. The new diabetic foot ulcer standard of care: Instant total contact cast plus polymeric membrane dressings. November 2012.

21. Dabiri G, Damstetter E, Phillips T. Choosing a wound dressing based on common wound characteristics. *Adv Wound Care (New Rochelle).* 2016;5(1):32–41.

22. Fowler E, Papen JC. Clinical evaluation of a polymeric membrane dressing in the treatment of dermal ulcers. *Ostomy Wound Manage.* 1991;35:35–38, 40–44.

23. Yastrub DJ. Relationship between type of treatment and degree of wound healing among institutionalized geriatric patients with stage II pressure ulcers. *Care Manag J.* 2004;5(4):213–218.

24. Benskin LL. Limitations of in vitro antimicrobial dressings study. *Burns.* 2016;42(5):1147–1148.

25. Larkö E, Blom K. Assessment of a Multifunctional Wound Dressing Using an Ex Vivo Wound Infection Healing Model. May 2012.

26. Boonkaew B, Barber PM, Rengpipat S, et al. Development and characterization of a novel, antimicrobial, sterile hydrogel dressing for burn wounds: single-step production with gamma irradiation creates silver nanoparticles and radical polymerization. *JPharmSci.* 2014;103(10):3244–3253.

27. Burd A, Kwok CH, Hung SC, et al. A comparative study of the cytotoxicity of silver-based dressings in monolayer cell, tissue explant, and animal models. *Wound Repair Regen.* 2007;15(1):94-104. doi:10.1111/j.1524-475X.2006.00190.x.

28. Tamir J. Mesh reinforced silver rope dressing for acute infected cavity wounds. April 2010.

29. Yeo ED, Yoon SA, Oh SR, et al. Degree of the hazards of silver- containing dressings on MRSAInfected wounds in Sprague-Dawley and streptozotocin-induced diabetic rats. *Wounds.* 2015;27(4):95–102.

30. Benskin L. Letter to the Editor: Degree of the hazards of silver-containing dressings on MRSA-infected wounds in Sprague-Dawley and streptozotocin-induced diabetic rats. *Wounds.* 2015;27(7):A10.

31. Rodeheaver GT, Kurtz L, Kircher BJ, et al. Pluronic F-68: a promising new skin wound cleanser. *Ann Emerg Med.* 1980;9(11):572–576.

32. Denyer JE, Pillay E. Best practice guidelines for skin and wound care in epidermolysis bullosa – International Consensus. 2012. http://www.woundsinternational.com/other-resources/view/best-practice-guidelines-for-skin-and-wound-care-in-epidermolysis-bullosa. Accessed March 30, 2015.

33. Davies SL, White RJ. Defining a holistic pain-relieving approach to wound care via a drug free polymeric membrane dressing. *J Wound Care.* 2011;20(5):250, 252, 254 passim.

34. Rafter L, Oforka E. Standard versus polymeric membrane finger dressing and outcomes following pain diaries. *Wounds UK.* 2014;10(2):40–49.

35. Cahn A, Kleinman Y. A novel approach to the treatment of diabetic foot abscesses—a case series. *J Wound Care.* 2014;23(8):394, 396–399.

36. Stoddart J. Circumferential Wrap Technique with Polymeric Membrane Dressings after Arthroscopic ACL Reconstruction Reduces Blistering, Inflammation and Bruising; Rapid Recovery and Improved Patient Satisfaction: 80 Prospective Patient Series. May 2013.

37. Fulton JA, Blasiole KN, Cottingham T, et al. Wound dressing absorption: a comparative study. *Adv Skin Wound Care.* 2012;25(7):315–320.

38. Bolhuis J. Evidence-based skin tear protocol. *Long-Term Living: For the Continuing Care Professional.* 2008;57(6):48–52.

39. Kahn AR, Sessions RW, Apasova EV. A superficial cutaneous dressing inhibits pain, inflammation and swelling in deep tissues. *Pain Medicine.* 2000;1(2):187.

40. Bauer J, Diem A, Ploder M. Efficiency and Safety of Using a Polymeric Membrane Wound Dressing in Patients with Epidermolysis Bullosa after a Release Operation. May 2013.

41. Bauer J, Brandtner G. Chirurgische Korrektur der Handfehlbildungen bei Epidermolysis bullosa dystrophicans. *Arzt+Kind.* 2013.

42. Rafter L, Oforka E. Trauma-free fingertip dressing changes. *Wounds UK.* 2013;9(1):96–100.

43. Hegarty F, Wong M. Polymeric membrane dressing for radiotherapy-induced skin reactions. *Br J Nurs.* 2014;23 Suppl 20:S38–S46.

44. Wilson D. Application of Polymeric Membrane Dressings to Stage I Pressure Ulcers Speeds Resolution, Reduces Ulcer Site Discomfort and Reduces Staff Time Devoted to Management of Ulcers. April 2010.

45. Carr RD, Lalagos DE. Clinical evaluation of a polymeric membrane dressing in the treatment of pressure ulcers. *Decubitus*. 1990;3(3):38–42.

46. Denyer JE. Wound management for children with epidermolysis bullosa. *Dermatol Clin*. 2010; 28(2):257–264.

47. Rahman S, Shokri A. Total Knee Arthroplasty (TKA) Infections Eliminated and Rehabilitation Improved Using Polymeric Membrane Dressing Circumferential Wrap Technique: 120 Patients at 12-month Follow-up. May 2013.

48. Edwards J, Mason S. An evaluation of the use of PolyMem Silver in burn management. *J Community Nurs*. 2010;24(6):16–19.

49. Denyer J. Managing pain in children with epidermolysis bullosa. *Nurs Times*. 2012;108(29):21–23.

50. Vanwalleghem G. A New Protocol for the Treatment of Pilonidal Cysts. May 2011.

51. Agathangelou C. Patients with Chronic Wound Pain Stop Hurting, Why? May 2011.

52. McGuiness W, Vella E, Harrison D. Influence of dressing changes on wound temperature. *J Wound Care*. 2004;13(9):383–385.

ANTIMICROBIALS

PolyMem® Silver™ Dressing

Ferris Mfg. Corp.

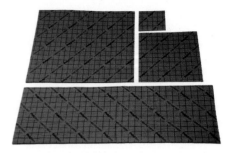

HOW SUPPLIED

Silver Nonadhesive PMD Pad	1.8″ × 1.8″, New Size	A6209
Silver Nonadhesive PMD Pad	4.25″ × 4.25″	A6210
Silver Nonadhesive PMD Pad	6.5″ × 7.5″	A6211
Silver Nonadhesive PMD Pad	4.25″ × 12.5″	A6211

ACTION

PolyMem Silver is an antimicrobial,[1] multifunctional,[2–5] interactive[6] polymeric membrane dressing (PMD) designed to decrease wound pain[5,7–10] and odor[4,6,10,11] while supporting brisk healing by continuously cleansing wounds,[10,12] balancing moisture,[4,6,13–15] and helping focus inflammation.[2,16–18] The silver kills pathogens in fluid and debris drawn into the dressings.[2,19–21] Rather than placing silver directly into the wound bed, the silver in PolyMem Silver is built into the dressing to help eliminate the bioburden and microbes in the dressing, doing potentially less damage to the healing wound.[2,19,22–25] Many new wound products are being developed to include small aspects of PolyMem dressings' many benefits, but none are able to furnish the integrated solutions PolyMem products have reliably provided for nearly three decades.[10]

Activated by moisture, PolyMem products gradually release a nontoxic surfactant cleanser and glycerin to loosen bonds between the wound bed and adherent substances that may impair healing.[2,6,26–28] Glycerin pulls nutrient-filled, enzyme-rich fluid from the body into the wound bed, enhancing healing and autolytic debridement while floating the contaminants.[4,6,15,29,30] The PolyMem membrane pulls in the undesirable substances along with the fluid, which are locked into the porous superabsorbent structure.[2,10,31,32] The wound contaminants are atraumatically removed and discarded when the PolyMem dressing is changed, eliminating the need for routine rinsing at dressing changes.[14,27,31,32]

The glycerin and surfactant in PolyMem products help moisturize dry areas of wounds while pulling fluid from the body into the wound bed and redistributing it.[4,6,13–15] Simultaneously, excess fluid from overly wet areas is absorbed into the dressing and is locked into a gel.[4,6,31,33] The "intelligent" backing allows excess fluid to evaporate while retaining the fluid needed to keep dry wounds moist.[34] Other available dressings have only portions of this complete moisture balancing system.[10]

All occlusive dressings provide some pain relief. However, PolyMem products are the only drug-free dressings with evidence showing that they also relieve pain by altering the response of the pain-sensing nerves (nociceptors).[13,16–18,28,35,36] PolyMem products' alteration of the nociceptor response occurs even on intact skin, and has been shown in clinical studies to decrease the excess inflammation that leads to excess swelling and often slows healing.[10,13,16–18,30,36]

PolyMem dressings are non-adherent while conforming to the wound bed.[6,14,15,29,31,35,37,38] They are flexible and comfortable to wear.[2,10,29,37–39]

INDICATIONS

Indicated for virtually all wounds at every stage of healing,[2,4,15,27,31] including closed tissue injuries,[17,36,40,41] multifunctional PolyMem dressings meet or exceed every criterion wound experts identify for an *Ideal Dressing*.[1,32,42] PolyMem dressings are safe for use over structures like tendon, bone, and exposed vessels because they can donate moisture.[2,6,15,29,30] PolyMem is suitable for use even when wounds are infected, provided that the infection is otherwise appropriately addressed.[2,6,10,43,44] PolyMem is especially suitable for chronic, trauma, and burn wounds because it helps subdue excess inflammation and is a pain relieving dressing.[3,7,10,13,16,33,44–46]

- PolyMem Silver dressings are especially suited for low to moderately exudating wounds when a wound displays signs of delayed healing or the patient is immune compromised, particularly when cutting dressings to size and taping is the preferred method of application.[47] See PolyMem Cutting Guides[48–50] for examples.

CONTRAINDICATIONS

- None.

APPLICATION

- Initially, irrigate or debride the wound bed as indicated or prescribed. Rinse with water or saline. Additional topical products are not necessary or recommended for use with PolyMem. Simply pat the periwound dry, leaving the wound bed slightly moist.
- Select a PolyMem Silver dressing with a membrane pad that is large enough to cover the open wound **AND** all of the surrounding inflamed (reddened, raw, tender, warm, itchy, or swollen) skin. Fill any deep cavities lightly with PolyMem WIC silver or WIC Silver Rope, allowing for about 30% expansion. Apply the PolyMem dressing with the moisture-barrier film (printed side) out.
- Secure PolyMem appropriately. Apply adhesives without tension.

How to know when to change PolyMem dressings

- Do NOT change PolyMem on a calendar schedule, especially in the first week of use; anticipate changes in exudate levels, which may dramatically increase initially.
- PolyMem is an indicator dressing: the backing will become a darker color when the membrane becomes saturated. Change the dressing when the darker color reaches any of the wound edges.

REMOVAL

- Simply, gently remove the PolyMem dressing and replace it with an appropriate new PolyMem configuration. In most cases, when using PolyMem, there is no need to rinse the wound.
- PolyMem is designed to continuously cleanse the wound and does not leave residue that needs to be removed. Excessive cleaning may injure regenerating tissue and delay wound healing.

Guidelines for optimal use

(See *Instructions for Use* provided in each box and **PolyMem.com for detailed information**.)

Independent wound experts have created a robust evidence base for PolyMem dressings by documenting their success in using PolyMem over the past 25+ years. Ferris has developed these guidelines based upon their documented experiences.

- Using PolyMem is simple. However, using PolyMem optimally (knowing which dressing configuration to use, and how) is an art.[10,51] PolyMem use saves time, giving wound specialists more time to address the whole patient, improving healing by optimizing offloading, compression, circulation, nutrition, medications, etc.[5,7,13,29,33,35,41,51–53]

- PolyMem dressings should be changed when indicated, rather than on a schedule. Changing PolyMem more frequently than necessary on a healthy, granulating wound bed may slow healing. Tracing the approximate wound borders on the outer film of the PolyMem dressing makes it easy to see when a change is needed without "peeking" at the wound.[42]
- PolyMem is an interactive dressing. PolyMem often recruits LARGE amounts of wound fluid, containing debris and metabolic wastes, for the first few days of use, which may prompt frequent dressing changes.[2,27,52] When the wound is clean and granulating, reduced exudate may allow PolyMem to be left in place for up to 7 days.[10]
- On first application, irrigate or debride the wound to remove causes of delayed healing that are easy to address; then allow PolyMem to remove the remainder of the contaminants atraumatically. The PolyMem membrane may become discolored or malodorous, but the wound bed itself will become cleaner and healthier.
- Experienced users gain the confidence to avoid routine rinsing at dressing changes.[4,5,10,53,54] Simply applying a PolyMem dressing **IS** wound cleansing.[10,51] Because rinsing cools the wound bed, washes away valuable nutrients, and can damage fragile new tissue, it is best to rinse only if loose contaminants are visible or the dressing has become dislodged prior to the dressing change, allowing the wound to become dirty and dry.[55]
- Patients with large surface area third degree burns must be carefully supervised by a burn specialist, especially when any absorptive dressing is used, including PolyMem.
- Healing wounds quickly is the most cost-saving choice. PolyMem is proven to help close wounds quickly.

*See package insert for complete information.

REFERENCES

PDFs of many of the footnoted references are available at www.polymem.com/clinicalguide/

1. Benskin L. PolyMem The Ideal Dressing. August 2015.
2. Benskin LL PolyMem Wic Silver Rope: A multifunctional dressing for decreasing pain, swelling, and inflammation. *Adv Wound Care (New Rochelle).* 2012;1(1):44–47.
3. Dawson, Lewis C, Boch R. Total Joint Replacement Surgical Site Infections Eliminated by Using Multifunctional Dressing. 900 Cases Report over 4 years. May 2010.
4. Cutting KF, Vowden P, Wiegand C. Wound inflammation and the role of a multifunctional polymeric dressing. *Inter Wounds J.* 2015;6(2):41–46.
5. White L. Optimal Management for Upper Extremity Wounds with a Multifunctional Polymeric Membrane Dressing. September 2015.
6. Denyer J, White R, Ousey K, et al. PolyMem dressings Made Easy. *Wounds International.* May 2015. http://www.woundsinternational.com/made-easys/view/polymem-dressings-made-easy. Accessed May 7, 2016.
7. Haik J, Weissman O, Demetrius S, et al. Polymeric Membrane Dressings* for Skin Graft Donor Sites: 6 Years Experience on 1200 Cases. April 2011.
8. Man D, Aleksinko P. Use of Polymeric Membrane Dressings After Occlusive Deep Facial and Neck Chemical Peel Improves Outcomes. April 2010.
9. Man D, Aleksinko P. Intra-Operative Use Followed with Post-Op Application of Polymeric Membrane Dressings Reduces Post-Op Pain, Edema and Bruising After Full Face Lift Surgery. April 2010.
10. Benskin LL. Polymeric Membrane Dressings for topical wound management of patients with infected wounds in a challenging environment: A protocol with 3 case examples. *Ostomy Wound Manage.* 2016;62(6):42–50. (OWM website adds evidence summaries, Tables 1 & 2)
11. Agathangelou C. Treating Fungating Breast Cancer Wounds with Polymeric Membrane Dressings, an Innovation in Fungating Wound Management. May 2015.
12. Blackman JD, Senseng D, Quinn L, et al. Clinical evaluation of a semipermeable polymeric membrane dressing for the treatment of chronic diabetic foot ulcers. *Diabetes Care.* 1994;17(4):322–325.
13. Weissman O, Hundeshagen G, Harats M, et al. Custom-fit polymeric membrane dressing masks in the treatment of second degree facial burns. *Burns.* 2013;39(6):1316–1320.
14. Scott A. Polymeric membrane dressings for radiotherapy-induced skin damage. *Br J Nurs.* 2014; 23(10):S24, S26–S31.

15. Dabiri G, Damstetter E, Phillips T. Choosing a wound dressing based on common wound characteristics. *Adv Wound Care (New Rochelle).* 2016;5(1):32–41.

16. Kim YJ, Lee SW, Hong SH, et al. The Effects of PolyMem(R) on the Wound Healing. *J Korean Soc Plast Reconstr Surg.* 1999;26(6):1165–1172.

17. Hayden JK, Cole BJ. The effectiveness of a pain wrap compared to a standard dressing on the reduction of postoperative morbidity following routine knee arthroscopy: a prospective randomized single-blind study. *Orthopedics.* 2003;26(1):59–63; discussion 63.

18. Beitz AJ, Newman A, Kahn AR, et al. A polymeric membrane dressing with antinociceptive properties: analysis with a rodent model of stab wound secondary hyperalgesia. *J Pain.* 2004;5(1):38–47.

19. Benskin LL Limitations of in vitro antimicrobial dressings study. *Burns.* 2016;42(5):1147–1148.

20. Larkö E, Blom K. Assessment of a Multifunctional Wound Dressing Using an Ex Vivo Wound Infection Healing Model. May 2012.

21. Boonkaew B, Kempf M, Kimble R, et al. Cytotoxicity testing of silver-containing burn treatments using primary and immortal skin cells. *Burns.* 2014;40(8):1562–1569.

22. Burd A, Kwok CH, Hung SC, et al. A comparative study of the cytotoxicity of silver-based dressings in monolayer cell, tissue explant, and animal models. *Wound Repair Regen.* 2007;15(1):94–104.

23. Tamir J. Mesh reinforced silver rope dressing for acute infected cavity wounds. April 2010.

24. Yeo ED, Yoon SA, Oh SR, et al. Degree of the hazards of silver- containing dressings on MRSAInfected wounds in Sprague-Dawley and streptozotocin-induced diabetic rats. *Wounds.* 2015;27(4):95–102.

25. Benskin L. Letter to the Editor: Degree of the hazards of silver-containing dressings on MRSA-infected wounds in Sprague-Dawley and streptozotocin-induced diabetic rats. *Wounds.* 2015;27(7):A10.

26. Rodeheaver GT, Kurtz L, Kircher BJ, et al. Pluronic F-68: a promising new skin wound cleanser. *Ann Emerg Med.* 1980;9(11):572–576.

27. Denyer JE, Pillay E. Best practice guidelines for skin and wound care in epidermolysis bullosa— International Consensus. 2012. http://www.woundsinternational.com/other-resources/view/best-practice-guidelines-for-skin-and-wound-care-in-epidermolysis-bullosa. Accessed March 30, 2015.

28. Davies SL, White RJ. Defining a holistic pain-relieving approach to wound care via a drug free polymeric membrane dressing. *J Wound Care.* 2011;20(5):250, 252, 254 passim.

29. Rafter L, Oforka E. Standard versus polymeric membrane finger dressing and outcomes following pain diaries. *Wounds UK.* 2014;10(2):40–49.

30. Cahn A, Kleinman Y. A novel approach to the treatment of diabetic foot abscesses—a case series. *J Wound Care.* 2014;23(8):394, 396–399.

31. Fowler E, Papen JC. Clinical evaluation of a polymeric membrane dressing in the treatment of dermal ulcers. *Ostomy Wound Manage.* 1991;35:35–38, 40–44.

32. Yastrub DJ. Relationship between type of treatment and degree of wound healing among institutionalized geriatric patients with stage II pressure ulcers. *Care Manag J.* 2004;5(4):213–218.

33. Stoddart J. Circumferential Wrap Technique with Polymeric Membrane Dressings after Arthroscopic ACL Reconstruction Reduces Blistering, Inflammation and Bruising; Rapid Recovery and Improved Patient Satisfaction: 80 Prospective Patient Series. May 2013.

34. Fulton JA, Blasiole KN, Cottingham T, et al. Wound Dressing Absorption: A Comparative Study. *Adv Skin Wound Care.* 2012;25(7):315–320.

35. Bolhuis J. Evidence-based skin tear protocol. *Long-Term Living: For the Continuing Care Professional.* 2008;57(6):48–52.

36. Kahn AR, Sessions RW, Apasova EV. A superficial cutaneous dressing inhibits pain, inflammation and swelling in deep tissues. *Pain Medicine.* 2000;1(2):187–187.

37. Bauer J, Diem A, Ploder M. Efficiency and Safety of Using a Polymeric Membrane Wound Dressing in Patients with Epidermolysis Bullosa after a Release Operation. May 2013.

38. Bauer J, Brandtner G. Chirurgische Korrektur der Handfehlbildungen bei Epidermolysis bullosa dystrophicans. *Arzt+Kind.* 2013.

39. Rafter L, Oforka E. Trauma-free fingertip dressing changes. *Wounds UK.* 2013;9(1):96–100.

40. Hegarty F, Wong M. Polymeric membrane dressing for radiotherapy-induced skin reactions. *Br J Nurs.* 2014;23 Suppl 20:S38–S46.

41. Wilson D. Application of Polymeric Membrane Dressings to Stage I Pressure Ulcers Speeds Resolution, Reduces Ulcer Site Discomfort and Reduces Staff Time Devoted to Management of Ulcers. April 2010.

42. Carr RD, Lalagos DE. Clinical evaluation of a polymeric membrane dressing in the treatment of pressure ulcers. *Decubitus.* 1990;3(3):38–42.

ANTIMICROBIALS

43. Denyer JE. Wound Management for Children with Epidermolysis Bullosa. *Dermatologic Clinics.* 2010;28(2):257–264.

44. Aaltonen M. Developing a Protocol For Burns in a Private Out-Patient Wound Clinic. May 2015.

45. Rahman S, Shokri A. Total Knee Arthroplasty (TKA) Infections Eliminated and Rehabilitation Improved Using Polymeric Membrane Dressing Circumferential Wrap Technique: 120 Patients at 12-month Follow-up. May 2013.

46. Edwards J, Mason S. An evaluation of the use of PolyMem Silver in burn management. *Journal of Community Nursing.* 2010;24(6):16–19.

47. Wilson D. Stalled diabetic ulcer closed in six weeks using PolyMem Silver dressings. June 2007.

48. Hegarty F, Scott A, Wong M, et al. PolyMem Cutting guide for dressing radiotherapy induced skin reactions. 2015.

49. Bostock S. Improving management of radiotherapy-induced skin reactions: a radiographer's perspective. *Wounds UK.* 2016;12(3). http://www.wounds-uk.com/journal-articles/improving-management-of-radiotherapy-induced-skin-reactions-a-radiographers-perspective. Accessed June 26, 2017.

50. Denyer J, Winblad R. PolyMem Dressings in the Management of Epidermolysis Bullosa. 2014. https://pages.cld.bz/data/tyEnNjo/common/downloads/publication.pdf.

51. Denyer J. Six Years' Experience Of PolyMem Dressings Used On Children With Epidermolysis Bullosa (EB). September 2015.

52. Denyer J. Managing pain in children with epidermolysis bullosa. *Nurs Times.* 2012;108(29):21–23.

53. Vanwalleghem G. A New Protocol for the Treatment of Pilonidal Cysts. May 2011.

54. Agathangelou C. Patients with Chronic Wound Pain Stop Hurting, Why? May 2011.

55. McGuiness W, Vella E, Harrison D. Influence of dressing changes on wound temperature. *J Wound Care.* 2004;13(9):383–385.

PolyMem® Silver™ Finger/Toe Dressing

Ferris Mfg. Corp.

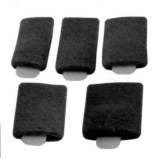

HOW SUPPLIED

#1 (Small) Finger/Toe PMD with Silver	1.8" × 2.2"	A6209
#2 (Medium) Finger/Toe PMD with Silver	2.2" × 2.6"	A6209
#3 (Large) Finger/Toe PMD with Silver	2.6" × 3.0"	A6209
#4 (Extra Large) Finger/ Toe PMD with Silver	3.0" × 3.4", New Size	A6209
#5 (XXL) Finger/Toe PMD with Silver	3.4" × 3.8", New Size	A6210

ACTION

PolyMem Silver Finger/Toe Dressings are antimicrobial multifunctional[1–4] polymeric membrane dressings (PMDs) designed to easily roll onto appendages or nearby joints, making dressing changes simple, atraumatic, and quick.[3,5,6] PolyMem helps diminish pain[3,7,8,9] and edema,[4,10–12] and promotes healing by continuously cleansing wounds,[9,13,14] balancing moisture,[2,15–18] helping to subdue and focus inflammation.[4,10–12]

PolyMem Silver dressings contain small particle silver.[19] All PolyMem dressings pull exudate, drainage, dirt, slough, and fibrin into the dressing matrix[9,20,21]; PolyMem Silver dressings also help manage bioburden by killing microbes as they come in contact with the dressing.[4,22–24] Rather than placing silver directly into the wound bed, the silver in PolyMem Silver is built into the dressing to help eliminate the bioburden and microbes in the dressing, doing potentially less damage to the healing wound.[4,22,25–28] Many new wound products are being developed to include small aspects of PolyMem dressings' many benefits, but none are able to furnish the integrated solutions PolyMem products have reliably provided for nearly three decades.[9]

Activated by moisture, PolyMem products gradually release a nontoxic surfactant cleanser and glycerin to loosen bonds between the wound bed and adherent substances that may impair healing.[4,15,29–31] Glycerin pulls nutrient-filled, enzyme-rich fluid from the body into the wound bed, enhancing healing and autolytic debridement while floating the contaminants.[2,5,15,18,32] The PolyMem membrane pulls in the undesirable substances along with the fluid, which are locked into the porous superabsorbent structure.[4,9,20,21] The wound contaminants are atraumatically removed and discarded when the PolyMem dressing is changed, eliminating the need for routine rinsing at dressing changes.[17,20,21,30]

The glycerin and surfactant in PolyMem products help moisturize dry areas of wounds while pulling fluid from the body into the wound bed and redistributing it.[2,15–18] Simultaneously, excess fluid from overly wet areas is absorbed into the dressing and is locked into a gel.[2,15,20,33] The "intelligent" backing allows excess fluid to evaporate while retaining the fluid needed to keep dry wounds moist.[34] Other available dressings have only portions of this complete moisture balancing system.[9]

All occlusive dressings provide some pain relief. However, PolyMem products are the only drug-free dressings with evidence showing that they also relieve pain by altering the response of the pain-sensing nerves (nociceptors).[10–12,16,31,35,36] PolyMem products' alteration of the nociceptor response occurs even on intact skin, and has been shown in clinical studies to decrease the excess inflammation that leads to excess swelling and often slows healing.[9–12,16,32,36]

PolyMem dressings are nonadherent while conforming to the wound bed.[5,15,17,18,20,35,37,38] They are flexible and comfortable to wear.[4–6,9,37,38]

INDICATIONS

Indicated for virtually all wounds at every stage of healing,[2,4,18,20,30] including closed tissue injuries,[11,36,39,40] multifunctional PolyMem dressings meet or exceed every criterion wound experts identify for an *Ideal Dressing*.[21,41,42] PolyMem dressings are safe for use over structures like tendon, bone, and exposed vessels because they can donate moisture.[4,5,15,18,32] PolyMem is suitable for use even when wounds are infected, provided that the infection is otherwise appropriately addressed.[4,9,15,43,44] PolyMem is especially suitable for chronic, trauma, and burn wounds because it helps subdue excess inflammation and is a pain-relieving dressing.[1,7,9,10,16,33,44–46]

- PolyMem Silver Finger/Toe dressings are especially suited for wounds on appendages[3,5,6] and adjacent joints when a wound displays signs of delayed healing or the patient is immune compromised.[4,42,47]

CONTRAINDICATIONS

- None.

APPLICATION

- Initially, irrigate or debride the wound bed as indicated or prescribed. Rinse with water or saline. Additional topical products are not necessary or recommended for use with PolyMem. Simply pat the periwound dry, leaving the wound bed slightly moist.
- Select a PolyMem Silver Finger/Toe dressing the appropriate diameter for the appendage. Trim excess length. Fill large voids lightly with PolyMem WIC silver. Insert tip of finger or toe into the rolled end of the dressing. Roll the PolyMem dressing onto the appendage with the moisture-barrier film (printed side) out.
- For joints, the dressing may be cut to form a ring or sleeve, and it may be split along seams with the ends secured with tape. See website and Instructions for Use for detailed application instructions.

How to know when to change PolyMem dressings

- Do NOT change PolyMem on a calendar schedule, especially in the first week of use; anticipate changes in exudate levels, which may dramatically increase initially.
- PolyMem is an indicator dressing: the backing will become a darker color when the membrane becomes saturated. Change the dressing when the darker color reaches any of the wound edges.

REMOVAL

- Simply, gently roll off the PolyMem Silver Finger/Toe dressing and replace it with an appropriate new PolyMem configuration. In most cases, when using PolyMem, there is no need to rinse the wound.
- PolyMem is designed to continuously cleanse the wound and does not leave residue that needs to be removed. Excessive cleaning may injure regenerating tissue and delay wound healing.

ANTIMICROBIALS

Guidelines for optimal use

(See *Instructions for Use* provided in each box and **PolyMem.com for detailed information.**)

Independent wound experts have created a robust evidence base for PolyMem dressings by documenting their success in using PolyMem over the past 25+ years. Ferris has developed these guidelines based upon their documented experiences.

- Using PolyMem is simple. However, using PolyMem optimally (knowing which dressing configuration to use, and how) is an art.[9,48] PolyMem use saves time, giving wound specialists more time to address the whole patient, improving healing by optimizing offloading, compression, circulation, nutrition, medications, and so forth.[3,5,7,16,33,35,40,48–50]
- PolyMem dressings should be changed when indicated, rather than on a schedule. Changing PolyMem more frequently than necessary on a healthy, granulating wound bed may slow healing. Tracing the approximate wound borders on the outer film of the PolyMem dressing makes it easy to see when a change is needed without "peeking" at the wound.[41]
- PolyMem is an interactive dressing. PolyMem often recruits LARGE amounts of wound fluid, containing debris and metabolic wastes, for the first few days of use, which may prompt frequent dressing changes.[4,30,49] When the wound is clean and granulating, reduced exudate may allow PolyMem to be left in place for up to 7 days.[9]
- On first application, irrigate or debride the wound to remove causes of delayed healing that are easy to address; then allow PolyMem to remove the remainder of the contaminants atraumatically. The PolyMem membrane may become discolored or malodorous, but the wound bed itself will become cleaner and healthier.
- Experienced users gain the confidence to avoid routine rinsing at dressing changes.[2,3,9,50,51] Simply applying a PolyMem dressing **IS** wound cleansing.[9,48] Because rinsing cools the wound bed, washes away valuable nutrients, and can damage fragile new tissue, it is best to rinse only if loose contaminants are visible or the dressing has become dislodged prior to the dressing change, allowing the wound to become dirty and dry.[52]
- Patients with large surface area third degree burns must be carefully supervised by a burn specialist, especially when any absorptive dressing is used, including PolyMem.
- Healing wounds quickly is the most cost-saving choice. PolyMem is proven to help close wounds quickly.

*See package insert for complete information.

REFERENCES

PDFs of many of the footnoted references are available at www.polymem.com/clinicalguide/

1. Dawson, Lewis C, Boch R. Total Joint Replacement Surgical Site Infections Eliminated by Using Multifunctional Dressing. 900 Cases Report over 4 years. May 2010.
2. Cutting KF, Vowden P, Wiegand C. Wound inflammation and the role of a multifunctional polymeric dressing. *Inter Wound J.* 2015;6(2):41–46.
3. White L. Optimal Management for Upper Extremity Wounds with a Multifunctional Polymeric Membrane Dressing. September 2015.
4. Benskin LL. PolyMem Wic Silver Rope: a multifunctional dressing for decreasing pain, swelling, and inflammation. *Adv Wound Care (New Rochelle).* 2012;1(1):44–47.
5. Rafter L, Oforka E. Standard versus polymeric membrane finger dressing and outcomes following pain diaries. *Wounds UK.* 2014;10(2):40–49.
6. Rafter L, Oforka E. Trauma-free fingertip dressing changes. *Wounds UK.* 2013;9(1):96–100.
7. Haik J, Weissman O, Demetrius S, et al. Polymeric Membrane Dressings® for Skin Graft Donor Sites: 6 Years Experience on 1200 Cases. April 2011.
8. Man D, Aleksinko P. Intra-Operative Use Followed with Post-Op Application of Polymeric Membrane Dressings Reduces Post-Op Pain, Edema and Bruising After Full Face Lift Surgery. April 2010.
9. Benskin LL. Polymeric Membrane Dressings for topical wound management of patients with infected wounds in a challenging environment: A protocol with 3 case examples. *Ostomy Wound Management.* 2016;62(6):42–50. (OWM website adds evidence summaries, Tables 1 & 2)

ANTIMICROBIALS

10. Kim YJ, Lee SW, Hong SH, et al. The Effects of PolyMem(R) on the Wound Healing. *J Korean Soc Plast Reconstr Surg.* 1999;26(6):1165–1172.

11. Hayden JK, Cole BJ. The effectiveness of a pain wrap compared to a standard dressing on the reduction of postoperative morbidity following routine knee arthroscopy: a prospective randomized single-blind study. *Orthopedics.* 2003;26(1):59–63; discussion 63.

12. Beitz AJ, Newman A, Kahn AR, et al. A polymeric membrane dressing with antinociceptive properties: analysis with a rodent model of stab wound secondary hyperalgesia. *J Pain.* 2004;5(1): 38–47.

13. Blackman JD, Senseng D, Quinn L, et al. Clinical evaluation of a semipermeable polymeric membrane dressing for the treatment of chronic diabetic foot ulcers. *Diabetes Care.* 1994;17(4):322–325.

14. Langemo DK, Black J; National Pressure Ulcer Advisory Panel. Pressure ulcers in individuals receiving palliative care: a National Pressure Ulcer Advisory Panel white paper. *Adv Skin Wound Care.* 2010;23(2):59–72.

15. Denyer J, White R, Ousey K, et al. PolyMem dressings Made Easy. *Wounds International.* May 2015. http://www.woundsinternational.com/made-easys/view/polymem-dressings-made-easy. Accessed May 7, 2016.

16. Weissman O, Hundeshagen G, Harats M, et al. Custom-fit polymeric membrane dressing masks in the treatment of second degree facial burns. *Burns.* 2013;39(6):1316–1320.

17. Scott A. Polymeric membrane dressings for radiotherapy-induced skin damage. *Br J Nurs.* 2014; 23(10):S24, S26–S31.

18. Dabiri G, Damstetter E, Phillips T. Choosing a Wound Dressing Based on Common Wound Characteristics. *Adv Wound Care (New Rochelle).* 2016;5(1):32–41.

19. Wilson D. Stalled diabetic ulcer closed in six weeks using PolyMem Silver dressings. June 2007.

20. Fowler E, Papen JC. Clinical evaluation of a polymeric membrane dressing in the treatment of dermal ulcers. *Ostomy Wound Manage.* 1991;35:35–38, 40–44.

21. Yastrub DJ. Relationship between type of treatment and degree of wound healing among institutionalized geriatric patients with stage II pressure ulcers. *Care Manag J.* 2004;5(4):213–218.

22. Benskin LL. Limitations of in vitro antimicrobial dressings study. *Burns.* 2016;42(5):1147–1148.

23. Larkö E, Blom K. Assessment of a Multifunctional Wound Dressing Using an Ex Vivo Wound Infection Healing Model. May 2012.

24. Boonkaew B, Barber PM, Rengpipat S, et al. Development and characterization of a novel, antimicrobial, sterile hydrogel dressing for burn wounds: single-step production with gamma irradiation creates silver nanoparticles and radical polymerization. *JPharmSci.* 2014;103(10):3244–3253.

25. Burd A, Kwok CH, Hung SC, et al. A comparative study of the cytotoxicity of silver-based dressings in monolayer cell, tissue explant, and animal models. *Wound Repair Regen.* 2007;15(1):94–104.

26. Tamir J. Mesh reinforced silver rope dressing for acute infected cavity wounds. April 2010.

27. Yeo ED, Yoon SA, Oh SR, et al. Degree of the hazards of silver- containing dressings on MRSAInfected wounds in Sprague-Dawley and streptozotocin-induced diabetic rats. *Wounds.* 2015;27(4):95–102.

28. Benskin L. Letter to the Editor: Degree of the hazards of silver-containing dressings on MRSA-infected wounds in Sprague-Dawley and streptozotocin-induced diabetic rats. *Wounds.* 2015;27(7):A10.

29. Rodeheaver GT, Kurtz L, Kircher BJ, et al. Pluronic F-68: a promising new skin wound cleanser. *Ann Emerg Med.* 1980;9(11):572–576.

30. Denyer JE, Pillay E. Best practice guidelines for skin and wound care in epidermolysis bullosa—International Consensus. 2012. http://www.woundsinternational.com/other-resources/view/best-practice-guidelines-for-skin-and-wound-care-in-epidermolysis-bullosa. Accessed March 30, 2015.

31. Davies SL, White RJ. Defining a holistic pain-relieving approach to wound care via a drug free polymeric membrane dressing. *J Wound Care.* 2011;20(5):250, 252, 254 passim.

32. Cahn A, Kleinman Y. A novel approach to the treatment of diabetic foot abscesses—a case series. *J Wound Care.* 2014;23(8):394, 396–399.

33. Stoddart J. Circumferential Wrap Technique with Polymeric Membrane Dressings after Arthroscopic ACL Reconstruction Reduces Blistering, Inflammation and Bruising; Rapid Recovery and Improved Patient Satisfaction: 80 Prospective Patient Series. May 2013.

34. Fulton JA, Blasiole KN, Cottingham T, et al. Wound Dressing Absorption: A Comparative Study. *Adv Skin Wound Care.* 2012;25(7):315–320.

35. Bolhuis J. Evidence-based skin tear protocol. *Long-Term Living: For the Continuing Care Professional.* 2008;57(6):48–52.

36. Kahn AR, Sessions RW, Apasova EV. A superficial cutaneous dressing inhibits pain, inflammation and swelling in deep tissues. *Pain Medicine.* 2000;1(2):187–187.

37. Bauer J, Diem A, Ploder M. Efficiency and Safety of Using a Polymeric Membrane Wound Dressing in Patients with Epidermolysis Bullosa after a Release Operation. May 2013.

38. Bauer J, Brandtner G. Chirurgische Korrektur der Handfehlbildungen bei Epidermolysis bullosa dystrophicans. *Arzt+Kind.* 2013.

39. Hegarty F, Wong M. Polymeric membrane dressing for radiotherapy-induced skin reactions. *Br J Nurs.* 2014;23 Suppl 20:S38–S46.

40. Wilson D. Application of Polymeric Membrane Dressings to Stage I Pressure Ulcers Speeds Resolution, Reduces Ulcer Site Discomfort and Reduces Staff Time Devoted to Management of Ulcers. April 2010.

41. Carr RD, Lalagos DE. Clinical evaluation of a polymeric membrane dressing in the treatment of pressure ulcers. *Decubitus.* 1990;3(3):38–42.

42. Benskin L. PolyMem The Ideal Dressing. August 2015.

43. Denyer JE. Wound management for children with epidermolysis bullosa. *Dermatologic Clinics.* 2010;28(2):257–264.

44. Aaltonen M. Developing a Protocol For Burns in a Private Out-Patient Wound Clinic. May 2015.

45. Rahman S, Shokri A. Total Knee Arthroplasty (TKA) Infections Eliminated and Rehabilitation Improved Using Polymeric Membrane Dressing Circumferential Wrap Technique: 120 Patients at 12-month Follow-up. May 2013.

46. Edwards J, Mason S. An evaluation of the use of PolyMem Silver in burn management. *Journal of Community Nursing.* 2010;24(6):16–19.

47. Benskin L. Combining Email Wound Consulting and Polymeric Membrane Dressings to Dramatically Improve Quality of Life. April 2009.

48. Denyer J. Six Years' Experience Of PolyMem Dressings Used On Children With Epidermolysis Bullosa (EB). September 2015.

49. Denyer J. Managing pain in children with epidermolysis bullosa. *Nurs Times.* 2012;108(29):21–23.

50. Vanwalleghem G. A New Protocol for the Treatment of Pilonidal Cysts. May 2011.

51. Agathangelou C. Patients with Chronic Wound Pain Stop Hurting, Why? May 2011.

52. McGuiness W, Vella E, Harrison D. Influence of dressing changes on wound temperature. *J Wound Care.* 2004;13(9):383–385.

ANTIMICROBIALS

PolyMem® WIC® Silver™ Rope and PolyMem® WIC® Silver™ Wound Fillers

Ferris Mfg. Corp.

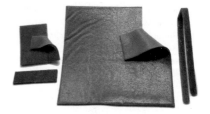

HOW SUPPLIED

PMD Wound Filler Rope with Silver	0.4" × 14" 3 g	A6215
PMD Wound Filler with Silver	1" × 3" 1.3 g	A6215
PMD Wound Filler with Silver	3" × 3" 4 g	A6215
PMD Wound Filler with Silver	8" × 8" 28 g, New Size	A6215

ACTION

PolyMem WIC Silver Rope is an antimicrobial,[1] multifunctional,[2–5] interactive[6] polymeric membrane dressing (PMD) designed to remain completely intact when filling tunnels.[2,7,8] PolyMem WIC Silver Rope wicks excess wound fluid into outer dressings[2,7] while helping reduce inflammation[2,9–11] and odor,[4,6,12,13] decreasing pain,[5,12,14–16] balancing moisture,[4,6,17–19] and continuously cleansing wounds.[2,7,12,20] PolyMem WIC Silver Wound Filler is a antimicrobial[1] multifunctional[2–5] wound filler that continuously cleanses[2,7,12,20,21] absorbs,[22] and moistens[1,22,23] as it expands to gently fill dead space.[7,22] PolyMem WIC Silver Wound Filler also helps reduce wound pain and odor.[1,21,22] All PolyMem dressings pull exudate, drainage, dirt, slough, and fibrin into the dressing matrix;[12,24,25] PolyMem Silver dressings also help manage bioburden by killing microbes as they come in contact with the dressing.[2,26–28] Rather than placing silver directly into the wound bed, the silver in PolyMem Silver wound fillers is built into the dressings to help eliminate the bioburden and microbes in the dressings, doing potentially less damage to the healing wound.[2,7,26,29–31] Many new wound products are being developed to include small aspects of PolyMem dressings' many benefits, but none are able to furnish the integrated solutions PolyMem products have reliably provided for nearly three decades.[12]

Activated by moisture, PolyMem products gradually release a nontoxic surfactant cleanser and glycerin to loosen bonds between the wound bed and adherent substances that may impair healing.[2,6,32–34] Glycerin pulls nutrient-filled, enzyme-rich fluid from the body into the wound bed, enhancing healing and autolytic debridement while floating the contaminants.[4,6,19,35,36] The PolyMem membrane pulls in the undesirable substances along with the fluid, which are locked into the porous superabsorbent structure.[2,12,24,25] The wound contaminants are atraumatically removed and discarded when the PolyMem dressing is changed, eliminating the need for routine rinsing at dressing changes.[18,24,25,33]

The glycerin and surfactant in PolyMem products help moisturize dry areas of wounds while pulling fluid from the body into the wound bed and redistributing it.[4,6,17–19] Simultaneously, excess fluid from overly wet areas is absorbed into the dressing and is locked into a gel.[4,6,24,37] The "intelligent" backing allows excess fluid to evaporate while retaining the fluid needed to keep dry wounds moist.[38] Other available dressings have only portions of this complete moisture balancing system.[12]

All occlusive dressings provide some pain relief. However, PolyMem products are the only drug-free dressings with evidence showing that they also relieve pain by altering the response of the pain-sensing nerves (nociceptors).[9–11,17,34,39,40] PolyMem products' alteration of the nociceptor response occurs even on intact skin, and has been shown in clinical studies to decrease the excess inflammation that leads to excess swelling and often slows healing.[9–12,17,36,40]

PolyMem dressings are non-adherent while conforming to the wound bed.[6,18,19,24,35,39,41,42] They are flexible and comfortable to wear.[2,12,35,41–43]

INDICATIONS

Indicated for virtually all wounds at every stage of healing,[2,4,19,24,33] including closed tissue injuries,[10,40,44,45] multifunctional PolyMem dressings meet or exceed every criterion wound experts identify for an *Ideal Dressing*.[1,25,46] PolyMem dressings are safe for use over structures like tendon, bone, and exposed vessels because they can donate moisture.[2,6,19,35,36] PolyMem is suitable for use even when wounds are infected, provided that the infection is otherwise appropriately addressed.[2,6,12,47,48] PolyMem is especially suitable for chronic, trauma, and burn wounds because it helps subdue excess inflammation and is a pain relieving dressing.[3,9,12,14,17,37,48–50]

- PolyMem WIC Silver Rope is designed especially for easy insertion and removal on tunneling wounds.[2,7,8] PolyMem WIC Silver wound filler is indicated to lightly fill dead space in dry to heavily exudating wounds when a wound displays signs of delayed healing or the patient is immune compromised.[21,22,51] PolyMem WIC Silver's unique properties make it ideal for use on heavily exudating wounds under absorptive compression wraps and as an absorptive layer under PolyMem secondary dressings.[52]

CONTRAINDICATIONS

- None.

APPLICATION

- Initially, irrigate or debride the wound bed as indicated or prescribed. Rinse with water or saline. Additional topical products are not necessary or recommended for use with PolyMem. Simply pat the periwound dry, leaving the wound bed slightly moist.
- Cut or tear PolyMem WIC Silver wound filler so that it lightly fills the cavity, allowing for about 30% expansion. For narrow spaces, use PolyMem WIC Silver Rope, which has a reinforced mesh to ensure one-piece removal, leaving the rope slightly longer than the wound. For use under secondary dressings or absorptive compression wraps, lay PolyMem WIC flat.
- Apply a PolyMem dressing with a membrane pad that is large enough to cover the wound filler **AND** all of the surrounding inflamed (reddened, raw, tender, warm, itchy, or swollen) skin, with the moisture-barrier film (printed side) out. Secure the secondary (outer) dressing appropriately. Apply adhesives without tension.

How to know when to change PolyMem dressings

- Do NOT change PolyMem on a calendar schedule, especially in the first week of use; anticipate changes in exudate levels, which may dramatically increase initially.
- PolyMem is an indicator dressing: the backing will become a darker color when the membrane becomes saturated. Change the dressing when the darker color reaches any of the wound edges.

REMOVAL

- Simply, gently remove the PolyMem dressing and PolyMem Silver WIC wound filler or PolyMem Silver Rope and replace them with an appropriate new PolyMem configuration. In most cases, when using PolyMem, there is no need to rinse the wound.
- PolyMem is designed to continuously cleanse the wound and does not leave residue that needs to be removed. Excessive cleaning may injure regenerating tissue and delay wound healing.

ANTIMICROBIALS

Guidelines for optimal use

(See *Instructions for Use* provided in each box and **PolyMem.com for detailed information**.)

Independent wound experts have created a robust evidence base for PolyMem dressings by documenting their success in using PolyMem over the past 25+ years. Ferris has developed these guidelines based upon their documented experiences.

- Using PolyMem is simple. However, using PolyMem optimally (knowing which dressing configuration to use, and how) is an art.[12,53] PolyMem use saves time, giving wound specialists more time to address the whole patient, improving healing by optimizing offloading, compression, circulation, nutrition, medications, and so forth.[5,14,17,35,37,39,45,53-55]
- PolyMem dressings should be changed when indicated, rather than on a schedule. Changing PolyMem more frequently than necessary on a healthy, granulating wound bed may slow healing. Tracing the approximate wound borders on the outer film of the PolyMem dressing makes it easy to see when a change is needed without "peeking" at the wound.[46]
- PolyMem is an interactive dressing. PolyMem often recruits LARGE amounts of wound fluid, containing debris and metabolic wastes, for the first few days of use, which may prompt frequent dressing changes.[2,33,54] When the wound is clean and granulating, reduced exudate may allow PolyMem to be left in place for up to 7 days.[12]
- On first application, irrigate or debride the wound to remove causes of delayed healing that are easy to address; then allow PolyMem to remove the remainder of the contaminants atraumatically. The PolyMem membrane may become discolored or malodorous, but the wound bed itself will become cleaner and healthier.
- Experienced users gain the confidence to avoid routine rinsing at dressing changes.[4,5,12,55,56] Simply applying a PolyMem dressing **IS** wound cleansing.[12,53] Because rinsing cools the wound bed, washes away valuable nutrients, and can damage fragile new tissue, it is best to rinse only if loose contaminants are visible or the dressing has become dislodged prior to the dressing change, allowing the wound to become dirty and dry.[57]
- Patients with large surface area third degree burns must be carefully supervised by a burn specialist, especially when any absorptive dressing is used, including PolyMem.
- Healing wounds quickly is the most cost-saving choice. PolyMem is proven to help close wounds quickly.

*See package insert for complete information.

REFERENCES

PDFs of many of the footnoted references are available at www.polymem.com/clinicalguide/

1. Benskin L. PolyMem The Ideal Dressing. August 2015.
2. Benskin LL. PolyMem Wic Silver Rope: a multifunctional dressing for decreasing pain, swelling, and inflammation. *Adv Wound Care (New Rochelle).* 2012;1(1):44–47.
3. Dawson, Lewis C, Boch R. Total Joint Replacement Surgical Site Infections Eliminated by Using Multifunctional Dressing. 900 Cases Report over 4 years. May 2010.
4. Cutting KF, Vowden P, Wiegand C. Wound inflammation and the role of a multifunctional polymeric dressing. *Wounds International Journal.* 2015;6(2):41–46.
5. White L. Optimal Management for Upper Extremity Wounds with a Multifunctional Polymeric Membrane Dressing. September 2015.
6. Denyer J, White R, Ousey K, et al. PolyMem dressings Made Easy. *Wounds International.* May 2015. http://www.woundsinternational.com/made-easys/view/polymem-dressings-made-easy. Accessed May 7, 2016.
7. Tamir J. Mesh reinforced silver rope dressing for acute infected cavity wounds. April 2010.
8. Harrison JE. An Independent Evaluation of a New Mesh-Reinforced Silver Rope Dressing. *J Wound Ostomy Continence Nurs.* 2009;36(Supplement):S35.

ANTIMICROBIALS

9. Kim YJ, Lee SW, Hong SH, et al. The Effects of PolyMem(R) on the Wound Healing. *J Korean Soc Plast Reconstr Surg.* 1999;26(6):1165–1172.
10. Hayden JK, Cole BJ. The effectiveness of a pain wrap compared to a standard dressing on the reduction of postoperative morbidity following routine knee arthroscopy: a prospective randomized single-blind study. *Orthopedics.* 2003;26(1):59–63; discussion 63.
11. Beitz AJ, Newman A, Kahn AR, et al. A polymeric membrane dressing with antinociceptive properties: analysis with a rodent model of stab wound secondary hyperalgesia. *J Pain.* 2004;5(1):38–47.
12. Benskin LL. Polymeric Membrane Dressings for topical wound management of patients with infected wounds in a challenging environment: A protocol with 3 case examples. *Ostomy Wound Management.* 2016;62(6):42–50. (OWM website adds evidence summaries, Tables 1 & 2)
13. Agathangelou C. Treating Fungating Breast Cancer Wounds with Polymeric Membrane Dressings, an Innovation in Fungating Wound Management. May 2015.
14. Haik J, Weissman O, Demetrius S, et al. Polymeric Membrane Dressings* for Skin Graft Donor Sites: 6 Years Experience on 1200 Cases. April 2011.
15. Man D, Aleksinko P. Use of Polymeric Membrane Dressings After Occlusive Deep Facial and Neck Chemical Peel Improves Outcomes. April 2010.
16. Man D, Aleksinko P. Intra-Operative Use Followed with Post-Op Application of Polymeric Membrane Dressings Reduces Post-Op Pain, Edema and Bruising After Full Face Lift Surgery. April 2010.
17. Weissman O, Hundeshagen G, Harats M, et al. Custom-fit polymeric membrane dressing masks in the treatment of second degree facial burns. *Burns.* 2013;39(6):1316–1320.
18. Scott A. Polymeric membrane dressings for radiotherapy-induced skin damage. *Br J Nurs.* 2014; 23(10):S24, S26–S31.
19. Dabiri G, Damstetter E, Phillips T. Choosing a wound dressing based on common wound characteristics. *Adv Wound Care (New Rochelle).* 2016;5(1):32–41.
20. Blackman JD, Senseng D, Quinn L, et al. Clinical evaluation of a semipermeable polymeric membrane dressing for the treatment of chronic diabetic foot ulcers. *Diabetes Care.* 1994;17(4):322–325.
21. Benskin LL. Dissecting Hand Abcess Wound Treated with Polymeric Membrane Dressings* Until Complete Wound Closure. May 2006.
22. Benskin L. Extensive tunneling lower leg wounds with exposed tendons closed quickly using various polymeric membrane dressing configurations. October 2008.
23. Agathangelou A. Deep Ulcer on Charcot Foot Closed After Treatment with Polymeric Membrane Silver Cavity Dressing. June 2008.
24. Fowler E, Papen JC. Clinical evaluation of a polymeric membrane dressing in the treatment of dermal ulcers. *Ostomy Wound Manage.* 1991;35:35–38, 40–44.
25. Yastrub DJ. Relationship between type of treatment and degree of wound healing among institutionalized geriatric patients with stage II pressure ulcers. *Care Manag J.* 2004;5(4):213-218.
26. Benskin LL. Limitations of in vitro antimicrobial dressings study. *Burns.* 2016;42(5):1147–1148. doi:10.1016/j.burns.2016.01.034.
27. Larkö E, Blom K. Assessment of a Multifunctional Wound Dressing Using an Ex Vivo Wound Infection Healing Model. May 2012.
28. Boonkaew B, Barber PM, Rengpipat S, et al. Development and Characterization of a Novel, Antimicrobial, Sterile Hydrogel Dressing for Burn Wounds: Single-Step Production with Gamma Irradiation Creates Silver Nanoparticles and Radical Polymerization. *JPharmSci.* 2014;103(10):3244–3253.
29. Burd A, Kwok CH, Hung SC, et al. A comparative study of the cytotoxicity of silver-based dressings in monolayer cell, tissue explant, and animal models. *Wound Repair Regen.* 2007;15(1):94–104.
30. Yeo ED, Yoon SA, Oh SR, et al. Degree of the hazards of silver- containing dressings on MRSAInfected wounds in Sprague-Dawley and streptozotocin-induced diabetic rats. *Wounds.* 2015;27(4):95–102.
31. Benskin L. Letter to the Editor: Degree of the hazards of silver-containing dressings on MRSA-infected wounds in Sprague-Dawley and streptozotocin-induced diabetic rats. *Wounds.* 2015;27(7):A10.
32. Rodeheaver GT, Kurtz L, Kircher BJ, et al. Pluronic F-68: a promising new skin wound cleanser. *Ann Emerg Med.* 1980;9(11):572–576.
33. Denyer JE, Pillay E. Best practice guidelines for skin and wound care in epidermolysis bullosa—International Consensus. 2012. http://www.woundsinternational.com/other-resources/view/best-practice-guidelines-for-skin-and-wound-care-in-epidermolysis-bullosa. Accessed March 30, 2015.
34. Davies SL, White RJ. Defining a holistic pain-relieving approach to wound care via a drug free polymeric membrane dressing. *J Wound Care.* 2011;20(5):250, 252, 254 passim.

35. Rafter L, Oforka E. Standard versus polymeric membrane finger dressing and outcomes following pain diaries. *Wounds UK*. 2014;10(2):40–49.

36. Cahn A, Kleinman Y. A novel approach to the treatment of diabetic foot abscesses—a case series. *J Wound Care*. 2014;23(8):394, 396–399.

37. Stoddart J. Circumferential Wrap Technique with Polymeric Membrane Dressings after Arthroscopic ACL Reconstruction Reduces Blistering, Inflammation and Bruising; Rapid Recovery and Improved Patient Satisfaction: 80 Prospective Patient Series. May 2013.

38. Fulton JA, Blasiole KN, Cottingham T, et al. Wound dressing absorption: a comparative study. *Adv Skin Wound Care*. 2012;25(7):315–320.

39. Bolhuis J. Evidence-based skin tear protocol. *Long-Term Living: For the Continuing Care Professional*. 2008;57(6):48–52.

40. Kahn AR, Sessions RW, Apasova EV. A superficial cutaneous dressing inhibits pain, inflammation and swelling in deep tissues. *Pain Medicine*. 2000;1(2):187–187.

41. Bauer J, Diem A, Ploder M. Efficiency and Safety of Using a Polymeric Membrane Wound Dressing in Patients with Epidermolysis Bullosa after a Release Operation. May 2013.

42. Bauer J, Brandtner G. Chirurgische Korrektur der Handfehlbildungen bei Epidermolysis bullosa dystrophicans. *Arzt+Kind*. 2013.

43. Rafter L, Oforka E. Trauma-free fingertip dressing changes. *Wounds UK*. 2013;9(1):96–100.

44. Hegarty F, Wong M. Polymeric membrane dressing for radiotherapy-induced skin reactions. *Br J Nurs*. 2014;23 Suppl 20:S38–S46.

45. Wilson D. Application of Polymeric Membrane Dressings to Stage I Pressure Ulcers Speeds Resolution, Reduces Ulcer Site Discomfort and Reduces Staff Time Devoted to Management of Ulcers. April 2010.

46. Carr RD, Lalagos DE. Clinical evaluation of a polymeric membrane dressing in the treatment of pressure ulcers. *Decubitus*. 1990;3(3):38–42.

47. Denyer JE. Wound management for children with epidermolysis bullosa. *Dermatologic Clinics*. 2010;28(2):257–264.

48. Aaltonen M. Developing a Protocol For Burns in a Private Out-Patient Wound Clinic. May 2015.

49. Rahman S, Shokri A. Total Knee Arthroplasty (TKA) Infections Eliminated and Rehabilitation Improved Using Polymeric Membrane Dressing Circumferential Wrap Technique: 120 Patients at 12-month Follow-up. May 2013.

50. Edwards J, Mason S. An evaluation of the use of PolyMem Silver in burn management. *Journal of Community Nursing*. 2010;24(6):16–19.

51. Agathangelou C. Huge sacral pressure ulcer closed in four months using silver polymeric membrane cavity filler and dressings. February 2009.

52. Harrison JE. Chronic Venous Ulcer Closing Steadily with Complete Elimination of Wound Pain Using Standard or Silver Polymeric Membrane Wound Filler Under Compression. June 2008.

53. Denyer J. Six Years' Experience Of PolyMem Dressings Used On Children With Epidermolysis Bullosa (EB). September 2015.

54. Denyer J. Managing pain in children with epidermolysis bullosa. *Nurs Times*. 2012;108(29):21–23.

55. Vanwalleghem G. A New Protocol for the Treatment of Pilonidal Cysts. May 2011.

56. Agathangelou C. Patients with Chronic Wound Pain Stop Hurting, Why? May 2011.

57. McGuiness W, Vella E, Harrison D. Influence of dressing changes on wound temperature. *J Wound Care*. 2004;13(9):383–385.

ANTIMICROBIALS

Shapes® by PolyMem® Oval and Sacral Silver™ Dressings

Ferris Mfg. Corp.

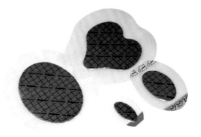

HOW SUPPLIED

#3 Oval-Shaped PMD with Silver	1″ × 2″ pad with 2″ × 3″ adhesive	A6212
#5 Oval-Shaped PMD with Silver	2″ × 3″ pad with 3.5″ × 5″ adhesive	A6212
#8 Oval-Shaped PMD with Silver	4″ × 5.7″ pad with 6.5″ × 8.2″ adhesive	A6213
Sacral (Heart-Shaped) PMD with Silver	4.5″ × 4.7″ pad with 7.2″ × 7.8″ adhesive	A6212

ACTION

Shapes by PolyMem Oval and Sacral Silver Dressings are wound-shaped water-resistant[1] multifunctional,[2–5] interactive[6] polymeric membrane dressings (PMDs) with a thin-film adhesive border.[7] These polymeric membrane dressings are designed to decrease pain,[5,8–11] odor,[4,6,11,12] and inflammation[2,13–15] and protect wounds[4,11] while promoting quick healing.[1] All PolyMem dressings pull exudate, drainage, dirt, slough, and fibrin into the dressing matrix[11,16,17]; PolyMem Silver dressings also help manage bioburden by killing microbes as they come in contact with the dressing.[2,18–20] Rather than placing silver directly into the wound bed, the silver in PolyMem Silver is built into the dressing to help eliminate the bioburden and microbes in the dressing, doing potentially less damage to the healing wound.[2,18,21–24] Many new wound products are being developed to include small aspects of PolyMem dressings' many benefits, but none are able to furnish the integrated solutions PolyMem products have reliably provided for nearly three decades.[11]

Activated by moisture, PolyMem products gradually release a nontoxic surfactant cleanser and glycerin to loosen bonds between the wound bed and adherent substances that may impair healing.[2,6,25–27] Glycerin pulls nutrient-filled, enzyme-rich fluid from the body into the wound bed, enhancing healing and autolytic debridement while floating the contaminants.[4,6,28–30] The PolyMem membrane pulls in the undesirable substances along with the fluid, which are locked into the porous superabsorbent structure.[2,11,16,17] The wound contaminants are atraumatically removed and discarded when the PolyMem dressing is changed, eliminating the need for routine rinsing at dressing changes.[16,17,26,31]

The glycerin and surfactant in PolyMem products help moisturize dry areas of wounds while pulling fluid from the body into the wound bed and redistributing it.[4,6,30–32] Simultaneously, excess fluid from overly wet areas is absorbed into the dressing and is locked into a gel.[4,6,16,33] The "intelligent" backing allows excess fluid to evaporate while retaining the fluid needed to keep dry wounds moist.[34] Other available dressings have only portions of this complete moisture balancing system.[11]

All occlusive dressings provide some pain relief. However, PolyMem products are the only drug-free dressings with evidence showing that they also relieve pain by altering the response of the pain-sensing nerves (nociceptors).[1,13–15,27,32,35] PolyMem products' alteration of the nociceptor response occurs even on intact skin, and has been shown in clinical studies to decrease the excess inflammation that leads to excess swelling and often slows healing.[11,13–15,29,32,35]

PolyMem dressings are non-adherent while conforming to the wound bed.[1,6,16,28,30,31,36,37] They are flexible and comfortable to wear.[2,11,28,36–38]

INDICATIONS

Indicated for virtually all wounds at every stage of healing,[2,4,16,26,30] including closed tissue injuries,[14,35,39,40] multifunctional PolyMem dressings meet or exceed every criterion wound experts identify for an *Ideal Dressing*.[17,41,42] PolyMem dressings are safe for use over structures like tendon, bone, and exposed vessels because they can donate moisture.[2,6,28–30] PolyMem is suitable for use even when wounds are infected, provided that the infection is otherwise appropriately addressed.[2,6,11,43,44] PolyMem is especially suitable for chronic, trauma, and burn wounds because it helps subdue excess inflammation and is a pain relieving dressing.[3,8,11,13,32,33,44–46]

- Shapes by PolyMem Silver dressings are especially suited to offer a secure fit for contoured areas of the body where the dressing needs to bend and conform when a wound displays signs of delayed healing or the patient is immune compromised.[1,47]

CONTRAINDICATIONS

- None.

APPLICATION

- Initially, irrigate or debride the wound bed as indicated or prescribed. Rinse with water or saline. Additional topical products are not necessary or recommended for use with PolyMem. Simply pat the periwound dry, leaving the wound bed slightly moist.
- Fill any deep cavities lightly with PolyMem WIC silver or WIC Silver Rope, allowing for about 30% expansion. Select a Shapes by PolyMem Silver dressing with a membrane pad that is large enough to cover the open wound **AND** all of the surrounding inflamed (reddened, raw, tender, warm, itchy, or swollen) skin.
- Apply the adhesive borders without tension. Smooth into place. See Instructions for Use for details.

How to know when to change PolyMem dressings

- Do NOT change PolyMem on a calendar schedule, especially in the first week of use; anticipate changes in exudate levels, which may dramatically increase initially.
- PolyMem is an indicator dressing: the backing will become a darker color when the membrane becomes saturated. Change the dressing when the darker color reaches any of the wound edges.

REMOVAL

- Simply, gently remove the Shapes by PolyMem Silver dressing and any PolyMem Silver WIC or Rope and replace it with an appropriate new PolyMem configuration. In most cases, when using PolyMem, there is no need to rinse the wound.
- PolyMem is designed to continuously cleanse the wound and does not leave residue that needs to be removed. Excessive cleaning may injure regenerating tissue and delay wound healing.

ANTIMICROBIALS

Guidelines for optimal use

(See *Instructions for Use* provided in each box and **PolyMem.com for detailed information.**)

Independent wound experts have created a robust evidence base for PolyMem dressings by documenting their success in using PolyMem over the past 25+ years. Ferris has developed these guidelines based upon their documented experiences.

- Using PolyMem is simple. However, using PolyMem optimally (knowing which dressing configuration to use, and how) is an art.[11,48] PolyMem use saves time, giving wound specialists more time to address the whole patient, improving healing by optimizing offloading, compression, circulation, nutrition, medications, and so forth.[1,5,8,28,32,33,40,48–50]

- PolyMem dressings should be changed when indicated, rather than on a schedule. Changing PolyMem more frequently than necessary on a healthy, granulating wound bed may slow healing. Tracing the approximate wound borders on the outer film of the PolyMem dressing makes it easy to see when a change is needed without "peeking" at the wound.[41]

- PolyMem is an interactive dressing. PolyMem often recruits LARGE amounts of wound fluid, containing debris and metabolic wastes, for the first few days of use, which may prompt frequent dressing changes.[2,26,49] When the wound is clean and granulating, reduced exudate may allow PolyMem to be left in place for up to 7 days.[11]

- On first application, irrigate or debride the wound to remove causes of delayed healing that are easy to address; then allow PolyMem to remove the remainder of the contaminants atraumatically. The PolyMem membrane may become discolored or malodorous, but the wound bed itself will become cleaner and healthier.

- Experienced users gain the confidence to avoid routine rinsing at dressing changes.[4,5,11,50,51] Simply applying a PolyMem dressing **IS** wound cleansing.[11,48] Because rinsing cools the wound bed, washes away valuable nutrients, and can damage fragile new tissue, it is best to rinse only if loose contaminants are visible or the dressing has become dislodged prior to the dressing change, allowing the wound to become dirty and dry.[52]

- Patients with large surface area third degree burns must be carefully supervised by a burn specialist, especially when any absorptive dressing is used, including PolyMem.

- Healing wounds quickly is the most cost-saving choice. PolyMem is proven to help close wounds quickly.

*See package insert for complete information.

REFERENCES

PDFs of many of the footnoted references are available at www.polymem.com/clinicalguide/

1. Bolhuis J. Evidence-based skin tear protocol. *Long-Term Living: For the Continuing Care Professional.* 2008;57(6):48–52.
2. Benskin LL. PolyMem Wic Silver Rope: a multifunctional dressing for decreasing pain, swelling, and inflammation. *Adv Wound Care (New Rochelle).* 2012;1(1):44–47.
3. Dawson, Lewis C, Boch R. Total Joint Replacement Surgical Site Infections Eliminated by Using Multifunctional Dressing. 900 Cases Report over 4 years. May 2010.
4. Cutting KF, Vowden P, Wiegand C. Wound inflammation and the role of a multifunctional polymeric dressing. *Wounds International Journal.* 2015;6(2):41–46.
5. White L. Optimal Management for Upper Extremity Wounds with a Multifunctional Polymeric Membrane Dressing. September 2015.
6. Denyer J, White R, Ousey K, et al. PolyMem dressings Made Easy. *Wounds International.* May 2015. http://www.woundsinternational.com/made-easys/view/polymem-dressings-made-easy. Accessed May 7, 2016.
7. Yastrub D. Heel Ulcer in Hospice Patient Closed Quickly Using Polymeric Membrane Dressings. June 2008.
8. Haik J, Weissman O, Demetrius S, et al. Polymeric Membrane Dressings® for Skin Graft Donor Sites: 6 Years Experience on 1200 Cases. April 2011.

9. Man D, Aleksinko P. Use of Polymeric Membrane Dressings After Occlusive Deep Facial and Neck Chemical Peel Improves Outcomes. April 2010.

10. Man D, Aleksinko P. Intra-Operative Use Followed with Post-Op Application of Polymeric Membrane Dressings Reduces Post-Op Pain, Edema and Bruising After Full Face Lift Surgery. April 2010.

11. Benskin LL. Polymeric Membrane Dressings for topical wound management of patients with infected wounds in a challenging environment: A protocol with 3 case examples. *Ostomy Wound Manage.* 2016;62(6):42–50. (OWM website adds evidence summaries, Tables 1 & 2)

12. Agathangelou C. Treating Fungating Breast Cancer Wounds with Polymeric Membrane Dressings, an Innovation in Fungating Wound Management. May 2015.

13. Kim YJ, Lee SW, Hong SH, et al. The Effects of PolyMem(R) on the Wound Healing. *J Korean Soc Plast Reconstr Surg.* 1999;26(6):1165–1172.

14. Hayden JK, Cole BJ. The effectiveness of a pain wrap compared to a standard dressing on the reduction of postoperative morbidity following routine knee arthroscopy: a prospective randomized single-blind study. *Orthopedics.* 2003;26(1):59–63; discussion 63.

15. Beitz AJ, Newman A, Kahn AR, et al. A polymeric membrane dressing with antinociceptive properties: analysis with a rodent model of stab wound secondary hyperalgesia. *J Pain.* 2004;5(1):38–47.

16. Fowler E, Papen JC. Clinical evaluation of a polymeric membrane dressing in the treatment of dermal ulcers. *Ostomy Wound Manage.* 1991;35:35–38, 40–44.

17. Yastrub DJ. Relationship between type of treatment and degree of wound healing among institution-alized geriatric patients with stage II pressure ulcers. *Care Manag J.* 2004;5(4):213–218.

18. Benskin LL. Limitations of in vitro antimicrobial dressings study. *Burns.* 2016;42(5):1147–1148.

19. Larkö E, Blom K. Assessment of a Multifunctional Wound Dressing Using an Ex Vivo Wound Infection Healing Model. May 2012.

20. Boonkaew B, Barber PM, Rengpipat S, et al. Development and characterization of a novel, antimi-crobial, sterile hydrogel dressing for burn wounds: single-step production with gamma irradiation creates silver nanoparticles and radical polymerization. *JPharmSci.* 2014;103(10):3244–3253.

21. Burd A, Kwok CH, Hung SC, et al. A comparative study of the cytotoxicity of silver-based dressings in monolayer cell, tissue explant, and animal models. *Wound Repair Regen.* 2007;15(1):94–104.

22. Tamir J. Mesh reinforced silver rope dressing for acute infected cavity wounds. April 2010.

23. Yeo ED, Yoon SA, Oh SR, et al. Degree of the hazards of silver- containing dressings on MRSAInfected wounds in Sprague-Dawley and streptozotocin-induced diabetic rats. *Wounds.* 2015;27(4):95–102.

24. Benskin L. Letter to the Editor: Degree of the hazards of silver-containing dressings on MRSA-infected wounds in Sprague-Dawley and streptozotocin-induced diabetic rats. *Wounds.* 2015;27(7):A10.

25. Rodeheaver GT, Kurtz L, Kircher BJ, et al. Pluronic F-68: a promising new skin wound cleanser. *Ann Emerg Med.* 1980;9(11):572–576.

26. Denyer JE, Pillay E. Best practice guidelines for skin and wound care in epidermolysis bullosa—International Consensus. 2012. http://www.woundsinternational.com/other-resources/view/best-practice-guidelines-for-skin-and-wound-care-in-epidermolysis-bullosa. Accessed March 30, 2015.

27. Davies SL, White RJ. Defining a holistic pain-relieving approach to wound care via a drug free poly-meric membrane dressing. *J Wound Care.* 2011;20(5):250, 252, 254 passim.

28. Rafter L, Oforka E. Standard versus polymeric membrane finger dressing and outcomes following pain diaries. *Wounds UK.* 2014;10(2):40–49.

29. Cahn A, Kleinman Y. A novel approach to the treatment of diabetic foot abscesses—a case series. *J Wound Care.* 2014;23(8):394, 396–399.

30. Dabiri G, Damstetter E, Phillips T. Choosing a Wound Dressing Based on Common Wound Character-istics. *Adv Wound Care (New Rochelle).* 2016;5(1):32–41.

31. Scott A. Polymeric membrane dressings for radiotherapy-induced skin damage. *Br J Nurs.* 2014; 23(10):S24, S26–S31.

32. Weissman O, Hundeshagen G, Harats M, et al. Custom-fit polymeric membrane dressing masks in the treatment of second degree facial burns. *Burns.* 2013;39(6):1316–1320.

33. Stoddart J. Circumferential Wrap Technique with Polymeric Membrane Dressings after Arthroscopic ACL Reconstruction Reduces Blistering, Inflammation and Bruising; Rapid Recovery and Improved Patient Satisfaction: 80 Prospective Patient Series. May 2013.

34. Fulton JA, Blasiole KN, Cottingham T, et al. Wound Dressing Absorption: A Comparative Study. *Adv Skin Wound Care.* 2012;25(7):315–320.

35. Kahn AR, Sessions RW, Apasova EV. A superficial cutaneous dressing inhibits pain, inflammation and swelling in deep tissues. *Pain Medicine.* 2000;1(2):187–187.

ANTIMICROBIALS

36. Bauer J, Diem A, Ploder M. Efficiency and Safety of Using a Polymeric Membrane Wound Dressing in Patients with Epidermolysis Bullosa after a Release Operation. May 2013.

37. Bauer J, Brandtner G. Chirurgische Korrektur der Handfehlbildungen bei Epidermolysis bullosa dystrophicans. *Arzt+Kind*. 2013.

38. Rafter L, Oforka E. Trauma-free fingertip dressing changes. *Wounds UK*. 2013;9(1):96-100.

39. Hegarty F, Wong M. Polymeric membrane dressing for radiotherapy-induced skin reactions. *Br J Nurs*. 2014;23 Suppl 20:S38–S46.

40. Wilson D. Application of Polymeric Membrane Dressings to Stage I Pressure Ulcers Speeds Resolution, Reduces Ulcer Site Discomfort and Reduces Staff Time Devoted to Management of Ulcers. April 2010.

41. Carr RD, Lalagos DE. Clinical evaluation of a polymeric membrane dressing in the treatment of pressure ulcers. *Decubitus*. 1990;3(3):38–42.

42. Benskin L. PolyMem The Ideal Dressing. August 2015.

43. Denyer JE. Wound management for children with epidermolysis bullosa. *Dermatologic Clinics*. 2010;28(2):257–264.

44. Aaltonen M. Developing a Protocol For Burns in a Private Out-Patient Wound Clinic. May 2015.

45. Rahman S, Shokri A. Total Knee Arthroplasty (TKA) Infections Eliminated and Rehabilitation Improved Using Polymeric Membrane Dressing Circumferential Wrap Technique: 120 Patients at 12-month Follow-up. May 2013.

46. Edwards J, Mason S. An evaluation of the use of PolyMem Silver in burn management. *Journal of Community Nursing*. 2010;24(6):16–19.

47. Wilson D. Stalled diabetic ulcer closed in six weeks using PolyMem Silver dressings. June 2007.

48. Denyer J. Six Years' Experience Of PolyMem Dressings Used On Children With Epidermolysis Bullosa (EB). September 2015.

49. Denyer J. Managing pain in children with epidermolysis bullosa. *Nurs Times*. 2012;108(29):21–23.

50. Vanwalleghem G. A New Protocol for the Treatment of Pilonidal Cysts. May 2011.

51. Agathangelou C. Patients with Chronic Wound Pain Stop Hurting, Why? May 2011.

52. McGuiness W, Vella E, Harrison D. Influence of dressing changes on wound temperature. *J Wound Care*. 2004;13(9):383–385.

ANTIMICROBIALS

SilvaKollagen Gel

DermaRite Industries, LLC

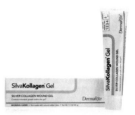

HOW SUPPLIED

Silver Collagen Wound Gel	1.5 oz	A6011

ACTION

SilvaKollagen® Gel is a hydrolyzed collagen gel wound dressing with silver oxide. The silver preservative in the dressing controls microbial growth within the gel. SilvaKollagen Gel provides a physiologically favorable environment that encourages wound healing while protecting the wound bed and its newly formed granulation tissue; soothes and deodorizes; conforms to any wound site; is naturally highly absorbent; is biocompatible and biodegradable, and is easy to use.

INDICATIONS

- For Over-the-Counter Use: Indicated for the management of minor burns, superficial cuts, lacerations, abrasions, and minor irritation of the skin.
- For Prescription Use: Under the supervision of a health care professional, it is indicated for partial- and full-thickness wounds, including:
  - pressure ulcers (Stages I–IV).
  - venous stasis ulcers.
  - diabetic ulcers.
  - abrasions.
  - lacerations.
  - donor sites.
  - skin tears.
  - first- and second-degree burns.
  - surgical wounds.
  - grafted wounds.

CONTRAINDICATIONS

- For individuals with a known sensitivity to silver.

APPLICATION

- Cleanse the wound with sterile water or normal saline. Leave the wound bed moist. Pat dry the periwound area.
- Apply gel directly to the wound site (approx. 1/4″ thickness).
- Cover the wound with an appropriate dressing such as a transparent film, foam, or composite dressing.
- Reapply as needed based on condition of wound, surrounding skin, and dressing, or as directed by a qualified health professional.

REMOVAL

- Dressing may be moistened with sterile water or normal saline to ease removal.

REFERENCE

1. http://dermarite.com/product/silvakollagen-gel/

SilvaSorb

Medline Industries, Inc.

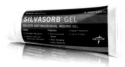

HOW SUPPLIED

Silver antimicrobial gel	0.25 oz 1.5 oz	A6248
Silver antimicrobial hydrogel sheet	3 oz 8 oz	A6243
Silver antimicrobial catheter site dressing	4.25″ × 4.25″ 1″ round	A6242

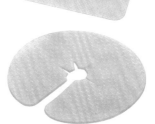

ANTIMICROBIALS

ACTION

SilvaSorb is a sterile, single-use wound dressing for use in moist wound management, combining patented MicroLattice technology with sustained-release silver. SilvaSorb's increased fluid management and antimicrobial performance make it ideal for chronic wounds. SilvaSorb is an effective barrier to bacterial penetration. The antimicrobial barrier function of the dressing may help reduce infection by inhibiting the growth of *Staphylococcus aureus,* methicillin-resistant *S. aureus, Pseudomonas aeruginosa, Escherichia coli, Candida albicans,* vancomycin-resistant *Enterococcus,* and other clinically significant microorganisms. SilvaSorb is biocompatible and will not stain or discolor tissue. It also does not require preconditioning or periodic irrigation.

SilvaSorb Amorphous Gel donates moisture to dry wound beds while providing ionic silver for antimicrobial protection. The thick, viscous formulation stays in contact with the wound bed to provide an optimally moist environment for up to 3 days.

The polyacrylate material in SilvaSorb Sheet helps maintain a moist wound environment, either by donating moisture to dry wounds, or absorbing at least five times its weight in exudating wounds. The dressing maintains its antimicrobial effectiveness for up to 7 days.

SilvaSorb Site offers ionic silver percutaneous site protection to help fight infection at pin, port, and catheter sites. The translucent, flexible material offers a snug fit around the indwelling device, reducing gaps that can otherwise grant bacteria access to the site, and is absorbent to help manage moisture. The dressing provides antimicrobial protection for up to 7 days.

INDICATIONS

To manage partial- and full-thickness wounds, such as pressure ulcers, diabetic foot ulcers, leg ulcers, skin tears, first- and second-degree burns, grafted wounds and donor sites, surgical wounds, and lacerations and abrasions.

CONTRAINDICATIONS

- Individuals with a known sensitivity to silver; Not for use over eschar. Eschar should be debrided before use.

APPLICATION

SilvaSorb amorphous gel

- Clean the wound using sterile saline or appropriate wound cleanser, such as Skintegrity Wound Cleanser.

- Dispense SilvaSorb to an appropriate clean applicator, such as a tongue blade or gauze, in sufficient quantities to liberally cover the wound.
- Cover the gel with an appropriate secondary dressing, such as a gauze pad, a film dressing, or nonwoven adhesive secondary dressing, such as Stratasorb.

SilvaSorb sheet

- Clean the wound using sterile saline or appropriate wound cleanser, such as Skintegrity Wound Cleanser.
- Remove the dressing from the package and blue liners.
- Place either side of the dressing in contact with the wound base, making sure that greater than 1/2″ (1.3 cm) is covering the periwound skin. If the sheet is too large for the wound, tear or cut the dressing to the appropriate size.
- Cover the dressing with an appropriate secondary cover like a transparent film, such as SureSite, or a composite island dressing, such as Stratasorb or Medline Bordered Gauze. Consider the amount of exudate, the condition of the periwound skin, and the desired wear time in the selection of a secondary dressing.
- The dressing may remain in place for up to 7 days, depending on the amount of exudate. Change the dressing if the wound exudate begins to pool within the wound or if significant strikethrough occurs.

SilvaSorb site

- Prepare the site per facility protocol.
- Wrap dressing around insertion site.
- Cover and secure with transparent film, such as SureView I.V.
- The dressing may remain in place for up to 7 days, depending on the amount of exudate.

REMOVAL

- Carefully remove the secondary dressing and SilvaSorb from the wound.
- SilvaSorb Sheet is normally nonadherent to the wound, but can be remoistened with saline or a wound cleanser to help ease removal if necessary.
- Gently clean the wound with sterile saline or an appropriate wound cleanser, such as Skintegrity Wound Cleanser.

REFERENCES

1. SilvaSorb Gel—http://www.medline.com/product/SilvaSorb-Antimicrobial-Wound-Gel/Gel/Z05-PF00181
2. SilvaSorb   Sheet—https://www.medline.com/product/SilvaSorb-Sheet-Dressings/Silver-Dressings/Z05-PF00207
3. SilvaSorb Site—http://www.medline.com/product/SilvaSorb-Site-Dressings/Z05-PF00208

New Product: Silver-Sept® Silver Antimicrobial Skin and Wound Gel

Anacapa Technologies, Inc.

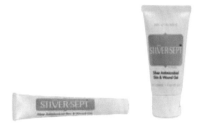

HOW SUPPLIED

Tube	3-oz	A6248
Tube	1.5-oz	A6248

ANTIMICROBIALS

PRODUCT DESCRIPTION

Silver-Sept Silver Antimicrobial Skin and Wound Gel containing 200 ug/gram total silver, is a clear, amorphous hydrogel wound dressing that helps to maintain a moist wound environment that is conducive to healing. Silver-Sept will not stain or discolor tissue. Silver-Sept gel functions as a long-lasting antimicrobial barrier inhibiting the growth of common bacteria such as *Staphylococcus aureus, Pseudomonas aeruginosa, Escherichia coli, Proteus mirabilis, Serratia marcescens*, including the antibiotic-resistant strains methicillin-resistant *S. aureus* (MRSA) and vancomycin-resistant *Enterococci* (VRE), as well as fungi such as, *Candida albicans* and *Aspergillus niger*.

INDICATIONS

Silver-Sept Gel is intended for OTC use for abrasions and lacerations and under the supervision of a health care professional in the management of stage I to IV pressure ulcers, partial- and full-thickness wounds, first- and second-degree burns, diabetic foot and leg ulcers, grafted and donor sites.

CONTRAINDICATIONS

- None.

APPLICATION

- Cleanse and debride the wound as necessary.
- Apply a generous amount of Silver-Sept Gel directly onto the wound bed (1/8″ to 3/16″ thick).
- Cover with a sterile gauze or other appropriate secondary dressing and secure in place.
- Maintain a moist environment between dressing changes.
  Note: Silver-Sept Silver Antimicrobial Skin and Wound Gel may remain in the wound bed for up to 3 days. More frequent dressing changes may be required depending upon the amount of wound exudate present and the condition of the secondary dressing.

REMOVAL

- Remove the secondary dressing.
- Cleanse with an appropriate skin or wound cleanser as necessary during dressing change.

OTHER CLINICAL INFORMATION

- **Bactericidal**: Including the antibiotic-resistant strains such as MRSA and VRE.
- **Fungicidal**: Effective against the well-known pathogenic fungi *C. albicans* and *A. niger*.

Biocompatibility and safety

Silver-Sept Gel has been subjected to rigorous biocompatibility and safety testing at independent laboratories and shown to be nonirritating, nonsensitizing, and noncytotoxic and meets the highest standards for safe use. Testing included:

- Cytotoxicity studies.
- ISO skin irritation studies.
- ISO sensitization studies.
- USP- and ISO-modified systemic toxicity studies.

Shelf-life

- 2 years when stored at room temperature: 15° to 30°C (59° to 86°F).

Other features and benefits

- Proudly manufactured in the United States in an FDA-registered and ISO-certified facility.
- Nonflammable and can be used in hyperbaric chambers.
- Long-lasting antimicrobial properties.
- Easy to apply and remove from wounds.
- No untoward or adverse reaction reported in over 10 years of use.

ANTIMICROBIALS

SILVERCEL™ NON-ADHERENT
Antimicrobial Alginate Dressing with EASYLIFT™ Precision Film Technology

Systagenix, An ACELITY™ Company

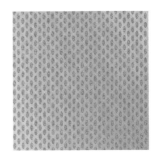

HOW SUPPLIED

SILVERCEL™ NON-ADHERENT Antimicrobial Alginate Dressing with EASYLIFT™ Precision Film Technology	2″ × 2″	A6196
SILVERCEL™ NON-ADHERENT Antimicrobial Alginate Dressing with EASYLIFT™ Precision Film Technology	4″ × 4″	A6197
SILVERCEL™ NON-ADHERENT Antimicrobial Alginate Dressing with EASYLIFT™ Precision Film Technology	4″ × 8″	A6197
SILVERCEL™ NON-ADHERENT Antimicrobial Alginate Dressing with EASYLIFT™ Precision Film Technology	1″ × 12″	A6199

ANTIMICROBIALS

ACTION

SILVERCEL™ NON-ADHERENT Antimicrobial Alginate Dressing with EASYLIFT™ Precision Film Technology is a sterile nonwoven pad composed of a high 6 (guluronic acid) alginate, carboxymethylcellulose (CMC), and silver coated nylon fibers, laminated to a perforated, non-adherent ethylene methyl acrylate (EMA) wound contact layer. The dressing absorbs exudate and allows intact removal, while maintaining a moist wound environment. A moist wound environment is optimal for wound healing. The silver ions within the dressing protect the dressing from bacterial contamination. Odor reduction results from the antibacterial effect.

INDICATIONS

SILVERCEL™ NON-ADHERENT Dressing is an effective barrier to bacterial penetration. The barrier functions of the dressing may help reduce infection in moderate to heavily exuding partial- and full-thickness wounds including: pressure ulcers, venous ulcers, diabetic ulcers, donor sites, traumatic wounds, surgical wounds. SILVERCEL™ NON-ADHERENT Dressing is indicated for external use only.

CONTRAINDICATIONS

- SILVERCEL™ NON-ADHERENT Dressing is not indicated for use on the following: third-degree burns, patients with a known sensitivity to alginates, ethylene methyl acrylate (EMA) or silver, surgical implantation, or to control heavy bleeding.

APPLICATION

- Cut or fold SILVERCEL™ NON-ADHERENT Dressing to fit the wound. (SILVERCEL™ NON-ADHERENT Dressing Rope should not be cut lengthwise).
- Cover the dressing with a nonocclusive secondary dressing, such as one of the Tielle Hydropolymer Dressings.
- Reapply SILVERCEL™ NON-ADHERENT Dressing when the secondary dressing has reached its absorbent capacity or whenever good wound care practice dictates that the dressing should be changed.

REMOVAL

- To remove the dressing, first gently remove the secondary dressing.
- Consistent with good wound care practice, always remove the dressing from the wound with gloved fingers or forceps.
- Grip both outer layers of SILVERCEL™ NON-ADHERENT Dressing and gently remove from the wound bed.
- If the wound appears dry, saturate the dressing with normal saline solution prior to removal.
- Irrigate the wound site with a suitable wound cleanser prior to application of a new dressing.
- Dressing change frequency will depend on wound condition and the level of exudate.

REFERENCE

1. Gray D. Silvercel Non-Adherent dressing: taking the pain out of antimicrobial use. *Wounds UK.* 2009;5(4):118–120.

ANTIMICROBIALS

SilverDerm 7

DermaRite Industries, LLC

HOW SUPPLIED

Silver Contact Layer Wound Dressing	4″ × 4″

ACTION

SilverDerm 7® Antimicrobial Wound Contact Silver Dressings are sterile, porous, nonadherent, knitted nylon dressings plated with 99% elemental silver and 1% silver oxide to deliver microbial silver ions in the dressing when activated by moisture. The silver ions in the dressing kill wound bacteria held in the dressing and provides an antimicrobial barrier from bacterial penetration of the dressing which may help reduce infection. SilverDerm 7 dressings have been tested in vitro and found effective against microorganisms such as *Staphylococcus aureus* (MRSA), *Vancomycin-resistant Enterococcus* (VRE), *Staphylococcus epidermidis, Escherichia Coli (E. coli), Shigella sonnei, Pseudomonas aeruginosa, Pseudomonas cepacia, Pseudomonas maltophilia, Acinetobacter calcoaceticus, Enterobacter cloacae, Salmonella typhimurium, Salmonella typhi,* Enterococcus sp., *Serratia marcescens, Listeria monocytogenes,* Staphylococcus, Streptococcus, Group B Streptococcus, *Candida albicans,* and *Aspergillus niger.*

SilverDerm 7 dressings have been subjected to independent in vitro and in vivo biocompatibility tests, including cytotoxicity, sensitization, and intracutaneous reactivity. All tests were performed in accordance with International Standard Organization (ISO) 10993 Standard Series for Biological Evaluation of Medical Devices.

INDICATIONS

- OTC USE.

Local management of superficial wounds, minor burns, abrasions, and lacerations.

- PRESCRIPTION INDICATIONS.
  - SilverDerm 7 is indicated for use up to 7 days for partial- and full-thickness wounds including traumatic wounds, surgical wounds (donor and graft sites, incisions), first- and second-degree burns, as well as dermal ulcers (stage I–IV pressure sores, venous stasis ulcers, arterial ulcers, diabetic ulcers), vascular access or peripheral IV sites, orthopedic external pin sites, and wound drain sites.
  - SilverDerm 7 dressings are indicated for the management of infected wounds, as the silver in the dressing provides an antimicrobial barrier that may be helpful in managing these wounds. In addition, the moist wound healing environment and control of wound bacteria within the dressing may help reduce the risk of wound infection and support the body's healing process.
  - SilverDerm 7 Dressings may be used for the management of painful wounds. SilverDerm 7 is a nonadherent wound contact layer that reduces pain during dressing changes and evaporation of moisture in the dressing may sooth the wound.

CONTRAINDICATIONS

- Avoid using SilverDerm 7 Antimicrobial Wound Contact Silver Dressing on patients with known sensitivity to silver or nylon.

ANTIMICROBIALS

APPLICATION

- Cleanse wound with sterile water, distilled water, or normal saline, removing necrotic debris or eschar as needed per local protocol.
- Activate SilverDerm 7 by thoroughly moistening with sterile water, distilled water, or normal saline.
- Position the SilverDerm 7 dressing directly over wound, with either silver side in contact with the skin; overlap the wound margins by 1 to 2 cm. Secure the dressing in place using a secondary dressing per local protocol:
  - For exudating wounds, use an absorbent secondary dressing of choice.
  - For dry wounds, use a moisture-donating secondary dressing such as hydrocolloid or premoistened foam or gauze.
- Periodically check the edges of the SilverDerm 7 dressing to ensure that it is maintained in a moist condition.

REMOVAL

- SilverDerm 7, first remove the outer secondary dressing per local protocol, and then gently depress surrounding skin while lifting the dressing edges. If sticking of the dressing to the wound occurs, moisten the dressing as needed with sterile water, distilled water or normal saline until it can be easily removed by gently lifting the corners.

REFERENCE

1. http://dermarite.com/product/silverderm-7/

UrgoCell Ag with TLC™ Technology*

Urgo Medical

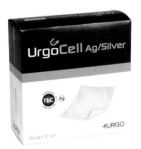

HOW SUPPLIED

Dressing	4″ × 4″	A6209
Dressing	6″ × 8″	A6210

ACTION

The proprietary TLC Technology is comprised of a nonocclusive polyester mesh impregnated with a polymer matrix containing hydrocolloid particles and petrolatum-based formulation. Upon contact with wound exudates, the hydrocolloid particles combine with the matrix to form a lipido-colloidal gel, providing a moist environment that promotes healing. Being nonadhesive, removal of Restore silver foam is virtually pain-free and helps minimize damage to newly formed surrounding skin. It is ideal for use on wound with fragile surrounding skin. Restore silver foam was shown to be particularly effective against bacteria most frequently associated with wound infections. Under a log reduction in vitro test, it has demonstrated an antibacterial activity (at least a 4 log reduction) against the following bacteria: *Staphylococcus aureus, Streptococcus pyogenes, Pseudomonas aeruginosa* (pyocyanic bacillus), and MRSA (strain ATCC 4300). The dressing sustains antibacterial activity for up to 7 days in *in vitro* studies.

The superabsorbent foam pad ensures drainage of exudates and helps protect the skin around the lesion from any maceration. The backing is soft, pliable, and very comfortable; it allows the dressing to be easily shaped to the anatomical contours of the wound. Restore silver foam with TLC Technology nonborder is suitable for use under compression bandaging, due to the ability of the dressing to retain exudates.

INDICATIONS

May help reduce infection in moderately to high exuding partial- and full-thickness wounds, including partial-thickness burns, pressure ulcers, venous stasis ulcers, diabetic ulcers, graft and donor sites.

CONTRAINDICATIONS

- Known sensitization to silver and/or other dressings components.

APPLICATION

- Cleanse the wound using sterile saline solution or an appropriate wound cleanser.
- Choose a dressing size that ensures the dressing will cover the entire wound.
- Remove the protective tabs from the dressing.
- Apply the dressing directly to wound.
- Hold in place using a fixing bandage. Use a compression bandage when prescribed.
- Duration of treatment is determined by the physician and depends on wound type and healing conditions.
- Concomitant use of other topical antimicrobial agent is not recommended.
- Use in pregnant or breastfeeding women and newborns has not been studied.
- Do not reuse the dressing.
- Store the dressing flat and at room temperature.

REMOVAL

- UrgoCell Ag foam dressing should be changed every 1 to 3 days, depending on the wound and the healing progression.

*See package insert for complete instructions for use.

ANTIMICROBIALS

UrgoTul™ Ag Contact Layer*

Urgo Medical

HOW SUPPLIED

Dressing	4″ × 5″	A6207
Dressing	6″ × 8″	A6207

ACTION

UrgoTul Ag contact layer with TLC Technology is comprised of a nonadhesive, nonocclusive, antimicrobial wound contact dressing composed of a polyester mesh impregnated with a polymer matrix containing hydrocolloid particles (carboxymethylcellulose), cohesion polymers, petrolatum and silver (2.25 mg/sq inch). Being nonadhesive, removal of Restore contact layer, silver is virtually pain-free and helps minimize damage to newly formed surrounding skin. It is ideal for use on wounds with fragile surrounding skin. Restore contact layer, silver was shown to be effective against bacteria most frequently associated with wound infections, *Staphylococcus aureus, Streptococcus pyogenes, Pseudomonas aeruginosa* (pyocyanic bacillus), and MRSA (strain ATCC 43300). The dressing sustains antibacterial activity for up to 7 days in *in vitro* studies.

INDICATIONS

The barrier functions of UrgoTul contact layer, silver may help reduce infection in low to moderate exuding partial- and full-thickness wounds, including second-degree burns, pressure ulcers, venous stasis ulcers, diabetic ulcers, and graft and donor sites.

CONTRAINDICATIONS

- Not for use on individuals who are sensitive to silver or who have had an allergic reaction to the dressing or one of its components.

APPLICATION

- Clean the wound using sterile saline solution.
- Choose a dressing size which ensures that the dressing will cover the entire wound.
- Remove the protective tabs from the dressing. (Note: UrgoTul Ag dressing tends to stick to latex gloves. Moisten latex gloves with normal sterile saline prior to use).
- Apply the dressing directly to wound.
- Cover with appropriate secondary dressing and hold in place using a fixating bandage.
- Remove gloves and wash hands after completing procedure.

REMOVAL

- UrgoTul Ag contact layer should be changed every 1 to 3 days. Dressing change frequency will depend on patient condition and the healing progression.
- Duration of treatment is determined by the physician and depends on wound type and healing conditions.

*See package insert for complete instructions for use.

3M™ Tegaderm™ Ag Mesh Dressing with Silver

3M™ Health Care

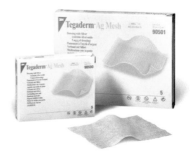

HOW SUPPLIED

Dressing	2" × 2"	A6402
Dressing	4" × 5"	A6403
Dressing	4" × 8"	A6403
Dressing	8" × 8"	A6404

ACTION

3M™ Tegaderm™ Ag Mesh Dressing with Silver is a non-woven gauze dressing that contains silver sulfate, 8 mg/g of dressing. Silver sulfate released as silver ions within the dressing creates an effective barrier for up to 7 days. The soft, absorbent dressing is supplied sterile and may be custom cut. The porous, non-occlusive dressing conforms to the wound base and wicks drainage into the dressing where the silver ions are available to reduce the number of bacteria and yeast that are absorbed into the dressing.

INDICATIONS

This dressing may be used as a primary wound dressing over abrasions; pressure injuries; arterial, neuropathic (diabetic), and venous leg ulcers; surgical and traumatic wounds; superficial and partial thickness burns and donor sites.

CONTRAINDICATIONS

- Not for use on individuals who have a known hypersensitivity to silver or cotton.
- For external use only.
- Not intended for use as a surgical sponge.
- Not for use on full-thickness burns.

APPLICATION

- Clean the wound and surrounding skin. If the patient's skin is fragile or wound drainage may contact the periwound skin, apply barrier film around the wound.
- Remove the dressing from the package. For dry to minimally draining wounds, the dressing should be moistened with a sterile normal saline or sterile water or liquid hydrogel, to provide a moist wound environment. For moderate to highly draining wounds, premoistening may not be required.
- If necessary, trim or fold the dressing to fit the wound site.
- Apply the dressing to the wound bed without overlap onto the surrounding skin.
- Secure with an appropriate secondary cover dressing to help manage the wound drainage. A moisture retentive barrier may be used as a cover dressing to help maintain a moist wound environment.

REMOVAL

- Change the dressing as needed. Frequency of changing will depend on factors such as the type of wound and volume of drainage. The dressing remains effective for up to 7 days.
- At the time of dressing change, if the dressing is adhered to the wound surface, saturate with sterile normal saline or sterile water, allow the dressing to soften, and gently remove.
- Avoid forceful removal of the dressing to minimize disruption of the wound.
- Do not reuse the dressing.
- Remove the dressing prior to magnetic resonance imaging (MRI) procedures.

REFERENCE

1. https://www.3m.com/3M/en_US/company-us/all-3m-products/~/3M-Tegaderm-Ag-Mesh-Dressing-with-Silver?N=5002385±3293321916&rt=rud

ANTIMICROBIALS

3M™ Tegaderm™ Alginate Ag Silver Dressing

3M™ Health Care

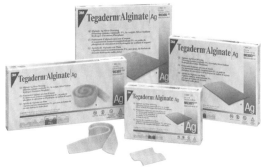

HOW SUPPLIED

Pad	2″ × 2″	A6196
Pad	4″ × 5″	A6197
Pad	6″ × 6″	A6197
Rope	1″ × 12″	A6199

ACTION

3M™ Tegaderm™ Alginate Ag Silver Dressing is a highly absorbent, sterile, nonwoven antimicrobial dressing composed of high G (guluronic acid), calcium alginate, carboxymethylcellulose (CMC), and an ionic silver complex (Silver Sodium Hydrogen Zirconium Phosphate), which releases silver ions in the presence of wound exudate. As exudate is absorbed, the dressing forms a gel, which aids in autolytic debridement while maintaining a moist environment for optimal wound healing and allows intact removal. The silver ions protect the dressing from a broad spectrum of microorganisms such as *Staphylococcus aureus* (including MRSA), *S. epidermidis* (including MRSE), *Streptococcus pyogenes*, and *Enterococcus faecalis* (VRE), *Pseudomonas aeruginosa, Escherichia coli*, and fungi such as *Candida albicans*. The dressing remains effective for up to 14 days, based on in vitro testing.

INDICATIONS

For use as a primary wound dressing in the management of moderate to heavily exuding, partial- to full-thickness wounds such as postoperative wounds, trauma wounds (dermal lesions, trauma wounds, or incisions), leg ulcers, pressure injuries, diabetic ulcers, graft and donor sites, and superficial, partial-thickness burns; for external use only; can be used under compression bandages; may assist in supporting the control of minor bleeding in superficial wounds.

CONTRAINDICATIONS

- Not for use on individuals with a known sensitivity to alginates or silver.
- Not for use as a surgical sponge or for surgical implantation to control heavy bleeding.

APPLICATION

- Clean the wound and surrounding area. If the patient's skin is fragile or wound drainage may contact the periwound skin, apply a barrier film around the wound.
- Remove the dressing from the package.
- For superficial wounds, the dressing may be cut or folded to fit the wound site. For use in wounds with depth, loosely fill the wound with the dressing making sure that the dressing does not overlap onto the wound margin or surrounding skin.
- Apply to the wound bed.
- Secure with an appropriate secondary dressing to help manage the wound drainage.
- The dressing performance may be impaired by used of petroleum-based ointments.

ANTIMICROBIALS

REMOVAL

- Dressing change frequency will depend on wound condition and level of exudate. Reapply 3M™ Tegaderm™ Alginate Ag Silver Dressing when the cover dressing has reached its absorbent capacity or per facility protocol. Initially it may be necessary to change the dressing every 24 hours. The dressing remains effective for up to 14 days.
- Gently remove the cover dressing.
- If the 3M™ Tegaderm™ Alginate Ag Silver Dressing appears dry, saturate the dressing with sterile saline solution prior to removal.
- Gently remove the 3M™ Tegaderm™ Alginate Ag Silver Dressing from the wound bed and discard.
- Do not reuse dressing.
- The dressing should be removed prior to magnetic resonance imaging (MRI) procedures.

REFERENCE

1. https://www.3m.com/3M/en_US/company-us/all-3m-products/~/3M-Tegaderm-Alginate-Ag-Silver-Dressing?N=5002385±3293321936&rt=rud

Cellular and Tissue-Based Products (CTPs)

It's the clinician's responsibility to understand the use of these products and verify coding of each product with the product's manufacturer or processor. Each product under this category description may be assigned a different code based on its physical size and characteristics; or the manufacturer hasn't yet received or applied for a code. Please refer to individual product listings for further information about each product and its reimbursement.[1]

There are currently a wide variety of products available for soft tissue coverage to affect closure. These products may be derived from allogeneic, xenogeneic, synthetic sources, or a combination of any or all of these types of materials.

Autologous skin grafts, also referred to as autografts, are permanent covers that use skin from different parts of the individual's body. These grafts consist of the epidermis and a dermal component of variable thickness. A split-thickness skin graft (STSG) includes the entire epidermis and a portion of the dermis. A full-thickness skin graft (FTSG) includes all layers of the skin. Although autografts are the optimal choice for full-thickness wound coverage, areas for skin harvesting may be limited, particularly in cases of large burns or venous stasis ulceration. Harvesting procedures are painful, disfiguring, and require additional wound care.

Allografts which use skin from another human (e.g., cadaver, placental-based products) and Xenografts which use skin from another species (e.g., porcine or bovine) may also be employed as temporary skin replacements, but they must later be replaced by an autograft or the ingrowth of the patient's own skin.

Bioengineered Skin/Cultured Epidermal Autografts (CEA) are autografts derived from the patient's own skin cells grown or cultured from very small amounts of skin or hair follicle. Production time is prolonged. One such product is grown on a layer of irradiated mouse cells, bestowing some elements of a xenograft. Wide spread usage has not been available due to limited availability or access to the technology.

Bioengineered Skin Substitutes or Cellular and Tissue-Based Products (CTPs), referred to as Skin Substitutes by CMS, The Current Procedural Terminology (CPT) and The Healthcare Common Procedure Coding Manuals, have been developed to further define autografts, allografts, and xenografts. These constitute biologic covers for refractory wounds with full-thickness skin loss. The production of these biologic skin substitutes or CTPs varies by company and product, but generally involves the preservation or creation of immunologically inert biologic products containing cells (including stem cells), proteins, hormones, or enzymes seeded into a matrix or delivered as an intact matrix which may provide extracellular matrix proteins (fibrous and nonfibrous) such as growth factors and collagen and are proposed to stimulate or facilitate healing by supplementing agents that are part of the normal acute wound healing process or promote epithelialization. A variety of biosynthetic and tissue-engineered skin substitution products marketed as Human Skin Equivalents (HSE) or Cellular or Tissue-based Products (CTP) are manufactured under an array of trade names and marketed for a variety of indications or uses. All are procured, produced, manufactured, processed, and promoted in sufficiently different manners to preclude direct product comparison for equivalency or superiority in randomized controlled trials.

Bioengineered skin substitutes or CTPs are classified into the following types:

- Human-Derived Allografts are processed from human skin components and human tissue which may have had intact cells removed or treated. They are available in different forms promoted to allow scaffolding, soft tissue filling, growth factors, and other bioavailable hormonal or enzymatic activity.

- Allogeneic Matrices are usually derived from human neonatal fibroblasts of the foreskin that may contain metabolically active or regenerative components primarily used for soft tissue support, though some have been approved for the treatment of full-thickness skin and soft tissue loss. Most are biodegradable and disappear after 3 to 4 weeks implantation.
- Composite Matrices are derived from human keratinocytes and fibroblasts supported by a scaffold of synthetic mesh or xenogeneic collagen. These are also referred to as human skin equivalent but are unable to be used as autografts due to immunologic rejection or degradation of the living components by the host. Active cellular components continue to generate bioactive compounds and protein(s) that may accelerate wound healing and epithelial regrowth.
- Acellular Matrices are derived from other than human skin and include the majority of bioengineered skin substitutes. All are composed of allogeneic- or xenogeneic-derived collagen, membrane, or cellular remnants proposed to simulate or exaggerate the characteristics of human skin. All propose to promote healing by the creation of localized intensification of an array of hormonal and enzymatic activity to accelerate closure by migration of native dermal and epithelial components, rather than function as distinctly incorporated tissue closing the skin defect.

REFERENCE

1. Local Coverage Determination (LCD): Application of Bioengineered Skin Substitutes to Lower Extremity Chronic Non-Healing Wounds. Available at https://www.cms.gov/medicare-coverage-database/details/lcd details.aspx?LCDId=35041&ver=69&name=331*1&UpdatePeriod=780&bc=AQAAEAAAAAAA& Accessed June 4, 2018.

ADDITIONAL REFERENCES

- Piaggesi A, Läuchli S, Bassetto F, et al. EWMA document: Advanced therapies in wound management: cell and tissue based therapies, physical and bio-physical therapies smart and IT based technologies. J Wound Care 2018; 27(6), Suppl 6.
- What's new in wound treatment: a critical appraisal. Available at https://onlinelibrary.wiley.com/doi/pdf/10.1002/dmrr.2747
- An update and review of cell-based wound dressings and their integration into clinical practice. Available at http://atm.amegroups.com/article/view/12913/html
- Wound Reference CTP guide. Available at https://woundreference.com/files/1588.pdf

AlloSkin™

AlloSource

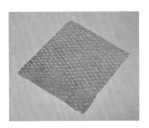

HOW SUPPLIED

Skin substitute	25 cm², 80 cm², 120 cm²	Q4115
Trunk, arms, legs (includes ankle)		15271–15274
	First 25 cm²	15271
	Each additional 25 cm² up to maximum 100 cm² area or 1% body area of infants/children	15272
	First 100 cm² or 1% of body area of infants/children	15273
	Each additional 100 cm² or 1% of body area	15724
Face, scalp, eyelids, mouth, neck, ears, orbits, genitalia, hands, feet, and/or multiple digits		15275–15278
	First 25 cm²	15275
	Each additional 25 cm² up to maximum 100 cm² area or 1% body area of infants/children	15276
	First 100 cm² or 1% of body area of infants/children	15277
	Each additional 100 cm² or 1% of body area	15278

ACTION

Scientific literature consistently lists these potential benefits of skin allograft use on chronic wounds: Minimizes infection and keeps the wound bed mechanically clean; acts as a bacterial barrier; decreases loss of protein, water, and electrolyte; reduces pain; decreases incidence of contractures; may provide a "dose pack" of growth factors to wound bed; prevents desiccation of bone and tendon; stimulates re-epithelialization and wound neovascularization.

(Snyder RJ. Treatment of nonhealing ulcers with allografts. *Clin Dermatol.* 2005;23:388–395; Spence RJ, Wong L. The enhancement of wound healing with human skin allograft. *Surg Clin North Am.* 1997;77:3,731–745.)

INDICATIONS

As a homologous-use allograft (FDA 21 CFR 1271), AlloSkin™ may be used to repair any integumental defect, such as those caused by ulcers and burns, and is appropriate for use over exposed substructures such as bone, tendon, ligament, and muscle.

CONTRAINDICATIONS

- The presence of gross infection at the transplantation site is a contraindication for use of skin allografts.

APPLICATION

- Ensure wound is adequately debrided and free of infection.
- Place AlloSkin or inner pouch in a sterile basin on a sterile field. Immerse the skin or inner pouch completely in sterile isotonic solution for a minimum of 1 minute and a maximum of 5 minutes until thawed. Avoid "soaking" tissue, as this may cause the dermal and epidermal layers to separate.
- Cryopreserved skin is preserved with 15% Glycerin in LR+ Gentamicin/RPMI 1640. Graft should be rinsed with sterile isotonic solution prior to transplant.
- Apply AlloSkin to wound dermal (shiny) side down. Stretch so graft has contact with all wound contours and trim excess graft to fit wound.
- Anchor graft as appropriate (can staple, suture, steristrip, or tack with silicone dressing) and dress graft as appropriate for amount of exudate and location of wound. Almost any dressing is appropriate for use over AlloSkin graft, including silver dressings and foams. May use in conjunction with NPWT and HBO therapy.

REMOVAL

- Inspect wound weekly, sooner if deemed necessary, to determine if AlloSkin is still in place or beginning to slough. Tissue sloughs in 7 to 14 days and wound bed granulation proceeds.
- Depending upon wound assessment, physician may leave graft in place, replace graft with new application of AlloSkin or apply a skin substitute if adequate granulation is present.

REFERENCE

1. Desman E, Barrow W, Anderson LH. Human Skin allografts for patients with diabetic foot ulcers, venous leg ulcers, or surgical/traumatic wounds: A retrospective, descriptive study. *Ostomy Wound Manage.* 2015;61(7):16–22.

AlloSkin™ AC (acellular dermal matrix)

AlloSource

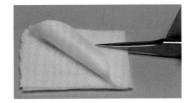

HOW SUPPLIED

Skin substitute	16 cm², 32 cm²	Q4141
Trunk, arms, legs (includes ankle)		15271–15274
	First 25 cm²	15271
	Each additional 25 cm² up to maximum 100 cm² area or 1% body area of infants/children	15272
	First 100 cm² or 1% of body area of infants/children	15273
	Each additional 100 cm² or 1% of body area	15724
Face, scalp, eyelids, mouth, neck, ears, orbits, genitalia, hands, feet, and/or multiple digits		15275–15278
	First 25 cm²	15275
	Each additional 25 cm² up to maximum 100 cm² area or 1% body area of infants/children	15276
	First 100 cm² or 1% of body area of infants/children	15277
	Each additional 100 cm² or 1% of body area	15278

ACTION

Through a proprietary process, viable cells and cellular elements that are capable of triggering an immunogenic response are removed from donated human dermal tissue, leaving a collagen elastin matrix behind. Upon transplantation (i.e., placement onto a prepared wound bed), the body's own cells infiltrate and repopulate this three-dimensional scaffold to begin the revascularization and remodeling processes.

AlloSkin™ AC is a meshed dermis-only human skin allograft that has been decellularized while preserving biologic components, including growth factors, and structure of the dermal matrix to provide a natural healing environment for wounds. AlloSkin AC is a sterile CTP (Cellular and/or Tissue Product), designed for a single application and ideal for acute and chronic wound therapy in the inpatient or outpatient setting.

(Eppley BL. Experimental assessment of the revascularization of acellular human dermis for soft-tissue augmentation. *Plast Reconstr Surg.* 2001; 107: 757–762.)

CELLULAR AND TISSUE-BASED PRODUCTS

INDICATIONS

As a homologous-use allograft (FDA 21 CFR 1271), AlloSkin AC may be used to repair any integumental defect, such as those caused by ulcers and burns, and is appropriate for use over exposed substructures, such as bone, tendon, ligament, and muscle. Sterile tissue should be stored at room temperature.

CONTRAINDICATIONS

- Patients exhibiting autoimmune connective tissue disease and the presence of gross infection at the transplantation site are contraindications for the use of AlloSkin AC.

APPLICATION

- Ensure wound is adequately debrided and free of infection.
- Adequately prepare the surgical site.
- Using atraumatic forceps remove AlloSkin AC from the inner pouch, keeping it in the moist gauze until ready for application.
- Rinse the graft with saline or sterile isotonic solution prior to applying to the wound.
- Remove and discard the larger gauze and apply graft to surgical site so the graft is in contact with all the contours of the surgical site.
- Remove the smaller gauze from the graft and discard, leaving the graft on the patient and trim to fit.
- Affix per clinician preference. AlloSkin AC can be secured using staples, sutures, or tacking.
- Apply any combination of nonadherent sterile dressing over AlloSkin AC.
  - May use in conjunction with VAC and HBO therapy.

REMOVAL

- Inspect weekly or sooner if deemed necessary.
- Depending upon periodic wound assessment, clinician may leave graft in place for incorporation and/or apply an additional application of AlloSkin AC where needed.

AlloSkin™ RT (room temperature)

AlloSource

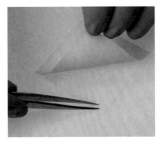

HOW SUPPLIED

Skin substitute	4 cm², 16 cm², 64 cm²	Q4123
Trunk, arms, legs (includes ankle)		15271–15274
	First 25 cm²	15271
	Each additional 25 cm² up to maximum 100 cm² area or 1% body area of infants/children	15272
	First 100 cm² or 1% of body area of infants/children	15273
	Each additional 100 cm² or 1% of body area	15724
Face, scalp, eyelids, mouth, neck, ears, orbits, genitalia, hands, feet, and/or multiple digits		15275–15278
	First 25 cm²	15275
	Each additional 25 cm² up to maximum 100 cm² area or 1% body area of infants/children	15276
	First 100 cm² or 1% of body area of infants/children	15277
	Each additional 100 cm² or 1% of body area	15278

ACTION

Scientific literature consistently lists these potential benefits of skin allograft use on chronic wounds: Minimizes infection and keeps the wound bed mechanically clean; acts as a bacterial barrier; decreases loss of protein, water, and electrolyte; reduces pain; decreases incidence of contractures; may provide a "dose pack" of growth factors to wound bed; prevents desiccation of bone and tendon; stimulates re-epithelialization and wound neovascularization.

(Snyder R J. Treatment of nonhealing ulcers with allografts. *Clin Dermatol.* 2005;23:388–395; Spence R J, Wong L. The enhancement of wound healing with human skin allograft. *Surg Clin North Am.* 1997;77:3,731—745.)

AlloSkin™ RT meshed human dermal graft is a sterile skin graft for acute and chronic wound therapy. Skin allografts may mechanically protect the wound and provide biologic factors native to human skin, which may help stimulate the wound healing process.

Our process uses e-beam irradiation to yield a pliable graft with broad clinical applications and room temperature storage, eliminating the need for costly cryo freezers. Extensive serological and microbiological testing increases safety of skin allografts.

INDICATIONS

As a homologous-use allograft (FDA 21 CFR 1271), AlloSkin may be used to repair any integumental defect, such as those caused by ulcers and burns, and is appropriate for use over exposed substructures, such as bone, tendon, ligament, and muscle. Sterile tissue should be stored at room temperature.

CONTRAINDICATIONS

- The presence of gross infection at the transplantation site is a contraindication for use of skin allografts.

APPLICATION

- Ensure wound is adequately debrided and free of infection.
- Remove AlloSkin RT from inner pouch, keeping it in moist gauze until ready for application. Rinse tissue with sterile saline or sterile isotonic solution prior to applying to wound. The graft is protected between two pieces of sterile gauze backing material. Remove the larger piece and apply graft to patient so graft has contact with all contours of the wound; remaining backing material should be facing away from patient. Remove remaining backing material from graft and discard, leaving graft on patient.
- Affix per clinician preference: staple, suture, glue, or tack.
- Apply any combination of nonadherent sterile dressing over AlloSkin RT. May use in conjunction with NPWT and HBO therapy.

REMOVAL

- Inspect wound weekly, sooner if deemed necessary, to determine if AlloSkin RT is still in place or beginning to slough. Tissue sloughs in 7 to 14 days as wound bed granulation proceeds. Depending upon wound assessment, clinician may leave graft in place. Replace graft with new application of AlloSkin RT or apply a skin substitute if adequate granulation is present.

AmnioFill® Placental Tissue Allograft

MiMedx Group, Inc.

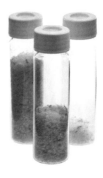

HOW SUPPLIED

AmnioFill	100 mg	J3590	15271–15278 possible for wound
AmnioFill	250 mg	J3590	15271–15278 possible for wound
AmnioFill	500 mg	J3590	15271–15278 possible for wound
AmnioFill	1,000 mg	J3590	15271–15278 possible for wound
AmnioFill	2,000 mg	J3590	15271–15278 possible for wound

ACTION

AmnioFill® is a placental connective tissue matrix allograft that may be used to replace or supplement damaged or inadequate integumental tissue and enhance healing. AmnioFill is minimally manipulated and contains non-viable cells.

USES

AmnioFill® is intended for homologous use as a placental connective tissue matrix to replace or supplement damaged or inadequate integumental tissue and modulate inflammation, enhance healing and reduce scar tissue formation.

CONTRAINDICATIONS

- AmnioFill® should not be used on areas with active or latent infection; on a patient with a disorder that would create an unacceptable risk of postoperative complications. This product is not intended for injection applications.

APPLICATION

Preparation, reconstitution and use

- Prior to implantation, carefully follow AmnioFill® allograft preparation steps below using aseptic technique:

Removing AmnioFill® from packaging

- The outer peel pouch is not sterile. The inner vial which contains the AmnioFill® allograft is sterile (unless the pouches are damaged or compromised). Using aseptic technique, slowly peel a corner of the peel pouch and remove the vial.

AmnioFill® preparation and application

- AmnioFill® can be applied by dispersing the product from the vial uniformly onto the treatment area. Take care to carefully apply the product evenly over the site. AmnioFill® can be hydrated while on the wound site with sterile saline solution. Simply apply several drops of sterile solution to the product.

Primary dressing

- AmnioFill® should be covered with a nonadherent contact layer when used to treat topical wounds. AmnioFill® should not be disturbed, if possible, for several days or before the next application, if needed. If an infection occurs at the graft site, treat infection per institution's protocol.

Secondary dressing

- AmnioFill® requires a moist wound environment. Use appropriate moisture management dressings for the wound type and treatment ideology.

Support therapies

- AmnioFill® allografts are compatible with offloading/compression/negative pressure therapies. AmnioFill® can be used in conjunction with hyperbaric oxygen therapy.
- It is recommended that AmnioFill® is applied weekly until wound epithelialization is achieved. However, clinician discretion should be used based on the patient and wound condition/progress. It is clinically acceptable to apply AmnioFill® on a biweekly basis if desired.

CELLULAR AND TISSUE-BASED PRODUCTS

DermaPure® Decellularized Dermal Allograft

TRX BioSurgery

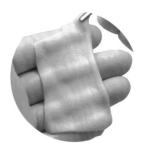

HOW SUPPLIED

DermaPure® Decellularized Dermal Allograft	1 cm × 2 cm	Q4152
DermaPure® Decellularized Dermal Allograft	2 cm × 2 cm	Q4152
DermaPure® Decellularized Dermal Allograft	2 cm × 3 cm	Q4152
DermaPure® Decellularized Dermal Allograft	3 cm × 4 cm	Q4152
DermaPure® Decellularized Dermal Allograft	4 cm × 6 cm	Q4152
DermaPure® Decellularized Dermal Allograft	7 cm × 10 cm	Q4152

ACTION

DermaPure® is a next generation decellularized dermal allograft that signals a new direction in soft tissue regeneration.

- Is minimally manipulated to preserve tissue structure.
- Signals cell migration and proliferation.
- Increases angiogenesis and reduces fibrosis.
- Provides optimal handling and biomechanical strength in a thin profile biologic.

INDICATIONS

DermaPure® Decellularized Dermal Allograft is intended to be used to provide reinforcement, repair, or replacement of damaged or inadequate integumental tissue or for other homologous uses of human integument.

CONTRAINDICATIONS

- No contraindications, please consult Instructions For Use (IFU) for Warnings, Precautions, and potential Adverse Effects associated with biologic use.

APPLICATION

- Place the DermaPure® onto the wound bed, with the basement membrane side outermost. Utilizing sterile scissors or scalpel, remove excess DermaPure®.
- Secure the DermaPure® with liquid skin adhesive, sterile adhesive strips, staples, or sutures if needed.
- Place a nonadherent contact layer over the DermaPure®, followed by an appropriate bolster to mitigate movement of the DermaPure® for 5 to 7 days.
- Cover with a secondary dressing to maintain a moist environment.
- Leave dressing in place for 5 to 7 days. Subsequent dressing management should provide a moist environment, taking care not to pull off the DermaPure® during the dressing change.

CELLULAR AND TISSUE-BASED PRODUCTS

REMOVAL

- Not applicable, biologics integrate with host over time.

REFERENCES

1. Greaves NS, Morris J, Benatar B, et al. Acute cutaneous wounds treated with human decellularised dermis show enhanced angiogenesis during healing. *PLoS ONE.* 2015;10(1):e0113209.
2. Greaves NS, Iqbal SA, Hodgkinson T, et al. Skin substitute-assisted repair shows reduced dermal fibrosis in acute human wounds validated simultaneously by histology and optical tomography. *Wound Repair Regen.* 2015;23(4):483–494
3. Kimmel H, Gittleman H. Retrospective observational analysis of the use of an architecturally unique dermal regeneration template (Derma Pure®) for the treatment of hard-to-heal wounds. *Int Wound J.* 2017;14(4):666–672.
4. Greaves NS, Benatar B, Baguneid M, et al. Single-stage application of a novel decellularized dermis for treatment-resistant lower limb ulcers: positive outcomes assessed by SIAscopy, laser perfusion, and 3D imaging, with sequential timed histological analysis. *Wound Repair Regen.* 2013;21(6):813–822.
5. Ashrafi M, Sebastian A, Shih B, et al. Whole genome microarray data of chronic wound debridement prior to application of dermal skin substitutes. *Wound Rep and Reg.* 2016;24:870–875.

CELLULAR AND TISSUE-BASED PRODUCTS

EpiFix® Dehydrated Human Amnion/Chorion Membrane Allograft

MiMedx Group, Inc.

HOW SUPPLIED

EpiFix Sheet	18 mm Disc	Q4186	15271–15278 possible for wound
EpiFix Sheet	2 cm × 2 cm	Q4186	15271–15278 possible for wound
EpiFix Sheet	2 cm × 3 cm	Q4186	15271–15278 possible for wound
EpiFix Sheet	2 cm × 4 cm	Q4186	15271–15278 possible for wound
EpiFix Sheet	3 cm × 4 cm	Q4186	15271–15278 possible for wound
EpiFix Sheet	4 cm × 4 cm	Q4186	15271–15278 possible for wound
EpiFix Sheet	5 cm × 6 cm	Q4186	15271–15278 possible for wound
EpiFix Sheet	7 cm × 7 cm	Q4186	15271–15278 possible for wound
EpiFix Mesh Sheet	2 cm × 3 cm	Q4186	15271–15278 possible for wound
EpiFix Mesh Sheet	3.5 cm × 3.5 cm	Q4186	15271–15278 possible for wound
EpiFix Mesh Sheet	4 cm × 4.5 cm	Q4186	15271–15278 possible for wound

CELLULAR AND TISSUE-BASED PRODUCTS

ACTION

Human amniotic membrane is a thin, collagenous membrane derived from the placenta, the area in which the human fetus grows and develops within the mother's uterus. Human amniotic membrane consists of multiple layers.

EpiFix® is a minimally manipulated, dehydrated, non-viable cellular amniotic membrane allograft that contains multiple extracellular matrix proteins, growth factors, cytokines and other specialty proteins present in amniotic tissue to provide a barrier membrane that enhances healing.

USES

EpiFix® is intended for homologous use in the treatment of acute and chronic wounds to provide a barrier, modulate inflammation, enhance healing, and reduce scar tissue formation.

CONTRAINDICATIONS

- EpiFix® should not be used on areas with active or latent infection and/or a patient with a disorder that would create an unacceptable risk of postoperative complications.

APPLICATION

- Prior to implantation, carefully follow the EpiFix® allograft preparation steps below using aseptic technique:

Wound bed preparation

- Ensure the wound is free from clinical signs of infection. Prepare wound bed as needed.

Removing EpiFix® from packaging

- The outer peel pouch is not sterile. The inner pouch that contains EpiFix® is sterile (unless the pouches are damaged or compromised). Carefully open the peelable corner of the outer pouch and extract the inner pouch using aseptic technique. Ensure the inner pouch does not come in contact with any portions of nonsterile surface of the outer pouch. Using aseptic technique, slowly peel a corner of the inner peel pouch and allow the authorized medical professional to grasp EpiFix® with fingers or nontoothed, sterile forceps.
- Use EpiFix® promptly after opening the inner, sterile pouch. Pleases take great care when removing EpiFix® from the internal pouch. EpiFix® is thin and extremely lightweight.

EpiFix® preparation

- In a dry state, use sterile dry scissors to cut EpiFix® to fit within the wound margins. It is acceptable to overlap the wound margins with EpiFix® by 1 mm. If needed, EpiFix® can be fenestrated to accommodate wounds that produce copious amounts of exudate.
- EpiFix® can be applied wet or dry.
- EpiFix® can be hydrated while on the wound site with sterile saline solution. Simply apply several drops of sterile solution to EpiFix®. During and following hydration, the embossment on EpiFix® will begin to fade.

EpiFix® orientation and application

- EpiFix® should be placed on the wound site, using the orientation of the embossment lettering as a guide. Proper orientation of EpiFix® can be noted when the embossment nomenclature reads correctly from left to right. Absorbable, nonabsorbable suture material and/or tissue adhesives can be used to fixate EpiFix® to the wound site.

Support therapies

- EpiFix® is compatible with offloading/compression/negative pressure therapies. EpiFix® can be used in conjunction with hyperbaric oxygen therapy.
- It is recommended that EpiFix® grafts be applied weekly until wound epithelialization is achieved. However, clinician discretion should be used based on patient and wound condition/progress. It is clinically acceptable to apply EpiFix® on a biweekly basis if desired.

REFERENCES

1. Koob TJ, Lim JJ, Massee M, et al. Properties of dehydrated human amnion/chorion composite grafts: Implications for wound repair and soft tissue regeneration. *J Biomed Mater Res B Appl Biomater*. 2014;102(6):1353–1362.
2. Lei J, Priddy LB, Lim JJ, et al. Identification of extracellular matrix components and biological factors in micronized dehydrated human amnion/chorion membrane. *Adv Wound Care (New Rochelle)*. 2017;6(2):43–53.
3. Koob TJ, Lim JJ, Massee M, et al. Angiogenic properties of dehydrated human amnion/chorion allografts: therapeutic potential for soft tissue repair and regeneration. *Vasc Cell*. 2014;6:10.
4. Maan ZN, Rennert RC, Koob TJ, et al. Cell recruitment by amnion chorion graft promotes neovascularization. *J Surg Res*. 2015;193(2):953–962.

5. Koob TJ, Rennert R, Zabek N, et al. Biological properties of dehydrated human amnion/chorion composite graft: implications for chronic wound healing. *Int Wound J.* 2013;10(5):493–500.

6. Massee M, Chinn K, Lei J, et al. Dehydrated human amnion/chorion membrane regulates stem cell activity in vitro. *J Biomed Mater Res B Appl Biomater.* 2016;104(7):1495–1503.

7. Massee M, Chinn K, Lim JJ, et al. Type I and II diabetic adipose-derived stem cells respond in vitro to dehydrated human amnion/chorion membrane allograft treatment by increasing proliferation, migration, and altering cytokine secretion. *Adv Wound Care (New Rochelle).* 2016;5(2):43–54.

8. Bianchi C, Cazzell S, Vayser D, et al.; EpiFix VLU Study Group. A multi-centre randomised controlled trial evaluating the efficacy of dehydrated human amnion/chorion membrane (EpiFix) allograft for the treatment of venous leg ulcers. *Int Wound J.* 2018;15(1):114–122.

9. Fetterolf DE, Istwan NB, Stanziano GJ. An evaluation of healing metrics associated with commonly used advanced wound care products for the treatment of chronic diabetic foot ulcers. *Manag Care.* 2014;23(7):31–38.

10. Fetterolf DE, Savage R. Dehydrated human amniotic membrane improves healing time, cost of care. *Today's Wound Clinic.* 2013;7(1):19–20.

11. Fetterolf DE, Snyder RJ. Scientific and clinical support for the use of dehydrated amniotic membrane in wound management. *Wounds.* 2012;24(10):299–307.

12. Forbes J, Fetterolf DE. Dehydrated amniotic membrane allografts for the treatment of chronic wounds: a case series. *J Wound Care.* 2012;21(6):290, 292, 294–296.

13. Koob TJ, Lim JJ, Zabek N, et al. Cytokines in single layer amnion allografts compared to multilayer amnion/chorion allografts for wound healing. *J Biomed Mater Res B Appl Biomater.* 2015;103(5):1133–1140.

14. Serena TE, Carter MJ, Le LT, et al.; EpiFix VLU Study Group. A multicenter, randomized, controlled clinical trial evaluating the use of dehydrated human amnion/chorion membrane allografts and multilayer compression therapy vs. multilayer compression therapy alone in the treatment of venous leg ulcers. *Wound Repair Regen.* 2014;22(6):688–693.

15. Serena TE, Yaakov R, DiMarco D, et al. Dehydrated human amnion/chorion membrane treatment of venous leg ulcers: correlation between 4-week and 24-week outcomes. *J Wound Care.* 2015;24(11):530–534.

16. Shah AP. Using amniotic membrane allografts in the treatment of neuropathic foot ulcers. *J Am Podiatr Med Assoc.* 2014;104(2):198–202.

17. Sheikh ES, Sheikh ES, Fetterolf DE. Use of dehydrated human amniotic membrane allografts to promote healing in patients with refractory non healing wounds. *Int Wound J.* 2014;11(6):711–717.

18. Zelen CM, Serena TE, Denozière G, et al. A prospective randomized comparative parallel study of amniotic membrane wound graft in the management of diabetic foot ulcers. *Int Wound J.* 2013;10(5):502–507.

19. Zelen CM. An evaluation of dehydrated human amniotic membrane allografts in patients with DFUs. *J Wound Care.* 2013;22(7):347–348, 350–351.

20. Zelen CM, Serena TE, Fetterolf DE. Dehydrated human amnion/chorion membrane allografts in patients with chronic diabetic foot ulcers: A long-term follow-up study. *Wound Medicine.* 2014;4:1–4.

21. Zelen CM, Serena TE, Snyder RJ. A prospective, randomised comparative study of weekly versus biweekly application of dehydrated human amnion/chorion membrane allograft in the management of diabetic foot ulcers. *Int Wound J.* 2014;11(2):122–128.

22. Zelen CM, Gould L, Serena TE, et al. A prospective, randomised, controlled, multi-centre comparative effectiveness study of healing using dehydrated human amnion/chorion membrane allograft, bioengineered skin substitute or standard of care for treatment of chronic lower extremity diabetic ulcers. *Int Wound J.* 2015;12(6):724–732.

23. Zelen CM, Serena TE, Gould L, et al. Treatment of chronic diabetic lower extremity ulcers with advanced therapies: a prospective, randomised, controlled, multi-centre comparative study examining clinical efficacy and cost. *Int Wound J.* 2016;13(2):272–282.

24. Garoufalis M, Nagesh D, Sanchez P, et al. Use of dehydrated human amnion/chorion membrane allografts in more than 100 patients with six major types of refractory nonhealing wounds. *J Am Pod Med Assoc.* 2018;108(2):84–89.

25. Tettelbach W, Cazzell S, Reyzelman AM, et al. A confirmatory study on the efficacy of dehydrated human amnion/chorion membrane dHACM allograft in the management of diabetic foot ulcers: A prospective, multicentre, randomised, controlled study of 110 patients from 14 wound clinics. *Int Wound J.* 2019;16:19–29.

CELLULAR AND TISSUE-BASED PRODUCTS

EpiFix® Micronized Dehydrated Human Amnion/Chorion Membrane Allograft

MiMedx Group, Inc.

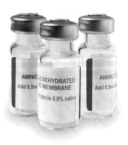

HOW SUPPLIED

EpiFix Micronized	40 mg	Q4145	15271–15278 possible for wound
EpiFix Micronized	100 mg	Q4145	15271–15278 possible for wound
EpiFix Micronized	160 mg	Q4145	15271–15278 possible for wound

ACTION

Human amniotic membrane is a thin, collagenous membrane derived from the placenta, the area in which the human fetus grows and develops within the mother's uterus. Human amniotic membrane consists of multiple layers.

EpiFix® Micronized is a dehydrated, non-viable cellular amniotic membrane allograft that contains multiple extracellular matrix proteins, growth factors, cytokines and other specialty proteins present in amniotic tissue.

USES

EpiFix® Micronized is intended for homologous use in the treatment of acute and chronic wounds to modulate inflammation, enhance healing, and reduce scar tissue formation.

CONTRAINDICATIONS

- EpiFix Micronized should not be injected into: (1) the spinal canal; (2) vital organs, including the heart; and/or (3) other areas of the circulatory system or the central nervous system. EpiFix Micronized should not be used: (1) on areas with active or latent infection; (2) on a patient with a disorder that would create an unacceptable risk of post-operative complications; (3) in intravenous, intra-arterial, or intrathecal applications.

APPLICATION

Removing EpiFix® micronized from packaging

- The outer peel pouch is not sterile. The inner pouch containing the EpiFix® Micronized vial is sterile (unless the pouches are damaged or compromised).
- Using aseptic technique, slowly peel a corner of the inner peel pouch and allow the authorized medical professional to remove the vial.

Injection preparation technique

Recommended Materials:
    Sterile 0.9% Saline Solution
    One (1) × 5 mL Syringe
    One (1) × 18–25G Needle
    Alcohol Swab

- Flip open the aluminum top of the vial. Wipe injection port with 70% isopropyl alcohol prep pad.
- Draw up the recommended volume of 0.9% sterile saline needed for rehydration as described below into a 5 mL syringe using an 18–25G needle. The volume used is left to the discretion of the authorized medical professional.
  - Amount of Material: 40 mg; Recommended Volume of Saline: 1 mL.
  - Amount of Material: 100 mg; Recommended Volume of Saline: 2.5 mL.
  - Amount of Material: 160 mg; Recommended Volume of Saline: 4 mL.
- Transfer a portion, 2 mL or less, of the recommended volume of 0.9% sterile saline into the vial of EpiFix® Micronized.
- Using a back and forth transfer with the plunger, mix the particulate to create a full suspension in the syringe. Because the reconstituted material is viscous, use proper preinjection techniques to reduce possible air introduction.
- Dispose of any material remaining after procedure is complete in accordance with biohazardous protocols. This product is for single patient use only.
- Use within 12 hours of reconstitution.
- If time elapses between rehydration and administration and product separates, resuspend by shaking.

Dry application

- Dry the wound surface to allow for even application of the powder. Remove the foil and stopper from the vial. Apply a thin even layer of the powder onto the wound area to be treated.

Rehydration and use as a paste

- Apply single drops of saline while mixing until desired consistency is achieved.

Support therapies

- EpiFix® Micronized is compatible with offloading/compression/negative pressure therapies and can be used in conjunction with hyperbaric oxygen therapy.
- Apply additional EpiFix® Micronized when the rate of wound healing slows.

REFERENCE

1. Lei J, Priddy LB, Lim JJ, et al. Identification of extracellular matrix components and biological factors in micronized dehydrated human amnion/chorion membrane. *Adv Wound Care (New Rochelle)*. 2017;6(2):43–53.

CELLULAR AND TISSUE-BASED PRODUCTS

EpiCord® Dehydrated Human Umbilical Cord Allograft

MiMedx Group, Inc.

HOW SUPPLIED

| EpiCord | 2 cm × 3 cm | Q4187 | 15271–15278 possible for wound |
| EpiCord | 3 cm × 5 cm | Q4187 | 15271–15278 possible for wound |

ACTION

EpiCord® is an allograft derived from umbilical cord, the structure that protects the arteries and vein that carry essential nourishment and oxygenated blood from mother to fetus. Human umbilical cord consists of amniotic epithelium and Wharton's jelly, containing extracellular matrix composed of collagen, proteoglycans and hyaluronic acid.

USES

EpiCord® is a minimally manipulated, dehydrated, non-viable cellular human umbilical cord allograft intended for homologous use to provide a protective environment for the healing process.

CONTRAINDICATIONS

- EpiCord® should not be used on areas with active or latent infection and/or a patient with a disorder that would create an unacceptable risk of postoperative complications.

APPLICATION

Preparation, reconstitution, and use

- Prior to implantation, carefully follow EpiCord® allograft preparation steps below using aseptic technique:

Removing EpiCord® from packaging

- The outer peel pouch is not sterile. The inner pouch which contains the EpiCord® allograft is sterile (unless the pouches are damaged or compromised). Carefully open the peelable corner of the outer pouch and present the inner pouch using aseptic technique. Ensure the inner pouch does not come in contact with any portions of nonsterile surface of the outer pouch. Using aseptic technique, slowly peel a corner of the inner peel pouch and grasp the allograft with fingers or nontoothed, sterile forceps. Use the EpiCord® allograft promptly after opening the inner, sterile pouch. Please take great care when removing the product from the internal pouch.

EpiCord® preparation and application

- In its dry state and prior to hydration, the allograft may be cut with sharp scissors to the appropriate and approximate size required. The allograft should then be placed on the site. The allograft can then be hydrated while on the site with sterile saline solution, if desired. Suture material (absorbable, nonabsorbable) and/or tissue adhesives can be used to fixate EpiCord® allografts to the site of application or to itself, if desired. Cover to maintain a moist wound environment. Use appropriate moisture management dressings for the wound type and treatment ideology.

- It is recommended that EpiCord® grafts are applied weekly until wound epithelialization is achieved. However, clinician discretion should be used based on patient and wound condition/progress. It is clinically acceptable to apply EpiCord® on a biweekly basis if desired.

REFERENCES

1. Bullard JD, Lei J, Lim JJ, et al. Evaluation of dehydrated human umbilical cord biological properties for wound care and soft tissue healing. *J Biomed Mater Res B Appl Biomater*. 2019;107(4):1035–1046.
2. Tettelbach W, Cazzell S, Sigal F, et al. A multicentre prospective randomised controlled comparative parallel study of dehydrated human umbilical cord (EpiCord) allograft for the treatment of diabetic foot ulcers. *Int Wound J*. 2019;16:122–130.

CELLULAR AND TISSUE-BASED PRODUCTS

New Product: Grafix CORE®

Osiris Therapeutics, Inc.

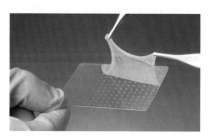

HOW SUPPLIED

Grafix CORE®	3 × 4 cm	Q4312
Grafix CORE®	5 × 5 cm	Q4312

ACTION

Grafix CORE® (cryopreserved placental membrane) is a cryopreserved chorion matrix retaining the extracellular matrix, growth factors, and endogenous neonatal mesenchymal stem cells and fibroblasts of the native tissue.

INDICATIONS

Grafix CORE may be used to repair acute and chronic wounds, including, but not limited to, diabetic foot ulcers, venous leg ulcers, pressure ulcers, dehisced surgical wounds, burns, acute surgical wounds, pyoderma gangrenosum, and epidermolysis bullosa. The product is limited to homologous use as a wound cover and may be used for acute and chronic wounds encompassing both upper extremity and lower extremity. Grafix CORE naturally conforms to complex anatomies and may be used over exposed bone, tendon, joint capsule, and muscle.

CONTRAINDICATIONS

- There are no known contraindications for this product.

APPLICATION

- You will need to thaw the graft following the package insert instructions. To apply, hold the plastic backing on the tab labeled CORE and remove the smaller, solid plastic cover from the top of the graft. The graft should remain on the plastic backing. Slide the graft from the plastic backing onto the wound.
- Grafix CORE does not require fixation (suturing, etc.), but these methods may be used by the physician or appropriate healthcare professional at his/her discretion. Cover the Grafix CORE-treated wound with nonadherent dressing followed by saline moistened gauze to fill but not pack the wound. Continue dressing appropriate for the wound type.

REMOVAL

- Grafix CORE does not need to be removed. The graft should be reapplied weekly at the discretion of the responsible physician for the duration of the treatment of the patient's wound.

REFERENCES

1. Regulski M, Jacobstein DA, Petranto RD, et al. A retrospective analysis of a human cellular repair matrix for the treatment of chronic wounds. *Ostomy Wound Manage.* 2013;59(12):38–43.
2. Lavery LA, Fulmer J, Shebetka KA, et al. The efficacy and safety of Grafix® for the treatment of chronic diabetic foot ulcers: Results of a multi-centre, controlled, randomised, blinded, clinical trial. *Int Wound J.* 2014;11(5):554–560.

3. Frykberg RG, Gibbons GW, Walters JL, et al. A prospective, multicentre, open-label, single-arm clinical trial for treatment of chronic complex diabetic foot wounds with exposed tendon and/or bone: Positive clinical outcomes of viable cryopreserved human placental membrane. *Int Wound J.* 2016;14(3):569–577.
4. Johnson E, Marshall J, Michael G. A comparative outcomes analysis evaluating clinical effectiveness in two different human placental membrane products for wound management. *Wound Repair Regen.* 2016;25(1):145–149.

CELLULAR AND TISSUE-BASED PRODUCTS

New Product: Grafix PRIME®

Osiris Therapeutics, Inc.

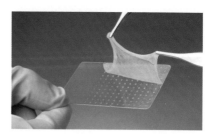

HOW SUPPLIED

Grafix PRIME®	16 mm disc	Q4133
Grafix PRIME®	1.5 × 2 cm	Q4133
Grafix PRIME®	2 × 3 cm	Q4133
Grafix PRIME®	3 × 4 cm	Q4133
Grafix PRIME®	5 × 5 cm	Q4133

ACTION

Grafix PRIME® (cryopreserved placental membrane) is a cryopreserved amnion matrix retaining the extracellular matrix, growth factors, and endogenous neonatal mesenchymal stem cells, fibroblasts, and epithelial cells of the native tissue.

INDICATIONS

Grafix PRIME may be used to repair acute and chronic wounds, including, but not limited to, diabetic foot ulcers, venous leg ulcers, pressure ulcers, dehisced surgical wounds, burns, acute surgical wounds, pyoderma gangrenosum, and epidermolysis bullosa. The product is limited to homologous use as a wound cover and may be used for acute and chronic wounds encompassing both upper extremity and lower extremity. Grafix PRIME naturally conforms to complex anatomies and may be used over exposed bone, tendon, joint capsule, and muscle.

CONTRAINDICATIONS

- There are no known contraindications for this product.

APPLICATION

- You will need to thaw the graft following the package insert instructions. To apply, hold the plastic backing on the tab labeled PRIME and remove the smaller, solid plastic cover from the top of the graft. The graft should remain on the plastic backing. Slide the graft from the plastic backing onto the wound.
- Grafix PRIME does not require fixation (suturing, etc.), but these methods may be used by the physician or appropriate healthcare professional at his/her discretion. Cover the Grafix PRIME-treated wound with nonadherent dressing followed by saline moistened gauze to fill but not pack the wound. Continue dressing appropriate for the wound type.

REMOVAL

- Grafix PRIME does not need to be removed. The graft should be reapplied weekly at the discretion of the responsible physician for the duration of the treatment of the patient's wound.

REFERENCES

1. Regulski M, Jacobstein DA, Petranto RD, et al. A retrospective analysis of a human cellular repair matrix for the treatment of chronic wounds. *Ostomy Wound Manage.* 2013;59(12):38–43.

CELLULAR AND TISSUE-BASED PRODUCTS

2. Lavery LA, Fulmer J, Shebetka KA, et al. The efficacy and safety of Grafix® for the treatment of chronic diabetic foot ulcers: Results of a multi-centre, controlled, randomised, blinded, clinical trial. *Int Wound J*. 2014;11(5):554–560.

3. Frykberg RG, Gibbons GW, Walters JL, et al. A prospective, multicentre, open-label, single-arm clinical trial for treatment of chronic complex diabetic foot wounds with exposed tendon and/or bone: Positive clinical outcomes of viable cryopreserved human placental membrane. *Int Wound J*. 2016;14(3):569–577.

4. Johnson E, Marshall J, Michael G. A comparative outcomes analysis evaluating clinical effectiveness in two different human placental membrane products for wound management. *Wound Repair Regen*. 2016;25(1):145–149.

CELLULAR AND TISSUE-BASED PRODUCTS

GrafixPL PRIME

Osiris Therapeutics, Inc.

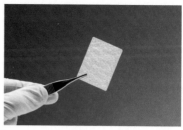

HOW SUPPLIED

GrafixPL PRIME	16-mm disc	Q4133
GrafixPL PRIME	1.5 × 2 cm	Q4133
GrafixPL PRIME	2 × 3 cm	Q4133
GrafixPL PRIME	3 × 3 cm	Q4133
GrafixPL PRIME	3 × 4 cm	Q4133
GrafixPL PRIME	5 × 5 cm	Q4133

ACTION

GrafixPL PRIME (lyopreserved placental membrane) is a lyopreserved amnion matrix retaining the extracellular matrix, growth factors, and endogenous neonatal mesenchymal stem cells, fibroblasts, and epithelial cells of the native tissue.

INDICATIONS

GrafixPL PRIME may be used to repair acute and chronic wounds, including, but not limited to, diabetic foot ulcers, venous leg ulcers, pressure ulcers, dehisced surgical wounds, burns, acute surgical wounds, pyoderma gangrenosum, and epidermolysis bullosa. The product is limited to homologous use as a wound cover and may be used for acute and chronic wounds encompassing both upper extremity and lower extremity. GrafixPL PRIME naturally conforms to complex anatomies and may be used over exposed bone, tendon, joint capsule, and muscle.

CONTRAINDICATIONS

- There are no known contraindications for this product.

APPLICATION

- GrafixPL PRIME can be applied in an office, hospital outpatient setting, or in an operating room. Always review and follow your facility's policy regarding sterile/aseptic/clean technique. Proper aseptic technique should be followed when applying the product.

APPLICATION PROTOCOL

- You will need to follow one of two application methods detailed in the package insert instructions, and summarized below.

Method #1

- Remove one mesh applicator from the graft.
- Apply the graft side directly onto the wound bed.
- Press and hold until the product is rehydrated by wound fluid or the addition of sterile saline.
- Remove the other mesh applicator. Do not leave the mesh on the wound.

Method #2

- Remove the mesh applicators from both sides of the graft. Do not leave the mesh on the wound.
- Apply the product directly onto the wound bed.
- Press and hold until the product is rehydrated by wound fluid or the addition of sterile saline.

APPLICATION NOTES FOR BOTH METHODS

- Ensure the graft is in direct contact with all surfaces of the wound bed.
- Apply sterile saline if needed to ensure the entire product is moistened and fold away any excess product into the wound bed.
- GrafixPL PRIME does not require fixation (suturing, etc.), but these methods may be used by the physician or the appropriate health care provider at his or her discretion. Cover the applied graft in the wound with a nonadherent dressing followed by saline moistened gauze to fill but not pack the wound, or use another dressing as appropriate for the wound type.

REMOVAL

- GrafixPL PRIME does not need to be removed, and should be reapplied weekly at the discretion of the responsible physician for the duration of the treatment of the patient's wound.

CELLULAR AND TISSUE-BASED PRODUCTS

New Product: Hyalomatrix

Medline Industries, Inc.

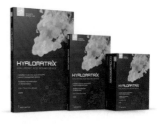

HOW SUPPLIED

Esterified Hyaluronic Acid Regenerative Matrix	2.5 × 2.5 cm	Q4117
Esterified Hyaluronic Acid Regenerative Matrix	5 × 5 cm	Q4117
Esterified Hyaluronic Acid Regenerative Matrix	10 × 10 cm	Q4117
Esterified Hyaluronic Acid Regenerative Matrix	10 × 20 cm	Q4117

ACTION

Hyalomatrix® is a bilayered, sterile, flexible and conformable hyaluronic acid regenerative matrix for advanced wound care. It is comprised of a non-woven pad made entirely of HYAFF®, a benzyl ester of hyaluronic acid, and a semi-permeable silicone membrane, which controls water vapor loss, provides a flexible covering for the wound surface, and adds increased tear strength to the device. The biodegradable matrix acts as a scaffold for cellular invasion and capillary growth. As Hyalomatrix is applied on the wound bed, the HYAFF wound contact layer provides a 3D scaffold able to be colonized by fibroblasts and onto which extracellular matrix components are regularly laid down, facilitating an ordered reconstruction of the dermal tissue.

INDICATIONS

- Chronic vascular ulcers.
- Diabetic ulcers.
- Draining wounds.
- Partial- and full-thickness wounds.
- Pressure ulcers.
- Second-degree burns.
- Surgical wounds (donor sites/grafts, post-Mohs surgery, post-laser surgery, podiatric, wound dehiscence).
- Trauma wounds (abrasions, lacerations, skin tears).
- Tunneled/undetermined wounds.
- Venous ulcers.

CONTRAINDICATIONS

- Individuals with a hypersensitivity to hyaluronan and/or its derivatives or silicone.

APPLICATION

- Use aseptic technique, open the outer pouch, and pass the inner tray into the sterile field (if applicable). Open the tray and gently remove the product from the protective sheet.
- Following wound bed preparation, immediately apply the device, keeping the fibrous HYAFF layer in contact with the wound bed. Hyalomatrix may be cut to size.
- Do not overlap Hyalomatrix units. Cover Hyalomatrix with an appropriate, nonadherent secondary dressing.

POST-APPLICATION

- Inspection of the wound bed is recommended every 3–4 days. During this timeframe, patients normally experience a significant reduction in local pain. Frequently, Hyalomatrix forms a yellow-green colored gel that is sometimes characterized by a bad odor. This is the result of the normal degradation process of HYAFF and is not necessarily indicative of a local infection.
- Change secondary dressing as needed—the frequency of secondary dressing change will be dependent upon volume of exudates produced and type of dressing used.
- After the first week, weekly inspections of the wound bed may be sufficient to monitor the repair process.
  Note: If excess exudates collect under the sheet, small openings can be cut in the sheet to allow fluid to drain.

REMOVAL

- Following formation of the new tissue, the silicone layer can be released.

CELLULAR AND TISSUE-BASED PRODUCTS

Kerecis Omega3 Wound

Kerecis LLC

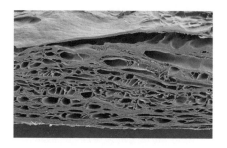

HOW SUPPLIED

Acellular Fish Skin	1.75 × 1.75 cm	Q4158
Acellular Fish Skin	3 × 3.5 cm	Q4158
Acellular Fish Skin	3 × 7 cm	Q4158
Acellular Fish Skin	7 × 10 cm	Q4158
Acellular Fish Skin	Circular 14 mm diamter	Q4158
Acellular Fish Skin	16 mm diameter	Q4158

ACTION

The Kerecis product with Omega-3 fatty acids help to progress the wound from the inflammatory stage of wound healing and recruits cellular ingrowth. The fish skin is highly porous and pore size is in the size range of cells (16.1 μm diameter on average) offering an optimum environment for cell ingrowth.[1] The fish skin is vascularized[2] and populated by the patient's own cells, and ultimately converted into living tissue. Kerecis Omega3 Wound also acts as a bacterial barrier.[3,4]

INDICATIONS

Partial- and full-thickness wounds, pressure ulcers, venous ulcers, chronic vascular ulcers, diabetic ulcers, trauma wounds (abrasions, lacerations, second-degree burns, skin tears), surgical wounds (donor sites/grafts, post-Mohs surgery, post-laser surgery, podiatric, wound dehiscence), draining wounds.

CONTRAINDICATIONS

- Kerecis Omega3 Wound is contraindicated in patients with known fish allergy.

APPLICATION

- Refer to the pouch inlay Instructions For Use before applying Kerecis Omega3 Wound.

PREPARATION

- When applying Kerecis Omega3 Wound for the first time, debride the wound bed by removing necrotic tissue to obtain a lightly bleeding fresh tissue surface. Irrigate.
- Remove the Kerecis Omega3 Wound sheet from the pouch using aseptic technique.
- Cut the sheet roughly to the size of the area to be covered and prehydrate in NaCl solution.

APPLICATION

- Kerecis has two sides; apply the sheet with the rough (scaly) side up.
- Apply sheet directly into the wound, making sure that the sheet does not overlap the wound edges.

- More than one sheet may be necessary for complete coverage. Overlap sheet edges slightly to assure coverage of the entire wound.
- Secure the product using steristrips, suture, or staples.

COVERING

- Apply a low-adherent wound contact layer such as Mepitel to protect the sheet.
- Use a covering dressing such as absorptive polyurethane dressing appropriate to the level of wound exudates. Note that exudates can increase during the first week of using Kerecis. Covering dressing can be changed between applications of Kerecis without changing the contact layer.
- Kerecis Omega3 Wound should be used along with necessary support devices such as compression wrappings and/or offloading devices.

FOLLOW-UP APPLICATIONS

- After starting treatment with Kerecis Omega3 Wound, the wound should be checked regularly to ensure that the cover dressing is maintaining a sufficient moist wound environment and if a reapplication of Kerecis Omega3 Wound is needed.
  - Inspect wound every 2 to 7 days. The duration between inspections may be extended as healing progresses.
  - Insert a new Kerecis Omega3 Wound sheet into the wound if the previously applied sheet has been absorbed and is no longer visible.
  - Change the cover dressing as needed to maintain a moist, clean wound area.
- As wound healing occurs, redness and swelling of wound edges will decrease and the level of exudate will be reduced. These are signs of wound healing and are often seen before epithelialization is obvious. Make sure to use an appropriate type of cover wound dressing at all times to maintain a moist, clean wound area.
- Should you suspect any adverse reaction from this product please report it to the e-mail adversereactions@kerecis.com leaving a phone number and e-mail address. Adverse reactions might also be subject to mandatory reporting to the authorities. Please submit the data on the package or pouch, that is, "lot number" and "use before" date.

REMOVAL

- Kerecis is permanently applied to the wound and does not need to be removed. The product gets integrated into the wound bed in 3 to 10 days depending on the enzymatic activity in the wound. A new sheet of the product can be re-applied when there are no visible remnants in the wound.

REFERENCES

1. Magnusson S, Baldursson BT, Kjartansson H, et al. Regenerative and antibacterial properties of acellular fish skin grafts and human amnion/chorion membrane: Implications for tissue preservation in combat casualty. *J Mil Med*. 2017;182(S1):383–388.
2. Magnusson S, Baldursson BT, Kjartansson H, et al. Decellularized fish skin: characteristics that support tissue repair. *The Icelandic Medical Journal*. 2015;101(12):567–573.
3. Baldursson BT, Kjartansson H, Konradsdottir F, et al. Healing rate and autoimmune safety of full-thickness wounds treated with fish skin acellular dermal matrix versus porcine small-intestine submucosa: a noninferiority study. *Int J Low Extrem Wounds*. 2015;14(1):37–43.
4. Winters C. Wound dehiscence on a diabetic patient with haemophilia and high risk of further amputation successfully healed with omega-3 rich fish skin: a case report. *The Diabetic Foot Journal*. 2018;21(3):186–190.

CELLULAR AND TISSUE-BASED PRODUCTS

New Product: MIRRAGEN® Advanced Wound Matrix

ETS Wound Care LLC

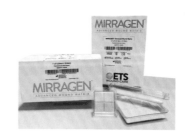

HOW SUPPLIED

Advanced Wound Matrix	1″ × 6″
Advanced Wound Matrix	2″ × 2″
Advanced Wound Matrix	4″ × 4″

ACTION

The MIRRAGEN® Advanced Wound Matrix is a next generation wound care solution composed of resorbable borate-based bioactive glass fibers and particulate. After a wound has been cleaned, MIRRAGEN® can be easily cut to shape and placed in the wound bed. The flexible nature of MIRRAGEN® allows it to be custom fit to a variety of wound shapes and sizes. Once placed at the wound site, the porous structure of MIRRAGEN® allows it to wick fluid away from the wound bed and control the moisture content (absorbs up to 400% by weight).

Due to the fibrous structure of MIRRAGEN®, the matrix facilitates the wound healing response and allows new tissue to regenerate at the site. New blood vessels also form in this area. During the healing process, MIRRAGEN® is absorbed by the surrounding tissue and simply needs to be reapplied every 3 to 7 days. Over time, the MIRRAGEN® matrix allows the wound to fully heal. With a unique structure and composition, the MIRRAGEN® Advanced Wound Matrix represents an innovative solution for acute and chronic wound management.

INDICATIONS

The MIRRAGEN® Advanced Wound Matrix is intended for use in the management of wounds. Wound types include partial- and full-thickness wounds, pressure ulcers, venous ulcers, diabetic ulcers, chronic vascular ulcers, tunneled/undermined wounds, surgical wounds (donor sites/grafts, post-Moh's surgery, postlaser surgery, podiatric, wound dehiscence), trauma wounds (abrasions, lacerations, first- and second-degree burns, skin tears), and draining wounds.

CONTRAINDICATIONS

- Discontinue use if adverse reactions are observed.

APPLICATION

- Apply MIRRAGEN® in a fashion which allows the soft moldable structure to come into direct contact with the wound surface. Loosely fill tunnels or areas of undermining—avoid temptation to "pack" or compact the product with application into these areas.
- Dead space may be filled with wound filler, gauze, or additional MIRRAGEN®, as desired.
- MIRRAGEN® Advanced Wound Matrix requires a cover dressing considering the wound exudate levels, as the matrix is highly absorptive. It is **important** to maintain moisture balance by addition of moisture or selecting a moisture retaining cover dressing as indicated.
- Secure outer dressings as desired/indicated.

REMOVAL

- Application may be left in place for up to 1 week, or reapplied every 3 to 7 days, as indicated.
- MIRRAGEN® may be applied under compression wraps or off-loading devices.
- MIRRAGEN® may remain intact until it is fully dissolved.
- To remove, gently flush, irrigate, or wash away any loose MIRRAGEN® matrix.
- **NOTE:** Any matrix incorporated into the wound tissue should not be disturbed. Do not aggressively debride or use sharp instruments to remove any integrated material from the wound base. Removal of callous or periwound debris is appropriate.
- MIRRAGEN® matrix incorporated into the wound tissue will be fully absorbed—does not need to be removed.

REFERENCE

1. ETS Website: www.etswoundcare.com

New Product: NEOX 100

Amniox Medical

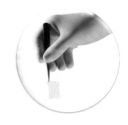

HOW SUPPLIED

NEOX 100	2 cm × 2 cm (4 sq. cm)	Q4156
NEOX 100	3 cm × 3 cm (9 sq. cm)	Q4156
NEOX 100	4 cm × 4 cm (16 sq. cm)	Q4156
NEOX 100	7 cm × 7 cm (49 sq. cm)	Q4156

ACTION

NEOX 100 Cryopreserved Amniotic Membrane allograft immunomodulates inflammation and orchestrates regenerative healing in chronic wounds.

INDICATIONS

NEOX 100 can be used as a wound covering for dermal ulcers or defects.

CONTRAINDICATIONS

- NEOX 100 should not be used on wounds that are actively infected.

APPLICATION

- Wound should be debrided to expose healthy bleeding wound edge, base, and granulation tissue. NEOX 100 is placed on the wound bed. A nonadherent contact layer is placed over the wound to protect and hold NEOX in place. The protective layer is then covered with an adsorptive pad or gauze layer to absorb any excess wound exudate.

REMOVAL

- NEOX 100 is absorbed into the wound bed. No removal of graft is required.

New Product: NEOX CORD 1K

Amniox Medical

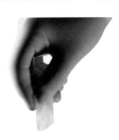

HOW SUPPLIED

NEOX CORD 1K	2 cm × 1 cm (2 sq. cm)	Q4148
NEOX CORD 1K	2 cm × 2 cm (4 sq. cm)	Q4148
NEOX CORD 1K	3 cm × 2 cm (6 sq. cm)	Q4148
NEOX CORD 1K	3 cm × 3 cm (9 sq. cm)	Q4148
NEOX CORD 1K	4 cm × 3 cm (12 sq. cm)	Q4148
NEOX CORD 1K	6 cm × 3 cm (18 sq. cm)	Q4148
NEOX CORD 1K	8 cm × 3 cm (24 sq. cm)	Q4148

ACTION

NEOX CORD 1K Cryopreserved Umbilical Cord allograft immunomodulates inflammation and orchestrates regenerative healing in chronic wounds.

INDICATIONS

NEOX CORD 1K can be used as a wound covering for dermal ulcers or defects.

CONTRAINDICATIONS

- NEOX CORD 1K should not be used on wounds that are actively infected.

APPLICATION

- Wound should be debrided to expose healthy bleeding wound edge, base, and granulation tissue. NEOX CORD 1K is placed on the wound bed and secured with steristrips, staples, or sutures. A nonadherent contact layer is placed over the wound to protect and hold NEOX in place. The protective layer is then covered with an adsorptive pad or gauze layer to absorb any excess wound exudate.

REMOVAL

- NEOX CORD 1K is absorbed into the wound bed. No removal of graft is required.

REFERENCES

1. Raphael A. A single centre, retrospective study of cryopreserved umbilical cord tissue for the treatment of diabetic foot ulcers. *J Wound Care*. 2016;25 Suppl 7:S10–S17.
2. Couture M. A single-center, retrospective study of cryopreserved umbilical cord for wound healing in patients suffering from chronic wounds of the foot and ankle. *Wounds*. 2016;28(7):217–225.
3. Caputo WJ, Vaquero C, Monterosa A, et al. A retrospective study of cryopreserved umbilical cord as an adjunctive therapy to promote the healing of chronic, complex foot ulcers with underlying osteomyelitis. *Wound Repair Regen*. 2016;24(5):885–893.

New Product: NEOX CORD RT

Amniox Medical

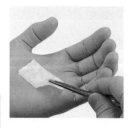

HOW SUPPLIED

NEOX CORD RT	2 cm × 1 cm (2 sq. cm)	Q4148
NEOX CORD RT	2 cm × 2 cm (4 sq. cm)	Q4148
NEOX CORD RT	3 cm × 2 cm (6 sq. cm)	Q4148
NEOX CORD RT	3 cm × 3 cm (9 sq. cm)	Q4148
NEOX CORD RT	4 cm × 3 cm (12 sq. cm)	Q4148
NEOX CORD RT	6 cm × 3 cm (18 sq. cm)	Q4148
NEOX CORD RT	8 cm × 3 cm (24 sq. cm)	Q4148

ACTION

NEOX CORD RT, a hydrated, shelf-stable umbilical cord allograft, immunomodulates inflammation and orchestrates regenerative healing in chronic wounds.

INDICATIONS

NEOX CORD RT can be used as a wound covering for dermal ulcers or defects.

CONTRAINDICATIONS

- NEOX CORD RT should not be used on wounds that are actively infected.

APPLICATION

- Wound should be debrided to expose healthy bleeding wound edge, base, and granulation tissue. NEOX CORD RT is placed on the wound bed and secured with steristrips, staples, or sutures. A nonadherent contact layer is placed over the wound to protect and hold NEOX in place. The protective layer is then covered with an adsorptive pad or gauze layer to absorb any excess wound exudate.

REMOVAL

- NEOX CORD RT is absorbed into the wound bed. No removal of graft is required.

OASIS® Wound Matrix and OASIS® Ultra Tri-Layer Matrix

Smith & Nephew, Inc.
Wound Management

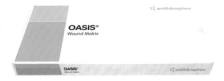

HOW SUPPLIED

OASIS® Wound Matrix	3 × 3.5 cm
OASIS® Wound Matrix	3 × 7 cm
OASIS Ultra Tri-Layer Matrix	3 × 3.5 cm
OASIS Ultra Tri-Layer Matrix	3 × 7 cm
OASIS Ultra Tri-Layer Matrix	5 × 7 cm
OASIS Ultra Tri-Layer Matrix	7 × 10 cm
OASIS Ultra Tri-Layer Matrix	7 × 20 cm

ACTION

OASIS Matrix provides a natural scaffold for host cells to repopulate and revascularize the wound. The ECM biomaterial in OASIS Matrix is infiltrated by the body's own host cells.

OASIS® Wound Matrix is an intact matrix naturally derived from porcine small intestinal submucosa (SIS), indicated for the management of wounds. SIS technology is proven to support the body's own tissue repair mechanisms critical to wound closure.

OASIS® Ultra Tri-Layer Matrix is three layers of bioresorbable extracellular matrix (ECM) that incorporate increased structure into the wound.

INDICATIONS

OASIS® Wound Matrix is indicated for the management of wounds including:
- Partial- and full-thickness wounds.
- Pressure ulcers.
- Venous ulcers.
- Chronic vascular ulcers.
- Tunneled, undermined wounds.
- Diabetic ulcers.
- Trauma wounds (abrasions, lacerations, second-degree burns, skin tears).
- Draining wounds.
- Surgical wounds (donor sites/grafts, post-Mohs surgery, postlaser surgery, podiatric, wound dehiscence).

CONTRAINDICATIONS

- This device is derived from a porcine source and should not be used in patients with known sensitivity to porcine material. This device is not indicated for use in third-degree burns.

APPLICATION

- For ease of handling, apply OASIS® Wound Matrix by placing it in a dry state over the wound.
- Position the dry OASIS® Wound Matrix to completely contact the entire surface of the wound bed and extend slightly beyond all wound margins. If multiple sheets are necessary to cover the wound, slightly overlap the edges of the sheets.

CELLULAR AND TISSUE-BASED PRODUCTS

- As required, securely anchor OASIS® Wound Matrix with physician's preferred fixation method (e.g., STERI-STRIPTM, tissue sealant, bolsters, dissolvable clips, sutures, staples, or other appropriate fixation method) based on the type of wound, location of wound, patient's mobility, and patient compliance.
- Thoroughly rehydrate OASIS® Wound Matrix by applying sterile saline.
- To protect OASIS® Wound Matrix from adhering to the secondary dressing, apply an appropriate nonadherent primary wound dressing over the OASIS® Wound Matrix.
- Apply an appropriate secondary dressing (multi-layer compression bandage system, total contact cast, or other appropriate dressing) that will manage the wound exudate, keep the OASIS® Wound Matrix moist, and keep all layers securely in place.

CELLULAR AND TISSUE-BASED PRODUCTS

New Product: Stravix®

Osiris Therapeutics, Inc.

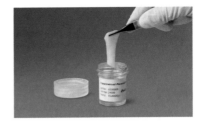

HOW SUPPLIED

Stravix®	2 × 4 cm
Stravix®	3 × 6 cm

PRODUCT DESCRIPTION

Stravix® is cryopreserved placental tissue. Composed of the umbilical amnion and Wharton's Jelly, Stravix retains the extracellular matrix, growth factors, and endogenous neonatal mesenchymal stem cells, fibroblasts, and epithelial cells of the native tissue.

INDICATIONS

Stravix is limited to the homologous use as a wound cover or surgical wrap. The product may be used to cover or wrap acute and chronic wounds, including, but not limited to, diabetic foot ulcers, venous leg ulcers, pressure ulcers, dehisced surgical wounds, burns, acute surgical wounds, pyoderma gangrenosum, and epidermolysis bullosa. Stravix may be used in wounds encompassing both upper extremity and lower extremity. Stravix naturally conforms to complex anatomies and may be used over exposed bone, nerves, tendon, joint capsule, muscle, hardware, and surgical mesh.

CONTRAINDICATIONS

• There are no known contraindications for this product.

APPLICATION

• You will need to thaw the graft following the package insert instructions. Stravix can be folded, trimmed, or cut as required to fit the surgical site using aseptic technique, ensuring allowance for overlap. When applying as a wound cover or surgical wrap, the Wharton's Jelly side (grooved side) should be placed in contact with the tissue being wrapped or covered.

REMOVAL

• Stravix may be trimmed away or removed at the discretion of the treating physician. In most cases it does not need to be removed, and may be reapplied as needed.

CELLULAR AND TISSUE-BASED PRODUCTS

Collagens

ACTION

Collagen, the most abundant protein in the body, is fibrous and insoluble and is produced by fibroblasts. Its fibers are found in connective tissues, including skin, bones, ligaments, and cartilage. During wound healing, collagen encourages the deposition and organization of newly formed collagen fibers and granulation tissue in the wound bed. It also stimulates new tissue development and wound debridement, creating an environment conducive to healing. Collagen dressings are manufactured as sheets, pads, particles, solutions, and gels.

INDICATIONS

Collagen dressings may be used as primary dressings for partial- and full-thickness wounds, infected and noninfected wounds, tunneling wounds, wounds with minimal to heavy exudate (depending on the form of collagen dressing), skin grafts, donor sites, and red or yellow wounds.

ADVANTAGES

- Are absorbent.
- Maintain a moist, wound-healing environment.
- May be used in combination with topical agents.
- Conform well to a wound surface.
- Are nonadherent.
- Are easy to apply and remove.

DISADVANTAGES

- Are not recommended for third-degree burns.
- Are not recommended for black wounds.
- Require a secondary dressing.

HCPCS CODE OVERVIEW

The HCPCS codes normally assigned to collagen dressings are:
A6021—pad size <16 in^2.
A6022—pad size >16 in^2 but <48 in^2.
A6023—pad size >48 in^2.
The HCPCS codes normally assigned to collagen wound fillers are:
A6010—wound filler, dry form, per gram of collagen.
A6011—wound filler, gel/paste, per gram of collagen.
A6024—wound filler, per 6 in.

CellerateRX® Hydrolyzed Collagen Gel

Wound Care Innovations, LLC

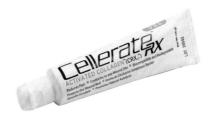

HOW SUPPLIED

Gel, Sterile	28 g	A6011

ACTION

CellerateRX® Hydrolyzed Collagen Gel is Type I bovine hydrolyzed collagen. The gel is approximately 65% hydrolyzed collagen and 35% purified water and contains no additives, synthetics, or fillers. The gel is biocompatible, bioabsorbable, nontoxic, and safe. CellerateRX Gel protects the wound bed and provides the ideal healing environment for newly formed granulation tissue and migrating cells, helping to establish the pace of normal wound healing. It may be used in all wound phases/states.

INDICATIONS

For use in the management of chronic and acute wounds including partial- and full-thickness wounds, pressure injuries 1–4, venous stasis ulcers, arterial ulcers, diabetic ulcers, surgical wounds, traumatic wounds, and first- and second-degree burns. Use the gel on dry or lightly to moderately exudative wounds.

CONTRAINDICATIONS

- Known sensitivities to bovine collagen.
- Not intended for use on third-degree burns.

APPLICATION

- It is recommended that the wound bed be debrided of slough and necrotic tissue.
- Cleanse the wound per protocol.
- Apply gel onto the wound bed approximately the thickness of a quarter (2–3 mm).
- The product should cover the entire wound bed and the edges of the wound, including any areas of undermining or tunneling.
- Cover with an appropriate dressing that maintains the optimum moisture level.
- Infected wounds are treated per physician direction.

REAPPLICATION

- Reapply CellerateRX Gel daily, with each dressing change, or a minimum of two to three times per week, taking care not to disrupt the wound site.

REFERENCE

1. www.Celleraterx.com

CellerateRX® Hydrolyzed Collagen Powder

Wound Care Innovations, LLC

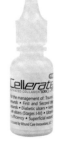

HOW SUPPLIED

Powder	1 g	A6010

ACTION

CellerateRX® Hydrolyzed Collagen Powder is Type I bovine hydrolyzed collagen and contains no additives, synthetics, or fillers. The powder is biocompatible, bioabsorbable, nontoxic, and safe. CellerateRX Powder protects the wound bed and provides the ideal healing environment for newly formed granulation tissue and migrating cells, helping to establish the pace of normal wound healing. It may be used in all wound phases/states.

INDICATIONS

For use in the management of chronic and acute wounds including partial- and full-thickness wounds, pressure injuries 1 to 4, venous stasis ulcers, arterial ulcers, diabetic ulcers, surgical wounds, traumatic wounds, and first- and second-degree burns. Use the powder on moderately to heavily exudative wounds.

CONTRAINDICATIONS

- Known sensitivities to bovine collagen.
- Not intended for use on third-degree burns.

APPLICATION

- It is recommended that the wound bed be debrided of slough and necrotic tissue.
- Cleanse the wound per protocol.
- Apply powder onto the wound bed approximately the thickness of a quarter (2 to 3 mm).
- The product should cover the entire wound bed and the edges of the wound, including any areas of undermining or tunneling.
- Cover with an appropriate dressing that maintains the optimum moisture level.
- Infected wounds are treated per physician direction.

REMOVAL

- Reapply CellerateRX Powder daily, with each dressing change, or a minimum of two to three times per week, taking care not to disrupt the wound site.

REFERENCE

1. www.Celleraterx.com

COLLAGENS

Collagen

Gentell

HOW SUPPLIED

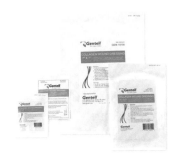

Pad	2″ × 2″	A6021
Pad	4″ × 4″	A6022
Pad	7″ × 7″	A6023
Particles	1 g	A6010

ACTION

Gentell Collagen is a primary dressing for management of pressure ulcers, diabetic ulcers, venous ulcers, arterial ulcers, burns, sores, blisters, and scrapes.

INDICATIONS

Gentell Collagen is a primary dressing for use on Stage 2–4 wounds with little to moderate exudate, diabetic skin ulcers, venous stasis ulcers, first and second-degree burns, post-surgical incisions, cuts and abrasions.

CONTRAINDICATIONS

- Do not use if allergic to bovine-derived materials.

APPLICATION

- Irrigate the wound with Gentell Wound Cleanser and gently dry the skin surrounding the wound site.
- Apply Gentell Collagen Wound Dressing directly to the wound bed. If the wound is dry (without exudate), Gentell Collagen may be moistened with Gentell Wound Cleanser before applying to the wound.
- Cover wound with a secondary dressing such as Gentell Bordered Gauze or Gentell Comfortell™.

REMOVAL

- Change daily or as ordered by a physician.

New Product: DermaCol

DermaRite Industries, LLC

HOW SUPPLIED

Collagen Matrix Dressing	2″ × 2″	A6021
Collagen Matrix Dressing	4″ × 4″	A6021

ACTION

DermaCol™ is an advanced wound dressing made from collagen, sodium alginate, carboxyl methylcellulose, and ethylenediaminetetraacetic acid (EDTA). DermaCol is a topically applied wound dressing that will transform into a soft gel sheet when in contact with wound exudates. The dressing maintains a moist wound environment that aids in the formation of granulation tissue and epithelialization. The EDTA in the dressing removes zinc to inhibit the activity of matrix metalloproteinases (MMP), thus creating a suitable environment for wound healing. DermaCol dressings may be trimmed and layered for the management of deep wounds.

INDICATIONS

DermaCol is indicated for management of full- and partial-thickness wounds including: pressure ulcers, diabetic ulcers, ulcers caused by mixed vascular etiologies, venous ulcers, donor and graft sites, abrasions, traumatic wounds healing by secondary intention, dehisced surgical wounds, and first- and second-degree burns.

CONTRAINDICATIONS

- DermaCol Dressing should not be used on patients with a known allergy or sensitivity to collagen, any other ingredient, or on third-degree burns.
- If sensitivity to DermaCol develops, discontinue use.
- DermaCol may be used under compression therapy under the supervision of a health care professional.

APPLICATION

- Debride and irrigate the wound bed with an appropriate wound cleanser or distilled water before application.
- Cut the dressing to fit the exact wound size. For heavily exuding wounds, apply the dressing directly to the wound bed. For dry wounds with very little exudate, moisten the wound bed with distilled water to begin the gelling process.
- Cover the DermaCol with an appropriate secondary dressing.
- Change dressings daily or as good nursing practice dictates.

REMOVAL

- Remove the secondary dressing with care. Gently remove DermaCol ensuring that the dressing removal does not damage any newly formed tissues.
- Use an appropriate wound cleanser or distilled water to cleanse the wound site prior to applying a new DermaCol dressing as per application instructions.

REFERENCE

1. http://dermarite.com/product/dermacol/

COLLAGENS

New Product: DermaCol 100

DermaRite Industries, LLC

HOW SUPPLIED

Type 1 Bovine Collagen Powder Wound Filler Dressing	1 gram	A6010

ACTION

DermaCol 100 is a Type 1 bovine collagen powder wound filler dressing.

DermaCol 100 is topically applied and designed to come into contact with wound exudate. It maintains a moist wound environment at the wound surface.

INDICATIONS

DermaCol™ 100 is intended for use in the management of partial and full thickness wounds, pressure (stage I to IV) and venous ulcers, ulcers caused by mixed vascular etiologies, venous stasis and diabetic ulcers, first- and second-degree burns, cuts, abrasions and surgical wounds.

CONTRAINDICATIONS

• Do not use on patients with a known allergy or sensitivity to bovine-derived materials.

APPLICATION

• Cleanse wound with advised liquid to remove residue according to local infection control protocol. Deep wounds should be well irrigated.
• Skin around wound should be clean and dry. Use skin barrier prep as needed.
• Apply DermaCol 100 in a layer approximately 1/4″ thick. Do not pack tightly.
• Cover with nonadherent dressing.
• Repeat process as needed.

REMOVAL

• Dressing may be moistened to ease removal.
• Carefully remove adhesive dressings by holding the edge of the dressing and slowly pulling it parallel to the skin.
• Dispose of in accordance with local guidance.

REFERENCE

1. http://dermarite.com/

COLLAGENS

New Product: Endoform® Natural Dermal Template*

Appulse
Aroa Biosurgery Limited Marketed in the US by Appulse

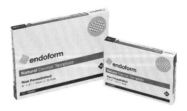

HOW SUPPLIED

Endoform Natural, Fenestrated	2" × 2"	A6021
Endoform Natural, Fenestrated	4" × 5"	A6022
Endoform Natural, Nonfenestrated	2" × 2"	A6021
Endoform Natural, Nonfenestrated	4" × 5"	A6022

ACTION

Endoform™ Natural Dermal Template is a collagen dressing with an intact extracellular matrix (ECM). Derived from ovine (sheep) forestomach tissue, this advanced wound care dressing is non-reconstituted collagen, thus it retains the innate biological structure of the native ECM associated macromolecules including elastin, fibronectin, glycosaminoglycans and laminin. When rehydrated with wound exudate or sterile saline, Endoform Natural Dermal Template transforms into a soft conforming sheet, which is naturally incorporated into the wound over time. Not made with natural rubber latex.

INDICATIONS

Endoform™ Natural Dermal Template is indicated for the management of wounds including:
- Partial- and full-thickness wounds.
- Pressure ulcers.
- Venous ulcers.
- Diabetic ulcers.
- Chronic vascular ulcers.
- Tunneled/undermined wounds.
- Surgical wounds (donor sites, grafts, post-Moh's surgery, post-laser surgery, podiatric, and wound dehiscence).
- Traumatic wounds (abrasions, lacerations, first- and second-degree burns, and skin tears).
- Draining wounds.

CONTRAINDICATIONS

- Endoform™ Natural Dermal Template is derived from an ovine (sheep) source and should not be used on patients with known sensitivity to ovine (sheep) derived material.
- Endoform™ Natural Dermal Template is not indicated for use on third-degree burns.

PRECAUTIONS

- Do not apply to wounds with uncontrolled clinical infection, acute inflammation, excessive exudate, or bleeding.
- Endoform™ Natural Dermal Template is supplied as a sterile dressing. Do not use if the pouch seal is broken.
- Discard the device if mishandling has caused possible damage or contamination.
- Single use product. Do not attempt to re-sterilize. Discard all unused portions. Do not reuse.
- Always handle Endoform™ Natural Dermal Template using aseptic technique.

COLLAGENS

APPLICATION

- These recommendations are designed to serve only as a general guideline. They are not intended to supersede institutional protocols or professional clinical judgment concerning patient care.
- **Wound Preparation.**
  - Prepare the wound bed by cleansing, irrigation and if necessary debridement to ensure the wound is free of debris, necrotic tissue or infected tissue.
- **Dressing Application.**
  - Select a sheet of the dermal template which is slightly larger than the wound and apply aseptically.
  - Endoform™ Natural Dermal Template can be applied as a wholensheet or trimmed so that it contacts the wound margins. Multiple sheets can be used to cover the entire wound bed.
  - For ease of handling, apply the dermal template by placing the dry material in the wound and rehydrating with exudate or sterile saline. When hydrated Endoform™ Natural Dermal Template transforms into a soft conforming sheet. Ensure that the dermal template conforms to the underlying wound bed.
  - To protect Endoform™ Natural Dermal Template from adhering to the secondary dressing, consider applying a non-adherent dressing over the dermal template to help protect the tissue while facilitating an optimal moist wound healing environment.
  - Secure the dermal template using an appropriate secondary dressing. The overlying dressing should be changed according to standard of care taking into account the level of exudate.
  - The biodegradable Endoform™ Natural Dermal Template is naturally absorbed and incorporated into the wound over time. Endoform™ Natural Dermal Template may last up to 7 days in the wound, depending on the wound environment.
  - Endoform™ Natural Dermal Template can be used in conjunction with compression therapy and negative pressure wound therapy under the supervision of a health care provider.
- **Dressing Changes.**
  - Duration of treatment and reapplication is determined by the physician and depends upon the wound type and conditions.
  - Reapply when the dermal template has been incorporated into the wound. It is recommended to assess the wound within 72 hours. Endoform™ Dermal Template may last up to 7 days in the wound, depending on the wound environment.
  - Carefully cleanse the wound surface in accordance with established procedures. Do not attempt to remove the off-white to golden gel that forms from residual Endoform™ Natural Dermal Template in the wound as it contains extracellular matrix components that assist in wound healing.
  - If areas of the dermal template are dry upon inspection, rehydrate with sterile saline and leave in place.
  - It is not necessary to remove any residual Endoform™ Natural Dermal Template during dressing changes. However, if the product has been overlapped onto the periwound area, the remaining loose product that has not incorporated into the wound may be gently removed around the edges if desired.
  - Change the secondary dressings as needed, and when Endoform™ Natural Dermal Template is re-applied.

DRESSING CHANGES

- Carefully cleanse the wound surface in accordance with established procedures. It is not necessary to remove the residual Endoform Natural that forms, as it contains ECM

COLLAGENS

components that assist in wound healing. Depending on the exudate color, the residual product may appear as an off-white to golden gel.

- Reapply Endoform Natural every 5 to 7 days or as needed, until the wound has reepithelialized. Duration of treatment is determined by the physician and depends upon the wound type and conditions.
- It is not necessary to remove any residual Endoform Natural during dressing changes. However, if the product has been overlapped onto the periwound area, and if desired, the remaining loose product that has not incorporated into the wound may be gently removed around the edges.
- Change the cover dressing as needed, and when Endoform Natural is reapplied.

*See package insert for complete instructions for use.

New Product: FIBRACOL™ Plus Collagen Wound Dressing with Alginate

Systagenix, An ACELITY™ Company

HOW SUPPLIED

FIBRACOL™ Plus Collagen Wound Dressing with Alginate	2" × 2"	A6021
FIBRACOL™ Plus Collagen Wound Dressing with Alginate	4" × 4 3/8"	A6022
FIBRACOL™ Plus Collagen Wound Dressing with Alginate	4" × 8 3/4"	A6022
FIBRACOL™ Plus Collagen Wound Dressing with Alginate	3/8" × 3/8" × 15 3/8"	A6024

ACTION

FIBRACOL™ Plus Collagen Wound Dressing with Alginate is an advanced wound care device composed of collagen and calcium alginate fibers. FIBRACOL™ Plus Dressing contains 80% more collagen than our traditional FIBRACOL™ Dressing. Its unique combination of natural biopolymers created by a patented process combines the structural support of collagen and the gel-forming properties of alginates into a sterile, soft, absorbent, and conformable topical wound dressing. In the presence of wound fluid, FIBRACOL™ Plus Dressing maintains a physiologically moist microenvironment at the wound surface that is conducive to granulation tissue formation, epithelialization, and enables healing to proceed at a rapid rate. FIBRACOL™ Plus Dressing is versatile as a primary wound dressing. It can be cut to the exact size of the wound, multilayered for the management of deep wounds, and used in combination with either a semi-occlusive or nonocclusive secondary dressing.

INDICATIONS

FIBRACOL™ Plus Dressing is indicated for the management of exuding wounds including:
- Full- and partial-thickness wounds.
- Pressure ulcers.
- Venous ulcers.
- Ulcers caused by mixed vascular etiologies.
- Diabetic ulcers.
- Second-degree burns.
- Donor sites and other bleeding surface wounds.
- Abrasions.
- Traumatic wounds healing by secondary intention.
- Dehisced surgical incisions.

FIBRACOL™ Plus Dressing may be used with visible signs of infection present in the wound area only when proper medical treatment addresses the underlying cause. FIBRACOL™ Plus Dressing may be used under compression therapy with health care professional supervision.

COLLAGENS

CONTRAINDICATIONS

- FIBRACOL™ Plus Dressing is not indicated for wounds with active vasculitis, third-degree burns, or patients with known sensitivity to collagen or alginates.

APPLICATION

- Debride when necessary and irrigate the wound site with normal saline solution.
- Remove excess solution from surrounding skin.
- For heavily exuding wounds, apply to wound bed directly. For wounds with minimal exudate, apply to moistened wound bed; this will initiate the gel-forming process.
- Pack deep wounds loosely. The dressing can be cut to size with sterile scissors. The amount of FIRBACOL™ Plus Dressing to be used depends on the size of the wound and the amount of exudate.
- FIBRACOL™ Plus Dressing may be covered with either a nonocclusive secondary dressing and fixed to the skin with a nonirritating tape or a semi-occlusive dressing (e.g., TIELLE™ Hydropolymer Adhesive Dressing or TIELLE™ Plus Hydropolymer Adhesive Dressing).
- Reapply FIBRACOL™ Plus Dressing when the secondary dressing has reached its absorbent capacity or whenever good wound care practice dictates that the dressing should be changed. A heavily exuding wound may require daily or twice daily dressing changes. More moderately exudating wounds will require less frequent changes (every 2 to 4 days or as directed by a health care professional). Following the initial application, irrigate the wound with saline solution. Reapply FIBRACOL™ Plus Dressing as previously instructed.

REMOVAL

- After gently removing the secondary dressing, lift any FIBRACOL™ Plus Dressing that has not formed a gel and discard. Using normal saline, gently irrigate the wound to remove any residual gel.
- Do not reuse.
- Do not resterilize.
- Do not use if the package is damaged.
- The use by date of this product is printed on the packaging.

REFERENCE

1. Van Gils CC, Roeder B, Chesler SM, Mason S. Improved healing with a collagen-alginate dressing in the chemical matricectomy. *J Am Podiatric Med Assoc.* 1998;88(9):452–456.

COLLAGENS

New Product: HELIX3-CM®
Collagen Matrix

AMERX Health Care Corp.

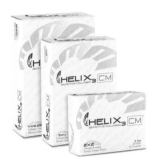

HOW SUPPLIED

Pads	2″ × 2″	A6021
Pads	3″ × 4″	A6021
Pads	4″ × 5.25″	A6022

ACTION

100% type-I bovine collagen, HELIX3® Bioactive Collagen provides moist healing of draining wounds and absorbs excess wound fluids.

INDICATIONS

Management of burns, sores, blisters, ulcers, and other wounds.

CONTRAINDICATIONS

- Do not use if allergic to bovine-derived materials.

APPLICATION

- Cleanse the wound with a sterile wound cleanser.
- Apply HELIX3-CM to the wound.
- Cover HELIX3-CM with a nonadherent dressing.
- Change the dressing daily or as indicated.

REMOVAL

- Gently remove the secondary dressing and any remaining HELIX3-CM. If the HELIX3-CM has become adhered to the wound, irrigate with sterile saline solution. Lift gently. If the HELIX3-CM is still adherent after irrigation, DO NOT attempt to remove.

REFERENCE

1. www.podiatrym.com/pdf/2015/11/Brenner1115web.pdf

COLLAGENS

New Product: HELIX3-CP® Collagen Powder

AMERX Health Care Corp.

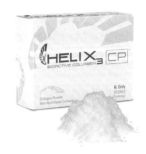

HOW SUPPLIED

Packets	10 1-g	A6010

ACTION

100% type I bovine collagen, HELIX3® Bioactive Collagen provides moist healing of draining wounds and absorbs excess wound fluids.

INDICATIONS

Management of burns, sores, blisters, ulcers, and other wounds.

CONTRAINDICATIONS

- Do not use if allergic to bovine-derived materials.

APPLICATION

- Cleanse the wound with a sterile wound cleanser.
- Apply HELIX3-CP in a layer approximately 1/4 inch thick to the wound surface.
- Do not pack the wound tightly.
- Cover with a non-adherent dressing.
- Change dressing daily or as indicated.

REMOVAL

- If secondary dressing is adhered to the wound, irrigate with sterile saline until dressing loosens. Lift gently. Irrigate wound with saline solution to cleanse the area thoroughly to remove all traces of foreign bodies present in the wound bed.

REFERENCE

1. www.podiatrym.com/pdf/2015/11/Brenner1115web.pdf

New Product: Puracol® Ultra Powder

Medline Industries, Inc.

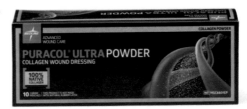

HOW SUPPLIED

100% collagen powder	1 gram	A6010

ACTION

Puracol® Ultra Powder is a powder-like fibrillar collagen microsponge, a native Type I porcine dermis collagen that is composed of specific amino acids. The building blocks that make up collagen are called amino acids. Collagen is primarily present in connective tissue and found in skin, tendon and ligament. Puracol® Ultra Powder is a sterile wound exudate absorber and filler. Puracol® Ultra Powder protects the wound bed and delicate newly regenerated granulation tissue. Puracol® Ultra Powder interacts with the wound by absorbing the wound's fluids forming a gel-like barrier and provides a moist healing environment.

INDICATIONS

Puracol® Ultra Powder is indicated for the management of full- and partial-thickness wounds including; pressure ulcers, diabetic ulcers caused by mixed vascular origin, venous ulcers, donor and graft sites, abrasions, traumatic wounds healing by secondary intention, dehisced surgical wounds, first- and second-degree burns.

CONTRAINDICATIONS

- Do not use on individuals with a known sensitivity to collagen.

APPLICATION

- Cleanse the burn or wound in accordance with normal procedures.
- Apply, from the product envelope, a uniform layer of Puracol® Ultra Powder directly onto the wound site.
- Cover the wound with an appropriate moisture retentive secondary dressing.
  Note: Superficial wounds such as cuts and abrasions may not require a secondary dressing due to the film that forms on the wound site if permitted to dry.
- Reapply Puracol® Ultra Powder and redress as needed.

REMOVAL

- Puracol Ultra Powder is 100% biodegradable and does not need to be removed from the wound bed.

REFERENCE

1. https://www.medline.com/product/Puracol-Ultra-Powder-Collagen-Wound-Dressing/Collagen-Dressings/Z05-PF150512?question=Puracol±Ultra±Powder&index=P1&indexCount=1

COLLAGENS

PROMOGRAN PRISMA™ Matrix

Systagenix, An ACELITY™ Company

HOW SUPPLIED

PROMOGRAN PRISMA™ Matrix	4.34 sq. in. Hexagon	A6021
PROMOGRAN PRISMA™ Matrix	19.1 sq. in. Hexagon	A6022

ACTION

PROMOGRAN PRISMA™ Matrix is comprised of a sterile, freeze-dried composite of 44% oxidized regenerated cellulose (ORC), 55% collagen, and 1% silver ORC. Silver ORC contains 25% w/w ionically bound silver, a well-known antimicrobial agent. In the presence of an exudate, the PROMOGRAN PRISMA™ Matrix transforms into a soft, conformable, biodegradable gel, and thus allows contact with all areas of the wound. PROMOGRAN PRISMA™ Matrix, when covered with a semi-occlusive dressing, maintains a physiologically moist microenvironment at the wound surface. This environment is conducive to granulation tissue formation, epithelialization, and optimal wound healing. PROMOGRAN PRISMA™ Matrix provides an effective antibacterial barrier as demonstrated by the in-vitro reduction of bacterial growth with common wound pathogens such as, *Pseudomonas aeruginosa, Staphylococcus aureus, Escherichia coli*, and *Streptococcus pyogenes*. Reduction of bacterial bioburden in the dressing may result in reduced risk of infection. Literature reports of in-vitro testing indicate that collagen fibers provide a biodegradable matrix for cellular invasion and capillary growth. In laboratory testing, collagen-ORC has been shown to absorb components of the wound exudate.

INDICATIONS

PROMOGRAN PRISMA™ Matrix is intended for the management of exuding wounds. Under the supervision of a health care professional, PROMOGRAN PRISMA™ Matrix may be used for the management of diabetic ulcers, venous ulcers, pressure ulcers, ulcers caused by mixed vascular etiologies, full- and partial-thickness wounds, donor site and other bleeding surface wounds, abrasions, traumatic wounds healing by secondary intention, and dehisced surgical wounds. PROMOGRAN PRISMA™ Matrix may be used under compression therapy with health care professional supervision.

CONTRAINDICATIONS

- PROMOGRAN PRISMA™ Matrix in not indicated for third-degree burns, or patients with known sensitivity to silver, ORC, or collagen.

APPLICATION

- Prepare the wound per your standard wound care protocol and debride when necessary.
- PROMOGRAN PRISMA™ Matrix may be used when visible signs of infection are present in the wound area only when proper medical treatment addresses the underlying cause.
- Hydrate with saline for wounds with low or no exudate.
- Apply directly to wound, covering the entire wound bed. PROMOGRAN PRISMA™ Matrix forms a gel on contact with exudate or through saline hydration.

COLLAGENS

- Cover PROMOGRAN PRISMA™ Matrix with a secondary dressing to maintain a moist wound healing environment.
- Choose a suitable secondary dressing depending on the level of the exudate.

REMOVAL

- It is not necessary to remove any residual PROMOGRAN PRISMA™ Matrix during dressing changes as it will be naturally absorbed into the body over time.
- After initial treatment, remove secondary dressing and retreat the wound with PROMOGRAN PRISMA™ Matrix up to every 72 hours depending upon the amount of exudates.
- Cover with new secondary dressing.

REFERENCES

1. Gottrup F, Cullen BM, Karlsmark T, Bischoff-Mikkelsen M, Nisbet L, Gibson MC. Randomized controlled trial on collagen/oxidized regenerated cellulose/silver treatment. *Wound Repair Regen* 2013; 21(2):216–225.
2. Duffy GP, McFadden TM, Byrne EM, Gill SL, Farrell E, O'Brien FJ. Towards in vitro vascularization of collagen-GAG scaffolds. *Eur Cell Mater* 2011;21:15–30.

COLLAGENS

PROMOGRAN™ Matrix Wound Dressing

Systagenix, An ACELITY™ Company

HOW SUPPLIED

PROMOGRAN™ Matrix Wound Dressing	4.34 sq. in. Hexagon	A6021
PROMOGRAN™ Matrix Wound Dressing	19.1 sq. in. Hexagon	A6022

ACTION

PROMOGRAN™ Matrix Wound Dressing is an advanced wound care device comprised of a sterile, freeze-dried composite of 45% oxidized regenerated cellulose (ORC) and 55% collagen. In the presence of exudate the PROMOGRAN™ Matrix transforms into a soft, conformable, biodegradable gel, and thus allows contact with all areas of the wound. PROMOGRAN™ Matrix maintains a physiologically moist microenvironment at the wound surface. This environment is conducive to granulation tissue formation, epithelialization, and rapid wound healing.

INDICATIONS

PROMOGRAN™ Matrix is intended for the management of exuding wounds. Under the supervision of a health care professional, PROMOGRAN™ Matrix may be used for the management of diabetic ulcers, venous ulcers, pressure ulcers, ulcers caused by mixed vascular etiologies, full- and partial-thickness wounds, donor site and other bleeding surface wounds, abrasions, traumatic wounds healing by secondary intention, and dehisced surgical wounds. PROMOGRAN™ Matrix may be used under compression therapy with health care professional supervision.

CONTRAINDICATIONS

- PROMOGRAN™ Matrix is not indicated for wounds with active vasculitis, third-degree burns, or patients with known sensitivity to ORC or collagen.

APPLICATION

- Prepare the wound per your standard wound care protocol and debride when necessary.
- PROMOGRAN™ Matrix may be used when visible signs of infection are present in the wound area only when proper medical treatment addresses the underlying cause.
- Hydrate with saline for wounds with low or no exudate.
- Apply directly to wound, covering the entire wound bed. PROMOGRAN™ Matrix forms a gel on contact with exudate or through saline hydration.
- Cover PROMOGRAN™ Matrix with a secondary dressing to maintain a moist wound healing environment.
- Choose a suitable secondary dressing depending on level of exudate.

REMOVAL

- It is not necessary to remove any residual PROMOGRAN™ Matrix during dressing changes as it will be naturally absorbed into the body over time.

COLLAGENS

- After initial treatment, remove secondary dressing and retreat the wound with PRO-MOGRAN™ Matrix up to every 72 hours depending upon the amount of exudates.
- Cover with new secondary dressing.

REFERENCES

1. Nisi G, Brandi C, Grimaldi L, Calabrò M, D'Aniello C. Use of a protease-modulating matrix in the treatment of pressure sores. *Chir Ital* 2005;57(4):465–468.
2. Veves A, Sheehan P, Pham HT. A randomized, controlled trial of Promogran (a collagen/oxidized regenerated cellulose dressing) vs standard treatment in the management of diabetic foot ulcers. *Arch Surg* 2002;137:822–827.
3. Vin F, Teot L, Meaume S. The healing properties of Promogran in venous leg ulcers. *J Wound Care* 2002;11(9):335–341.

COLLAGENS

Stimulen™

Southwest Technologies, Inc.

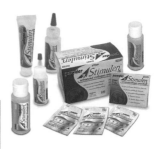

HOW SUPPLIED

Powder	1 g (10 packs/box, 10 boxes/case)	A6010
Powder	10 g (12 bottles/case)	A6010
Powder	20 g (12 bottles/case)	A6010
Collagen Gel	0.5 oz (12 tubes/case)	A6011
Collagen Gel	1 oz (12 tubes/case)	A6011
Lotion	2 oz (12 bottles/case)	

ACTION

Stimulen™ is a new collagen line that comes in various forms: powder (which is 100% collagen), collagen gel, and lotion are that contains collagen and glycerin. These collagen products are combined with long and short polypeptides. The long strands offer a "bridge" to connect wound edge to wound edge, providing a lattice, and the short are broken down into the amino acid form so that the body can readily create and use a healing environment especially suited for the rapid regeneration of cells and tissue.

INDICATIONS

Stimluen® products used for stalled wounds or wounds in compromised patients, for full- and partial-thickness wounds, pressure ulcers (stages I to IV), venous and diabetic ulcers, partial-thickness burns, acute and chronic wounds, and traumatic wounds healing by secondary intention.

CONTRAINDICATIONS

- Allergies to bovine.

APPLICATION

Powder

- Prepare the wound site using the standard protocol. If the wound is highly contaminated, a preliminary treatment to reduce bioburden may be appropriate.
- Open the package, and apply Stimulen to the wound site. Apply a generous covering of powder over the entire wound surface, to 1/8" deep. The nature of the wound will be a factor to consider when applying the product.
- Cover the dressing with a nonadherent secondary dressing, and secure with tape or appropriate covering.
- Maintain a moist, not wet, wound healing environment.
- Change the secondary dressing, and reapply the Stimulen powder daily or as needed.

Collagen gel

- Before use, remove cap and peel off the safety seal.
- Cleanse the wound using standard protocol.
- Apply a generous coating of the collagen gel onto wound site, or fill wound cavity.

- Cover the dressing with a nonadherent secondary dressing, and secure with tape or appropriate covering.
- Change the secondary dressing, and reapply the collagen gel daily or as needed.

Lotion

- Before use, remove cap and peel off the safety seal.
- Cleanse the wound using standard protocol.
- Apply 2 to 4 drops of the lotion, and spread evenly over the affected area.

REMOVAL

- Remove the dressing, gel, or lotion according to your facility's policy.

COLLAGENS

Composites

ACTION

Composite dressings combine two or more physically distinct products and are manufactured as a single dressing with several functions. Features must include a physical (not chemical) bacterial barrier that is present over the entire dressing pad and extends out into the adhesive border; an absorptive layer other than an alginate or other fiber-gelling dressing, foam, hydrocolloid, or hydrogel; and either a semiadherent or nonadherent property over the wound site.

INDICATIONS

Composite dressings may be used as primary or secondary dressings for partial- and full-thickness wounds with minimal to heavy exudate, healthy granulation tissue, or necrotic tissue (slough or moist eschar), or mixed wounds (granulation and necrotic tissue).

ADVANTAGES

- May facilitate autolytic debridement.
- Allow for exchange of moisture vapor.
- Mold well.
- May be used on infected wounds.
- Are easy to apply and remove.
- Include an adhesive border.

DISADVANTAGES

- Require a border of intact skin for anchoring the dressing.

HCPCS CODE OVERVIEW

The HCPCS codes normally assigned to composite dressings with an adhesive border are:
A6203—pad size ≤ 16 in^2.
A6204—pad size >16 in^2 but ≤ 48 in^2.
A6205—pad size >48 in^2.

Comfortell Water-Resistant Composite Dressing

Gentell

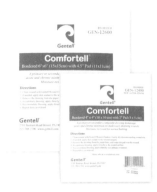

HOW SUPPLIED

Dressing	4″ × 4″	A6203
Dressing	6″ × 6″	A6203
Dressing	8″ × 8″	A6204

ACTION

Gentell Comfortell™ is a composite wound dressing with four distinct layers and a waterresistant border. Comfortell combines an absorbent layer with a selectively permeable barrier that enables the wound to breathe while keeping out contaminants. Comfortell™ can be a primary dressing over a postoperative site, sutures, or skin tears, and can also be applied as a secondary dressing with impregnated gauzes, wound fillers, and enzymatic ointments.

INDICATIONS

Apply Gentell's Comfortell as a cover dressing for any primary or secondary treatment.

CONTRAINDICATIONS

- None.

APPLICATION

- Irrigate the wound with Gentell Wound Cleanser and gently dry the skin surrounding the wound site.
- As a primary dressing, apply directly to the wound surface.
- As a secondary dressing, apply directly over primary treatment.

REMOVAL

- Change daily or as ordered by a physician.

Covaderm® Composite Dressing

DeRoyal

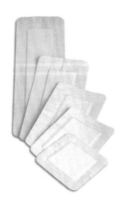

HOW SUPPLIED

Multilayered Pad with Fabric Tape Border	2 1/2" × 2 1/2" with 4" × 4"	A6254
Multilayered Pad with Fabric Tape Border	2 1/2" × 4" with 4" × 6"	A6254
Multilayered Pad with Fabric Tape Border	2" × 5 1/2" with 4" × 8"	A6254
Multilayered Pad with Fabric Tape Border	2" × 7 1/2" with 4" × 10"	A6254
Multilayered Pad with Fabric Tape Border	2" × 11" with 4" × 14"	A6255

ACTION

Covaderm® Composite Dressing is an absorbent island dressing with a protective, air-permeable, adhesive fabric tape border for aseptic, one-step application. Rounded edges conform to jointed, curved, or irregular wound areas.

INDICATIONS

For use as a primary or secondary dressing to manage surgical incisions, superficial lacerations, and abrasions; may also be used as an all-purpose dressing.

CONTRAINDICATIONS

- None provided by the manufacturer.

APPLICATION

- Peel back the edge of the folded release liner.
- Anchor the exposed edge of the tape to the skin and then peel off the remaining release paper.
- Smooth all the tape edges onto the skin.

REMOVAL

- Carefully lift the edges of the tape and peel off the dressing.

COMPOSITES

Covaderm Plus

DeRoyal

HOW SUPPLIED

Multilayered Pad with Fabric Tape Border	1″ pad with 2″ tape	A6203
Multilayered Pad with Fabric Tape Border	1 1/2″ pad with 2 1/2″ tape	A6203
Multilayered Pad with Fabric Tape Border	2 1/2″ pad with 4″ tape	A6203
Multilayered Pad with Fabric Tape Border	2 × 7 1/2″ pad with 4″ × 10″ tape	A6203
Multilayered Pad with Fabric Tape Border	4″ pad with 6″ tape	A6203
Multilayered Pad with Fabric Tape Border	2 1/2″ diameter pad with 4″ diameter tape with 2″ radial slit	A6203
Multilayered Pad with Fabric Tape Border	2″ × 11″ pad with 4″ × 14″ tape	A6204
Multilayered Pad with Fabric Tape Border	4″ × 6″ pad with 6″ × 8″ tape	A6204

ACTION

Covaderm Plus is an adhesive barrier composite wound dressing that consists of a protective, nonadherent wound contact layer; a soft drainage absorption pad; a semiocclusive polyurethane film (to maintain moisture, prevent contamination, and allow vapor transmission); and a conformable adhesive tape border.

INDICATIONS

For use as a primary or secondary dressing to manage pressure ulcers (stages 1 to 4), leg ulcers, IV sites, chronic wounds, and surgical wounds; may also be used on partial- and full-thickness wounds, burns, tunneling wounds, infected and noninfected wounds, wounds with moderate drainage, wounds with serosanguineous or purulent drainage, and red, yellow, or black wounds; may also be used to cover orthopedic incisions and joint pins under casts.

CONTRAINDICATIONS

- None provided by the manufacturer.

APPLICATION

- Peel the dressing's backing from the center to expose the pad.
- Apply the pad over the cleansed wound, making sure that adhesive tape does not touch the wound site.
- Remove the product's backing one side at a time, and smooth the dressing into place.

REMOVAL

- Carefully lift the edges of the tape, and peel off the dressing.

COMPOSITES

Covaderm Plus VAD

DeRoyal

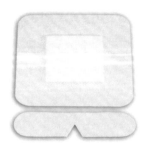

HOW SUPPLIED

Multilayered Dressing	4" × 4"	A6203
Multilayered Dressing	6" × 6"	A6203

ACTION

The Covaderm Plus Vascular Access Device (VAD) dressing is a multilayered dressing that provides protection, bacterial barrier, absorption, cushioning, and conformability and also has an extra tape that is uniquely shaped to seal around the vascular access catheter extension.

INDICATIONS

For use with central venous catheter sites (subclavian, jugular, femoral, and antecubital); peripheral IV sites; implanted parts; and midline catheters.

CONTRAINDICATIONS

- None provided by the manufacturer.

APPLICATION

- Peel the dressing's backing from the center to expose the pad.
- Apply the pad over the cleansed wound, making sure that adhesive tape does not touch the wound site.
- Remove the product's backing one side at a time, and smooth the dressing into place.

REMOVAL

- Carefully lift the edges of the tape, and peel off the dressing.

DermaDress™

DermaRite Industries, LLC

HOW SUPPLIED

Dressing	4″ × 4″	A6203
Dressing	4″ × 10″	A6203
Dressing	4″ × 14″	A6204
Dressing	6″ × 6″	A6203
Dressing	6″ × 8″	A6204

ACTION

DermaDress™ is a multilayered waterproof composite dressing. Its low adherent pad absorbs exudate and protects the wound. A nonwoven waterproof backing with adhesive tape holds the dressing in place and provides a bacterial barrier.

INDICATIONS

May be used as a primary or secondary dressing for the management of acute or chronic partial- and full-thickness wounds/ulcers with minimal to moderate drainage.

CONTRAINDICATIONS

- DermaDress should not be used on people who are sensitive or allergic to the dressing and its components.

APPLICATION

- Cleanse wound with advised liquid to remove residue according to local infection control protocol. Deep wounds should be well irrigated.
- Skin around wound should be clean and dry; use skin barrier prep as needed.
- Remove dressing from package.
- Remove backing paper from dressing.
- Apply sticky side of dressing to moist wound bed overlapping 1 to 2 inches of dry skin; gently smooth into place.

REMOVAL

- Dressing may be moistened to ease removal.
- Carefully remove adhesive dressings by holding the edge of the dressing and slowly pulling it parallel to the skin.
- Dispose of in accordance with local guidance.

REFERENCE

1. http://dermarite.com/product/dermadress/

COMPOSITES

New Product: DermaView™ II Island

DermaRite Industries, LLC

HOW SUPPLIED

Transparent Film Island Wound Dressing	2.75″ × 4″	
Transparent Film Island Wound Dressing	2″ × 2.75″	
Transparent Film Island Wound Dressing	3.5″ × 4″	
Transparent Film Island Wound Dressing	3.5″ × 10″	A6203
Transparent Film Island Wound Dressing	6″ × 6″	A6203

ACTION

DermaView™ II Island is a semipermeable transparent composite wound dressing with a nonadherent absorbent pad. The waterproof outer film is permeable to moisture vapor and oxygen, and helps keep contaminants out. Picture frame border allows for easy application. Conforms easily to awkward to dress wound sites.

INDICATIONS

May be used as a primary or secondary dressing. For the management of lightly exuding wounds, including noninfected wounds, partial-thickness ulcers, and full-thickness ulcers.

CONTRAINDICATIONS

- DermaView II Island should not be used on people who are sensitive or allergic to the dressing and its components.

APPLICATION

- Cleanse wound with advised liquid to remove residue according to local infection control protocol. Deep wounds should be well irrigated.
- Skin around wound should be clean and dry; use skin barrier prep as needed.
- Remove dressing from package.
- If applicable, remove middle paper panel from the front (nonsticky) side of dressing.
- Remove backing paper from dressing.
- Apply sticky side of dressing to moist wound bed overlapping 1 to 2 inches of dry skin; gently smooth into place.
- If applicable, remove paper frame from front (nonsticky) side of dressing.

REMOVAL

- Dressing may be moistened to ease removal.
- Carefully remove adhesive dressings by holding the edge of the dressing and slowly pulling it parallel to the skin.
- Dispose of in accordance with local guidance.

REFERENCE

1. http://dermarite.com/product/dermaview-ii-island/

Mepore® Pro Showerproof, Self-Adhesive Absorbent Dressing

Mölnlycke Health Care

Mepore® Pro

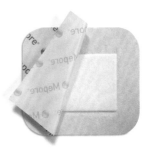

HOW SUPPLIED

Mepore® Pro	2.5″ × 3″	A6203
Mepore® Pro	3.6″ × 4″	A6203
Mepore® Pro	3.6″ × 6″	A6203
Mepore® Pro	3.6″ × 8″	A6203
Mepore® Pro	3.6″ × 10″	A6203
Mepore® Pro	3.6″ × 12″	A6203
Mepore® Pro	3″ × 3″	A6212
Mepore® Pro	4″ × 4″	A6212
Mepore® Pro	6″ × 6	A6213
Mepore® Pro	6″ × 8″	A6213

ACTION

Mepore® Pro self-adherent, absorbent and breathable dressing for low to moderately exuding wounds. The outer film layer protects the wound from both water and contamination so it can be worn while showering. The absorbent wound pad has a low-adherent wound contact layer so that it's comfortable to wear and stays in place. Its skin-friendly, water- based, solvent-free adhesive provides a gentle and secure fixation. Protects the wound against water and outside contamination and serves as a viral and bacterial barrier.

INDICATIONS

Designed for wounds with low to moderate exudate, surgical wounds, minor burns, cuts and abrasions.

CONTRAINDICATIONS

• Not for use on patients that have a sensitivity to acrylic adhesives.

APPLICATION

• Clean the wound area. Make sure the surrounding skin is dry.
• Remove the release film, exposing adhesive surface allowing initial fixation of the dressing.
• Position the dressing on the skin without stretching and gently remove the rest of the release papers. Firmly smooth adhesive border to obtain proper adhesion. Do not stretch the dressing when applying.

REMOVAL

• The frequency of dressing changes for Mepore Pro should be governed by the condition of the wound in accordance with accepted clinical practice.

COMPOSITES

OPSITE Post-Op Composite Dressing

Smith & Nephew, Inc.
Wound Management

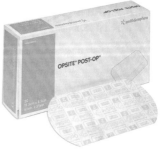

HOW SUPPLIED

Dressing	2 1/2″ × 2″ with 1 1/2″ × 1/2″ pad	A6203
Dressing	3 1/4″ × 3 3/8″ with 3″ × 1″ pad	A6203
Dressing	4 3/4″ × 4″ with 3″ × 2″ pad	A6203
Dressing	6 1/8″ × 3 1/8″ with 5″ × 1 1/2″ pad	A6203
Dressing	8″ × 4″ with 6″ × 2″ pad	A6203
Dressing	10″ × 4″ with 8″ × 2″ pad	A6203
Dressing	11 3/4 × 4″ with 10″ × 2″ pad	A6204
Dressing	13 1/4″ × 4″ with 11 3/4″ × 2″ pad	A6204

ACTION

OPSITE Post-Op Composite Dressings combine OPSITE transparent film with an absorbent, nonadherent pad. Drainage can be monitored without disturbing the dressing. Moisture vapor permeability combined with nonsensitizing adhesive allows the wound and the skin under the dressing to breathe. The dressing stays in place, reducing the risk of maceration. The OPSITE film is impermeable to water and body fluids. The pad is highly absorbent, minimizing the number of dressing changes. Its nonadherent surface leaves the wound site undisturbed, reducing pain and wound trauma during dressing changes.

INDICATIONS

For use as primary dressings for skin tears, pressure ulcers (stages 1 to 3), postoperative and arthroscopic wounds, minor cuts, and lacerations; may also be used as secondary dressings over gels and alginates.

CONTRAINDICATIONS

- None provided by the manufacturer.

APPLICATION

- Remove one backing tab and place the dressing over the wound.
- Peel off the remaining backing while smoothing the dressing onto the skin.
- Remove the film carrier.

REMOVAL

- Grasp a corner of the dressing's clear film and pull it parallel to the skin. This stretching action releases the adhesive for gentle removal.
- Continue stretching around the circumference of the dressing and then lift it off.

COMPOSITES

Stratasorb

Medline Industries, Inc.

HOW SUPPLIED

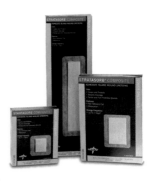

Island Dressing, Pad	4″ × 4″ (2.5″ × 2″)	A6203
Island Dressing, Pad	6″ × 6″ (4″ × 4″)	A6203
Island Dressing, Pad	4″ × 10″ (2″ × 8″)	A6203
Island Dressing, Pad	6″ × 7.5″ (4″ × 6″)	A6204
Island Dressing, Pad	4″ × 14″ (2″ × 12″)	A6204

ACTION

Stratasorb is a four-layer composite island dressing that absorbs exudate, protects the wound, and keeps it moist. It consists of a nonadherent wound contact layer, an absorbent soaker, a nonwoven adhesive border, and a waterproof, bacteria-resistant outer layer.

INDICATIONS

To manage pressure ulcers (stages 1 to 4), partial- and full-thickness wounds, tunneling wounds, infected and noninfected wounds, wounds with minimal to heavy drainage, wounds with serosanguineous or purulent drainage, and red, yellow, or black wounds.

CONTRAINDICATIONS

- None provided by the manufacturer.

APPLICATION

- Clean the application site with normal saline solution or an appropriate cleanser, such as Skintegrity Wound Cleanser. Dry the surrounding area to ensure that it is free from any greasy substance.
- If using Stratasorb as a secondary dressing, apply the appropriate primary dressing.
- Select the appropriate dressing size for the wound. Make sure the dressing extends 1 1/4″ to 1 1/2″ (3 to 4 cm) beyond the wound, so the dressing can attach to healthy tissue.
- Remove one side of the dressing's paper backing, and apply the exposed adhesive to the skin.
- Remove the second side of the paper backing, and apply the remaining adhesive, being careful not to stretch the dressing.

REMOVAL

- Change the dressing as indicated by the wound's condition and the amount of exudate or as the primary dressing indicates.
- Lift the dressing by one edge, and peel it back while holding the skin edge.
- Repeat cleansing procedure before applying a new dressing.

REFERENCE

1. http://www.medline.com/product/Stratasorb-Composite-Dressings/Composite-Dressings/Z05-PF00144

3M™ Tegaderm™ Absorbent Clear Acrylic Dressing

3M™ Health Care

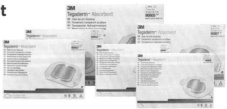

HOW SUPPLIED

Oval	3″ × 3 3/4″ (1 1/2″ × 2 1/4″ pad)	A6203
Oval	4 3/8″ × 5″ (2 3/8″ × 3″ pad)	A6203
Oval	5 3/8″ × 6 1/4″ (3 3/8″ × 4 1/4″ pad)	A6203
Square	5 7/8″ × 6″ (3 7/8″ × 4″ pad)	A6203
Square	7 7/8″ × 8″ (5 7/8″ × 6″ pad)	A6204
Sacral	6 5/8″ × 7 1/2″ (4 1/2″ × 5 5/8″ pad)	A6204

ACTION

3M™ Tegaderm™ Absorbent Clear Acrylic Dressing is a sterile wound dressing. It consists of a conformable acrylic pad enclosed between two layers for transparent film. The film in contact with the wound surface is perforated to allow uptake of the wound fluid by the absorbent acrylic pad. The nonperforated film backing is moisture vapor permeable, but impermeable to liquids such as urine and feces, bacteria, and viruses.[1]

INDICATIONS

It is indicated for partial- and full-thickness dermal ulcers including skin tears, pressure injuries, superficial wounds, abrasions, superficial and partial-thickness burns, donor sites, and clean, closed approximated surgical incisions or laparoscopic incisions. It may also be used as a protective dressing on at-risk, undamaged skin or skin beginning to show signs of damage from friction or shear.

CONTRAINDICATIONS

- The dressings are not to be designed, sold or, intended for use except as indicated.

APPLICATION

- Cleanse wound and surrounding skin according to facility policy. If periwound skin is fragile or exposure to wound exudate is likely, apply a barrier film. Allow the barrier film to dry before dressing application.
- Hold the dressing by a tab, and peel the liner from the dressing, exposing the adhesive surface.
- Hold the dressing by the tabs, and center the dressing over the wound, adhesive side down. Avoid stretching the dressing or skin.
- Gently position the dressing in place, smoothing from the center outward.
- Slowly remove the paper frame while pressing down and smoothing the film border to ensure good adhesion.

- Note: During use, it is normal for wound fluid to be absorbed throughout the pad. Movement of drainage to the edge of the pad does not create a need to change the dressing. The dressing should be changed if it is leaking, lifting off, or if wound fluid is under the adhesive border.

REMOVAL

- Carefully lift the film edges from the skin. If there is difficulty lifting the dressing, apply tape to the edge and use tape to lift.
- Continue lifting the film until all edges are free from the skin surface.
- Remove the dressing slowly, folding it over itself. Pull carefully in the direction of hair growth.

REFERENCE

1. https://www.3m.com/3M/en_US/company-us/all-3m-products/~/3M-Tegaderm-Absorbent-Clear-Acrylic-Dressing?N=5002385+3293321937&rt=rud

COMPOSITES

3M™ Tegaderm™ +Pad Film Dressing with Non-Adherent Pad

3M™ Health Care

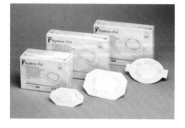

HOW SUPPLIED

Island	2" × 2 3/4" (1" × 1 1/2" pad)	A6203
Island	2 × 3/8" × 4" (1" × 2 3/8" pad)	A6203
Island	3 1/2" × 4" (1 3/4" × 2 3/8" pad)	A6203
Island	6" × 6" (4" × 4" pad)	A6203
Island	3 1/2" × 6" (1 3/4" × 4" pad)	A6203
Island	3 1/2" × 8" (1 3/4" × 4" pad)	A6203
Island	3 1/2" × 10" (1 3/4" × 8" pad)	A6203
Island	3 1/2" × 13 3/4" (1 3/4" × 11 3/4" pad)	A6203
Oval	3 1/2" × 4 1/8" (1 3/4" × 11 3/4" pad)	A6204

ACTION

The 3M™ Tegaderm™ +Pad Film Dressing with Non-Adherent Pad is a sterile, waterproof, bacterial and viral* barrier dressing, which consists of a nonadherent absorbent pad bonded to a larger, thin film transparent dressing.

INDICATIONS

The 3M™ Tegaderm™ +Pad Film Dressing with Non-Adherent Pad is designed for covering superficial and partial-thickness wounds, surgical incisions and IV catheter sites. Follow your "tape and gauze" protocol for use.

CONTRAINDICATIONS

- This product is not designed, sold, or intended for use except as indicated.
- Not for replacing sutures or other primary wound closures.

APPLICATION

- Prepare the site for wound dressing or catheter insertion according to facility policy. To ensure dressing adhesion, clip excess hair at the site, but do not shave. Allow all preparation liquids to dry completely before applying the dressing.
- Peel the paper liner from the paper-framed dressing, exposing the adhesive surface. Position the framed window over the wound site or catheter insertion site; apply the dressing.
- Remove the paper frame from the dressing while smoothing down the dressing edges and sealing them securely around the wound or catheter.

COMPOSITES

REMOVAL

- Grasp the edge gently, and slowly peel the dressing from the skin in the direction of hair growth. Avoid skin trauma by peeling the dressing back, rather than pulling it up from the skin.

REFERENCES

1. https://www.3m.com/3M/en_US/company-us/all-3m-products/~/3M-Tegaderm-Pad-Film-Dressing-with-Non-Adherent-Pad?N=5002385±3293321914&rt=rud

2. www.3M.com/postopcare

COMPOSITES

Contact Layers

ACTION

Contact layers are manufactured as single layers of a woven (polyamide) net that acts as a low-adherence material when placed in contact with the base of the wound. These materials allow wound exudate to pass to a secondary dressing. They may be used with topical medications. Contact layers are not intended to be changed with each dressing change.

INDICATIONS

Contact layers may be used as primary dressings for partial- and full-thickness wounds; wounds with minimal, moderate, and heavy exudate; donor sites; and split-thickness skin grafts.

ADVANTAGES

- Can protect wound bases from trauma during dressing changes.
- May be applied with topical medications, wound fillers, or gauze dressings.

DISADVANTAGES

- Are not recommended for stage 1 pressure ulcers; wounds that are shallow, dehydrated, or covered with eschar; or wounds that are draining a viscous exudate.
- Require secondary dressings.

HCPCS CODE OVERVIEW

The HCPCS codes normally assigned to contact layer dressings are:
A6206—pad size ≤ 16 in^2.
A6207—pad size >16 in^2 but ≤ 48 in^2.
A6208—pad size >48 in^2.

New Product: ADAPTIC TOUCH™ Non-Adhering Silicone Dressing

Systagenix, An ACELITY™ Company

HOW SUPPLIED

ADAPTIC TOUCH™ Non-Adhering Silicone Dressing	2" × 3"	A6206
ADAPTIC TOUCH™ Non-Adhering Silicone Dressing	3" × 4 1/4"	A6206
ADAPTIC TOUCH™ Non-Adhering Silicone Dressing	5" × 6"	A6207
ADAPTIC TOUCH™ Non-Adhering Silicone Dressing	8" × 12 3/4"	A6208

ACTION

Silicone assists dressing application and atraumatic removal; advanced mesh design means minimized risk of exudates pooling and secondary dressing adherence to wounds, reduced chance of maceration.

INDICATIONS

Indicated for use in the management of dry to heavily exuding, partial- and full-thickness chronic wounds, including venous ulcers, decubitus (pressure) ulcers, diabetic ulcers, traumatic and surgical wounds, donor sites and first- and second-degree burns. It can be used under compression and in conjunction with negative pressure wound therapy (NPWT).

CONTRAINDICATIONS

- Not indicated for use with patients with a known sensitivity to silicone or cellulose acetate fabric or surgical implantation.

APPLICATION

- To prevent potential adherence of silicone to gloves, moisten gloves with a sterile solution to facilitate handling.
- Prepare the wound according to wound management protocol.
- Ensure that skin surrounding the wound is dry.
- If needed, ADAPTIC TOUCH™ Non-Adhering Silicone Dressing may be cut to size with sterile scissors—leave one or two of the release papers in place when cutting.
- Remove protective films from ADAPTIC TOUCH™ Dressing.
- Place ADAPTIC TOUCH™ Dressing directly over the wound and smooth in place around the wound.
- ADAPTIC TOUCH™ Dressing should be applied as a single layer (no folding), as this will allow exudates to easily flow through into secondary layer.

- If more than one piece of ADAPTIC TOUCH™ Dressing is required, ensure dressings overlap completely covering entire wound bed and surrounding edges to avoid secondary dressing adherence to the wound; however, overlap should be minimized to prevent occlusion of mesh.
- Cover with an appropriate semiocclusive secondary dressing, for example, TIELLE™ Hydropolymer Adhesive Dressing.

REMOVAL

- ADAPTIC TOUCH™ Dressing may be left in place for several days depending on wound condition and exudate level.

REFERENCE

1. Pierrefeu-Lagrange A, Mari K, Hoss C, et al. A randomized controlled study evaluating the clinical benefits of a cellulose acetate mesh coated with a soft silicone in the management of acute wounds. *Wounds*. 2018;30(4):84–89.

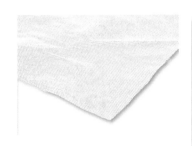

Conformant 2 Wound Veil

Smith & Nephew, Inc.
Wound Management

HOW SUPPLIED

Sterile Sheet	4" × 4"	A6206
Sterile Sheet	4" × 12"	A6207
Sterile Sheet	12" × 12"	A6208
Sterile Sheet	12" × 24"	A6208
Sterile Sheet	24" × 36"	A6208
Sterile Roll	3" × 5 yards	A6206
Sterile Roll	4" × 3 yards	A6206
Sterile Roll	6" × 2 yards	A6206
Sterile Roll	6" × 4 yards	A6206

ACTION

Conformant 2 is a single, transparent, nonadherent wound veil made of perforated high-density polyethylene. It is used to line wounds or to place under packing materials. It is easy to remove and assists in the removal of other products placed over the veil. Because it is transparent, Conformant 2 allows visualization of the wound bed.

INDICATIONS

To prevent skin breakdown and to manage pressure ulcers (stages 1 to 4), partial- and full-thickness wounds, infected and uninfected wounds, draining wounds, and red, yellow, or black wounds; may also be applied directly to the wound as a liner or used with any topical preparation or ointment.

CONTRAINDICATIONS

- Contraindicated for tunneling wounds.

APPLICATION

- Place the sheet over the wound and surrounding tissue, and affix it with tape or roll gauze.

REMOVAL

- Remove the tape or roll gauze.
- Gently lift one corner of the sheet, and peel it back from the wound.

New Product: ComfiTel

DermaRite Industries, LLC

HOW SUPPLIED

Silicone Contact Layer Wound Dressing	2″ × 3″	A6206
Silicone Contact Layer Wound Dressing	3″ × 4″	A6206
Silicone Contact Layer Wound Dressing	4″ × 7″	A6207

ACTION

ComfiTel™ is a silicone wound dressing that adheres gently to intact skin, but not to wounds. Porous mesh design allows wound exudate to pass through to absorbent secondary dressing materials. Allows for more frequent dressing changes while protecting from wound trauma. Comfortable and conformable.

INDICATIONS

Use as a primary dressing for a protective barrier between wound and outer dressing for dry to heavily exuding partial- or full-thickness wounds such as venous pressure; neuropathic ulcers; traumatic wounds such as abrasions, cuts, and lacerations, surgical wounds, and first- or second-degree burns.

CONTRAINDICATIONS

- ComfiTel should not be used on people who are sensitive or allergic to silicone and/or any other contents of the dressing.

APPLICATION

- Cleanse wound with advised liquid to remove residue according to local infection control protocol. Deep wounds should be well irrigated.
- Skin around wound should be clean and dry, use skin barrier prep as needed.
- Remove dressing from package.
- Dressing may be cut to size prior to application.
- Remove backing paper from dressing.
- Apply sticky side of dressing to moist wound bed overlapping 1 to 2 inches of dry skin; gently smooth into place.
- Cover with appropriate secondary dressing that manages drainage and maintains a moist wound environment.

REMOVAL

- Dressing may be moistened to ease removal.
- Carefully remove adhesive dressings by holding the edge of the dressing and slowly pulling it parallel to the skin.
- Dispose of in accordance with local guidance.

REFERENCE

1. http://dermarite.com/product/comfitel/

DERMANET Wound Contact Layer

DeRoyal

HOW SUPPLIED

Sheet	3" × 3"	A6206
Sheet	5" × 4"	A6207
Sheet	8" × 10"	A6208
Sheet	20" × 15"	A6208
Sheet	24" × 36"	A6208
Roll	6" × 72"	A6208

ACTION

DERMANET Wound Contact Layer is a lightweight net made from high-density polyethylene that forms a porous fine-mesh structure. It is nonlinting, inert (totally nonreactive), soft, air- and fluid-permeable, and nonadherent. It conforms to the shapes of wounds and may be used as a primary dressing, coated with ointment for burns, or used as a liner for deep wounds that need to be packed (thus allowing easy removal of packing material).

INDICATIONS

For use as a primary dressing to protect burns, graft sites, donor sites, and granulating dermal ulcers and to line deep wounds before packing.

CONTRAINDICATIONS

- None provided by the manufacturer.

APPLICATION

- After cleaning the wound and applying topical medications, as prescribed, carefully apply DERMANET Wound Contact Layer.
- Cover the contact layer with a secondary dressing.
- Alternatively, apply medications directly to DERMANET Wound Contact Layer, and place it over the wound before applying a cover dressing.
- For deep, open wounds, line the wound with DERMANET Wound Contact Layer, pack the wound with appropriate packing material, and then apply a cover dressing.

REMOVAL

- Gently lift the dressing off or out of the wound.

Mepitel® One Wound Contact Layer

Mölnlycke Health Care

Mepitel® One

HOW SUPPLIED

Single Sided Sheet	2" × 3"	A6206
Single Sided Sheet	3" × 4"	A6206
Single Sided Sheet	4" × 7"	A6207
Single Sided Sheet	6.8" × 10"	A6208
Single Sided Sheet	10.8" × 20"	A6208
Single Sided Sheet	3.75" × 59"	

ACTION

Mepitel® One is a soft silicone wound contact layer featuring a Safetac technology layer on one side and a transparent, flexible, thin, and perforated polyurethane film. The Safetac technology layer tacks gentle to dry surfaces but not to moist ones such as open wound, therefore reducing trauma and pain to the patient during dressing changes. Mepitel One is a nonabsorbent dressing that allows for exudate to pass vertically into a secondary absorbent pad. It may also be used under compression bandages and may be cut to suit various wound shapes and sizes.

INDICATIONS

- For the management of a wide range of exuding wounds such as painful wounds, skin tears, skin abrasions, surgical incisions, partial-thickness burns, traumatic wounds, blistering, lacerations, partial- and full-thickness grafts, radiated skin, leg and foot ulcers, as well as for a protective layer on nonexuding wounds or fragile skin.

CONTRAINDICATIONS

- When used on epidermolysis bullosa patients, please consult with a qualified health care professional.
- Avoid unnecessary pressure upon the dressing when Mepitel One is used on burns treated with mesh grafts, or after facial resurfacing.
- When Mepitel One is used for the fixation of skin grafts, the dressing should not be changed before the fifth day post application.

APPLICATION

- Clean the wound in accordance with clinical practice and dry the surrounding skin.
- Choose a size of Mepitel One that covers the wound and the surrounding skin by at least 2 cm. For larger wounds, more overlap is required. If more than one piece of Mepitel One is required, overlap the dressings, making sure that the holes are not blocked.
- Remove the protective film by using the overlapping grip edge and apply Mepitel One with the tacky side to the wound.
- Remove the remaining protective film and smooth Mepitel One in place onto the surrounding skin, ensuring a good seal.
- Apply a secondary absorbent dressing on top of Mepitel One and fixate.

REMOVAL

- Gently lift one corner of the sheet, and peel back from the wound.

Mepitel® Wound Contact Layer

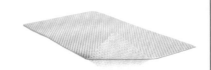

Mölnlycke Health Care

HOW SUPPLIED

Sheet	2″ × 3″	A6206
Sheet	3″ × 4	A6206
Sheet	4″ × 7″	A6207
Sheet	8″ × 12″	A6208

ACTION

Mepitel® is a soft silicone wound contact layer featuring double-sided Safetac® technology that is nonadherent to moist the wound bed, yet adheres gently to dry skin. Mepitel prevents the outer dressing from sticking to the wound and therefore minimizes trauma and pain associated with dressing changes. This results in less trauma to the wound and less pain to the patient, which ensures undisturbed wound healing.

INDICATIONS

To manage a wide range of painful wounds and wounds with compromised or fragile surrounding skin, such as skin tears, chronic wounds, traumatic wounds, contact layer for protection of fragile granulation tissue, fixation of grafts, partial-thickness burns, and painful skin conditions with blisters such as epidermolysis bullosa.

CONTRAINDICATIONS

- None provided by the manufacturer.

APPLICATION

- Clean the wound area.
- If necessary, cut the dressing to the appropriate shape.
- Remove the release film. (*Note:* To avoid sticking when handling Mepitel once the backing has been removed, moisten gloves with saline or water.)
- Apply Mepitel to the wound, overlapping dry skin by at least 2 cm.
- Apply outer absorbent dressing. Mepitel can be left in place through several outer-dressing changes.

REMOVAL

- Gently lift one corner of the sheet, and peel back from the wound.

Profore WCL

Smith & Nephew, Inc.
Wound Management

HOW SUPPLIED

Sheet	5 1/2" × 8"	A6207

ACTION

PROFORE WCL (wound contact layer) is a dressing made of knitted viscose rayon. It provides physical separation between the wound and external environments to assist in preventing bacterial contamination of the wound. It also aids in the creation and maintenance of a moist wound environment. Moist wound environments have been established as optimal environments for the management of the wound.

INDICATIONS

To act as a nonadherent interface between the granulating wound surface and conventional absorbent dressings; also for use in conjunction with PROFORE, PROFORE LF, and PRO-FORE Lite, the Multi-Layer Compression Bandage Systems.

CONTRAINDICATIONS

- Not for use if reddening or sensitization occurs; discontinue use and consult a health care professional.

APPLICATION

- CAUTION: Do not use contents if pouch is opened or damaged.
- Use a clean technique to remove the wound contact layer from the pack and apply directly to the wound.
- Either side of the WCL can be placed in contact with the wound.
- Make sure that the ulcerated area is covered.
- Use extra WCL as required.

REMOVAL

- Gently lift the layer out of the wound.

New Product: Silflex® Silicone Contact Layer

Advancis Medical/DUKAL Corporation

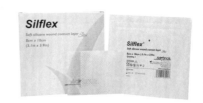

HOW SUPPLIED

Silflex® Silicone Contact Layer	2" × 3"	A6206
Silflex® Silicone Contact Layer	3" × 4"	A6206
Silflex® Silicone Contact Layer	5" × 6"	A6207
Silflex® Silicone Contact Layer	8" × 12"	A6208
Silflex® Silicone Contact Layer	14" × 24"	A6208

ACTION

- An atraumatic, soft silicone wound contact layer designed to prevent secondary dressings adhering to fragile skin and delicate wound beds.
- Pain-free removal, adheres to healthy tissue and not the secondary dressing.
- Large open pores allow the passage of exudate.
- Can be used in conjunction with topical negative pressure.
- Highly conformable and can be cut to size.

INDICATIONS

- Skin tears.
- Skin abrasions.
- Surgical wounds.
- Second degree burns.
- Lacerations.
- Leg and pressure ulcers.
- Topical negative pressure (primary dressing).

CONTRAINDICATIONS

- Do not use if allergic to silicone.

APPLICATION

- Remove the clear liners on each side of the dressing and place directly over the wound.
- Silflex® may overlap the wound edges.
- Can be cut to size ensuring sharp scissors are used.
- Cover with a secondary dressing of choice which may be an absorbent pad or film dressing.

REMOVAL

- Up to 14 days.

UrgoTul™ Contact Layer*

Urgo Medical

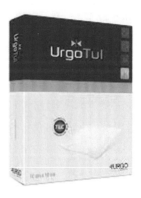

HOW SUPPLIED

Dressing	2″ × 2″	A6206
Dressing	4″ × 5″	A6207
Dressing	6″ × 8″	A6207

ACTION

The proprietary TLC Technology is comprised of a nonadhesive, nonocclusive polyester mesh impregnated with a polymer matrix containing hydrocolloid particles and petrolatum-based formulation. Upon contact with wound exudates, the hydrocolloid particles combine with the matrix to form a lipido-colloid gel, providing a moist environment that promotes healing. Being nonadhesive, removal of UrgoTul Contact Layer dressing is virtually pain-free and helps minimize damage to newly formed surrounding skin. It is ideal for use on wounds with fragile surrounding skin.

INDICATIONS

Indicated in low to moderate exuding partial- and full-thickness wounds, including minor cuts, abrasions, scalds and burns, leg ulcers, diabetic ulcers, pressure ulcers, surgical wounds, graft and donor sites, second-degree burns, and skin tears.

CONTRAINDICATIONS

- Should not be used on individuals who are sensitive to or who have had an allergic reaction to the dressing or one of its components.

APPLICATION

- Cleanse the wound using sterile saline solution or an appropriate wound cleanser.
- Choose a dressing size which ensures that the dressing will cover the entire wound.
- Remove the protective clear tabs from both sides of the UrgoTul Contact Layer dressing.
- Apply UrgoTul Contact Layer dressing to cover the entire wound.
- Cover with appropriate secondary dressing. Secure secondary dressing with tape or other material.

REMOVAL

- Remove secondary dressing.
- Remove UrgoTul Contact Layer dressing.
- Irrigate wound base using Vashe® Wound Solution or sterile saline.
- Reapply dressing if necessary.
- UrgoTul should be changed depending on the wound and the healing progression or after a maximum of 7 days.

*See package insert for complete instructions for use.

3M™ Tegaderm™ Non-Adherent Contact Layer

3M™ Health Care

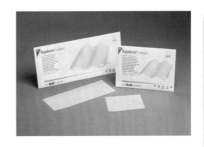

HOW SUPPLIED

Sheet	3″ × 4″	A6206
Sheet	3″ × 8″	A6207
Sheet	8″ × 10″	A6208

ACTION

3M™ Tegaderm™ Non-Adherent Contact Layer primary dressing that protects the wound bed while reducing pain of dressing changes. A woven nylon fabric with sealed edges that is a lint-free, nonadherent, nontoxic, nonirritating, and hypoallergenic material. The wound contact material is placed over the wound and under gauze or other absorbent dressing, while allowing exudates to pass through to an absorbent outer barrier. Clinical studies show that Tegaderm Contact Layer can be left on the wound for up to 7 days. The additional secondary dressing may need to be changed more frequently. The nonadherence of this material will minimize disruption of healthy granulation tissue and re-epithelialized surfaces.

INDICATIONS

For use directly over wounds, including partial- and full-thickness wounds, clean closed surgical incisions, superficial partial-thickness burns, donor sites, graft fixation sites, skin tears, traumatic and chronic wounds, and dermatologic lesions. Use of this wound contact material should be part of a well-defined protocol for wound management and prevention for infection.

CONTRAINDICATIONS

- Not designed, sold, or intended for use except as indicated.

APPLICATION

- Debride, clean, or irrigate the wound and surrounding skin as necessary according to facility policy.
- Topical treatment with ointments or medicaments, if indicated, can be applied to the wound surface before applying the wound contact material, or they can be applied on top of the material after it has been placed on the wound.
- If the dressing material must be cut to fit, remove all frayed or loose fibers.
- When wound drainage is minimal, moisten the dressing's wound contact material with sterile saline solution to facilitate positioning and to ensure complete contact with the wound surface.
- Gently position the material over the entire wound, including a margin of healthy skin. The material should extend at least 1/2″ (1.3 cm) beyond the edge of the wound, and the cut edges of the material should not be placed directly over the wound bed.
- Dress the wound with an outer dressing of gauze, a transparent dressing, a hydrocolloid, or other suitable wound dressing.

REMOVAL

- Dressing may remain undisturbed on the wound for up to 7 days. If the wound is infected, change the dressing according to facility policy for infected wounds.
- Change gauze dressings as needed, or at least every 24 hours. During gauze dressing changes, moisten 3M™ Tegaderm™ Non-Adherent Contact Layer, if necessary, to maintain a moist healing environment.
- When a transparent or hydrocolloid dressing is used as the outermost dressing, follow facility policy for dressing changes.
- Gently lift 3M™ Tegaderm™ Non-Adherent Contact Layer off the wound. When this material is maintained in a moist environment, it is nonadherent and its removal is virtually pain free.
- If the wound surface is dry, soak the dressing with normal saline solution, and then gently remove it.

REFERENCE

1. https://www.3m.com/3M/en_US/company-us/all-3m-products/~/3M-Tegaderm-Non-Adherent-Contact-Layer?N=5002385±3293321975&rt=rud

Drugs

OVERVIEW

In this section, you will find a list of products that are considered drugs because their administration provokes a series of physiochemical events within the body. The drugs listed in this section each have unique actions, indications, and contraindications specific to the individual product. This information can also be found on the product's package insert. The clinician holds responsibility for understanding how each of these products affects the cascade of wound-healing events.

Products listed in this section are reimbursed as prescription drugs. The clinician must contact the appropriate payor regarding specific payment information for a given drug.

Collagenase Santyl Ointment

Smith & Nephew, Inc.
Wound Management

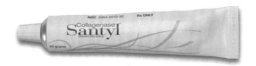

HOW SUPPLIED

Product Number	
NDC Number	30g tube NDC 50484-010-30 90g tube NDC 50484-010-90
Size	15 g, 30 g
CPT/HCPCS	CPT Code = 97602 HCPCS Code = J3590

Collagenase Santyl Ointment is a sterile enzymatic debriding ointment which contains 250 collagenase units per gram of white petrolatum USP. The enzyme collagenase is derived from the fermentation by *Clostridium histolyticum*. It possesses the unique ability to digest collagen in necrotic tissue.

ACTION

Collagenase Santyl Ointment is a sterile enzymatic debriding ointment which contains 250 collagenase units per gram of white petrolatum USP. The enzyme collagenase is derived from the fermentation by *Clostridium histolyticum*. It possesses the unique ability to digest collagen in necrotic tissue.

Because collagen accounts for 75% of the dry weight of skin tissue, the ability of collagenase to digest collagen in the physiological pH and temperature range makes it particularly effective in the removal of detritus. Collagenase thus contributes to the formation of granulation tissue and subsequent epithelialization of dermal ulcers and severely burned areas. Collagen in healthy tissue or in newly formed granulation tissue is not attacked. No information is available on collagenase absorption through skin or its concentration in body fluids associated with therapeutic and/or toxic effects, degree of binding to plasma proteins, degree of uptake by a particular organ or in the fetus, and passage across the blood–brain barrier.

INDICATIONS

For debriding chronic dermal ulcers and severely burned areas.

CONTRAINDICATIONS

- Contraindicated on patients who have local or systemic hypersensitivity to collagenase.

APPLICATION

- Before application, wound should be cleansed of debris and digested material by gently rubbing with a gauze pad saturated with normal saline solution, or with the desired cleansing agent compatible with Collagenase Santyl Ointment, followed by a normal saline solution rinse.
- Whenever infection is present, it is desirable to use an appropriate topical antibiotic powder. The antibiotic should be applied to the wound prior to the application of Collage-

nase Santyl Ointment. Should the infection not respond, therapy with Collagenase Santyl Ointment should be discontinued until remission of the infection.

- Collagenase Santyl Ointment may be applied directly to the wound or to a sterile gauze pad, which is then applied to the wound and properly secured.

REMOVAL

- Use of Collagenase Santyl Ointment should be terminated when debridement of necrotic tissue is complete and granulation tissue is well established.

REFERENCES

1. Mandl I. Collagenases and elastases. *Adv Enzymol*. 1961;23:163.
2. Boxer AM, Gottesman N, Bernstein H, et al. Debridement of dermal ulcers and decubiti with collagenase. *Geriatrics*. 1969;24(7):75–86.
3. Mazurek I. *Med Welt*. 1971;22:150.
4. Zimmermann WE. "Collagenase". In I Mandl., ed. Gordon & Breach, Science Publishers, New York; 1971:131, 185.
5. Vetra H, Whittaker D. Hydrotherapy and topical collagenase for decubitus ulcers. *Geriatrics*. 1975;30(8):53–58.
6. Rao DB, Sane PG, Georgiev EL. Collagenase in the treatment of dermal and decubitus ulcers. *J Am Geriatr Soc*. 1975;23(1):22.
7. Vrabec R, Moserova J, Konickova Z, et al. Clinical experience with enzymatic debridement of burned skin with the use of collagenase. *J Hyg Epidemiol Microbiol Immunol*. 1974;18(4):496–498.
8. Lippmann HI. *Arch Phys Med Rehabil*. 1973;54:588.
9. German FM. "Collagenase." In: I Mandl., ed. Gordon & Breach, Science Publishers. New York;1971;165.
10. Haimovici H, Strauch B. "Collagenase." In: I Mandl., ed. Gordon & Breach, Science Publishers. New York;1971:177.
11. Lee LK, Ambrus JL. Collagenase therapy for decubitus ulcers. *Geriatrics*. 1975;30(5):91–93, 97–98.
12. Locke RK, Heifitz NM. Collagenase as an aid in healing. *J Am Podiatry Assoc*. 1975;65(3):242–247.
13. Varma AO, Bugatch E, German FM. Debridement of dermal ulcers with collagenase. *Surg Gynecol Obstet*. 1973;136(2):281–282.
14. Barrett D Jr., Klibanski A. Collagenase debridement. *Am J Nurs*. 1973;73(5):849–851.
15. Bardfeld LA, *J Pod Ed*. 1970;1:41.
16. Blum G, Schweiz, Rundschau Med Praxis. 1973;62:820. *Abstr. in Dermatology Digest*, Feb. 1974;36.
17. Zaruba F, Lettl A, Brozkova L, et al. Collagenase in the treatment of ulcers in dermatology. *J Hyg Epidemiol Microbiol Immunol*. 1974;18(4):499–500.
18. Altman MI, Goldstein L, & Horwitz S, *J Am Pod Assoc*. 1978;68:11.
19. Rehn VJ. [Treatment of burns]. *Med Klin*. 1963;58:799–802.
20. Krauss H, Koslowski L, Zimmermann WE. [Recent findings on metabolic changes in burns and shock]. *Langenbecks Arch Klin Chir Ver Dtsch Z Chir*. 1963;303:23–40.
21. Gruenagel HH. [Collagenase treatment of necrolysis in thermal injuries]. *Med Klin*. 1963;58: 442–445.

DRUGS

REGRANEX (becaplermin) Gel 0.01%

Smith & Nephew, Inc.
Wound Management

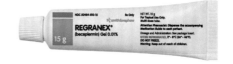

HOW SUPPLIED

REGRANEX Gel Tube	15-g	140384-0814

REGRANEX Gel contains becaplermin, a recombinant human-platelet–derived growth factor for topical administration. Becaplermin is produced by recombinant DNA technology by insertion of the gene for the B chain of platelet-derived growth factor (PDGF) into the yeast, *Saccharomyces cerevisiae*. Becaplermin has a molecular weight of approximately 25 kD and is a homodimer composed of two identical polypeptide chains that are bound together by disulfide bonds. REGRANEX Gel is a nonsterile, low bioburden, preserved, sodium carboxymethylcellulose-based (CMC) topical gel, containing the active ingredient becaplermin and the following inactive ingredients: CMC sodium, glacial acetic acid, l-lysine hydrochloride, m-cresol, methylparaben, propylparaben, sodium acetate trihydrate, sodium chloride, and water for injection. Each gram of REGRANEX Gel contains 100 mcg of becaplermin.

ACTION

REGRANEX Gel has biological activity similar to that of endogenous PDGF, which includes promoting the chemotactic recruitment and proliferation of cells involved in wound repair and enhancing the formation of granulation tissue.

INDICATIONS

REGRANEX (becaplermin) Gel is indicated for the treatment of lower-extremity diabetic neuropathic ulcers that extend into the subcutaneous tissue or beyond and have an adequate blood supply, when used as an adjunct to, and not a substitute for, good ulcer-care practices including initial sharp debridement, pressure relief, and infection control.

CONTRAINDICATIONS

- REGRANEX Gel is contraindicated in patients with known neoplasm(s) at the site(s) of application.

APPLICATION

- To apply REGRANEX Gel, the calculated length of gel should be squeezed on to a clean measuring surface, for example, wax paper. The measured REGRANEX Gel is transferred from the clean measuring surface using an application aid and then spread over the entire ulcer area to yield a thin continuous layer of approximately 1/16 of an inch thickness. The site(s) of application should then be covered by a saline moistened dressing and left in place for approximately 12 hours. The dressing should then be removed and the ulcer rinsed with saline or water to remove residual gel and covered again with a second moist dressing (without REGRANEX Gel) for the remainder of the day. REGRANEX Gel should be applied once daily to the ulcer until complete healing has occurred. If the ulcer does not decrease in size by approximately 30% after 10 weeks of treatment or complete healing has not occurred in 20 weeks, continued treatment with REGRANEX Gel should be reassessed.

REMOVAL

- REGRANEX Gel is a nonsterile, low bioburden preserved product. Therefore, it should not be used in wounds that close by primary intention.

REFERENCES

1. *J. Enterostomal Ther.* 1988;15:4.
2. Pressure ulcers prevalence, cost and risk assessment: consensus development conference statement—The National Pressure Ulcer Advisory Panel. *Decubitus.* 1989;2:24.

DRUGS

Foams

ACTION

Foam dressings are nonlinting and absorbent and have a wide range of functional attributes. They vary in thickness and have a nonadherent layer, allowing nontraumatic removal. Some have an adhesive border and may have a film coating as an additional bacterial barrier. Foam dressings provide a moist environment and thermal insulation. They are manufactured as pads, sheets, and pillow (cavity) dressings.

INDICATIONS

Foam dressings are versatile in their use and may be used as primary and secondary dressings for partial- and full-thickness wounds with minimal, moderate, or heavy drainage, as primary dressings for absorption and insulation, or as secondary dressings for wounds with packing. They may also be used to provide additional absorption and to absorb drainage around tubes. Some foam dressings, such as silicone adhesive dressings, hydrofiber interface dressings, and polymeric membrane dressings (PMD), have additional indications. Some foam dressings are designed for specific anatomical areas.

ADVANTAGES

- Are nonadherent.
- May repel or absorb contaminants.
- Are easy to apply and remove.
- Absorb light to heavy amounts of exudate.
- May be used under compression.
- Provide thermal insulation.

DISADVANTAGES

- Most are not effective for wounds with dry eschar.
- May macerate periwound skin if they become overly saturated.
- Some may require secondary dressing, tape, wrap, or net.

HCPCS CODE OVERVIEW

The HCPCS codes normally assigned to foam wound covers without an adhesive border are:
A6209—pad size $\leq$16 in^2.
A6210—pad size >16 in^2 but $\leq$48 in^2.
A6211—pad size >48 in^2.
The HCPCS codes normally assigned to foam wound covers with an adhesive border are:
A6212—pad size $\leq$16 in^2.
A6213—pad size >16 in^2 but $\leq$48 in^2.
A6214—pad size >48 in^2.
The HCPCS code normally assigned to foam wound filler is:
A6215—per gram.

New Product: Advazorb® Border Hydrophilic Foam Dressing

Advancis Medical/DUKAL Corporation

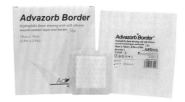

HOW SUPPLIED

Advazorb® Border Hydrophilic Foam Dressings	3″ × 3″	A6212
Advazorb® Border Hydrophilic Foam Dressings	4″ × 4″	A6212
Advazorb® Border Hydrophilic Foam Dressings	5″ × 5″	A6212
Advazorb® Border Hydrophilic Foam Dressings	6″ × 6″	A6213
Advazorb® Border Hydrophilic Foam Dressings	4″ × 8″	A6213
Advazorb® Border Hydrophilic Foam Dressings	8″ × 8″	A6213
Advazorb® Border Hydrophilic Foam Dressings	4″ × 12″	A6213

ACTION

- Hydrophilic foam dressing with soft silicone wound contact layer and border.
- Soft silicone layer extends across entire surface area of the dressing, providing secure but gentle adhesion.
- Large open pores enable passage of exudate through the foam while providing optimal adherence to the skin.

INDICATIONS

- Suitable for acute and chronic wounds.
- Cuts and abrasions.
- Superficial burns.
- Surgical wounds.
- Leg ulcers.
- Pressure ulcers.
- Diabetic ulcers.

CONTRAINDICATIONS

- Do not use on arterial bleeds, heavily bleeding wounds, or vascular fungating tumors.

APPLICATION

- Remove clear liners and apply (pink side up) to the wound ensuring the dressing covers the entire wound area and a minimum overlap of 2 cm around the edges of the wound.

REMOVAL

- Up to 7 days.

FOAMS

New Product: Advazorb® Border Lite Hydrophilic Foam Dressings

Advancis Medical/DUKAL Corporation

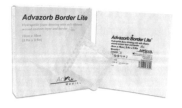

HOW SUPPLIED

Advazorb® Border Lite Hydrophilic Foam Dressings	3" × 3"	A6212
Advazorb® Border Lite Hydrophilic Foam Dressings	4" × 4"	A6212
Advazorb® Border Lite Hydrophilic Foam Dressings	4" × 8"	A6213
Advazorb® Border Lite Hydrophilic Foam Dressings	5" × 5"	A6212
Advazorb® Border Lite Hydrophilic Foam Dressings	6" × 6"	A6213
Advazorb® Border Lite Hydrophilic Foam Dressings	8" × 8"	A6213
Advazorb® Border Lite Hydrophilic Foam Dressings	4" × 12"	A6123

ACTION

- Hydrophilic foam dressing with soft silicone wound contact layer and border.
- Soft silicone layer extends across entire surface area of the dressing, providing secure but gentle adhesion.
- Large open pores enable passage of exudate through the foam while providing optimal adherence to the skin.

INDICATIONS

- Suitable for acute and chronic wounds.
- Cuts and abrasions.
- Superficial burns.
- Surgical wounds.
- Leg ulcers.
- Pressure ulcers.
- Diabetic ulcers.

CONTRAINDICATIONS

- Do not use on arterial bleeds, heavily bleeding wounds, and vascular fungating tumors.

APPLICATION

- Remove clear liners and apply (pink side up) to the wound ensuring the dressing covers the entire wound area and a minimum overlap of 2 cm around the edges of the wound.

REMOVAL

- Up to 7 days.

New Product: Advazorb®
Hydrophilic Foam Dressings

Advancis Medical/DUKAL Corporation

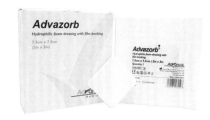

HOW SUPPLIED

Advazorb® Hydrophilic Foam Dressings	3″ × 3″	A6209
Advazorb® Hydrophilic Foam Dressings	4″ × 4″	A6209
Advazorb® Hydrophilic Foam Dressings	5″ × 5″	A6210
Advazorb® Hydrophilic Foam Dressings	6″ × 6″	A6210
Advazorb® Hydrophilic Foam Dressings	8″ × 8″	A6211
Advazorb® Hydrophilic Foam Dressings	4″ × 8″	A6210

ACTION

- Soft and conformable, low-adherent, hydrophilic, polyurethane foam dressings with a breathable film backing.
- Ideal for use under compression bandaging with its fluid retention, low profile, and low-friction film backing.

INDICATIONS

- Suitable for acute and chronic wounds.
- Cuts and abrasions.
- Superficial burns.
- Surgical wounds.
- Leg ulcers.
- Pressure ulcers.
- Diabetic ulcers.

CONTRAINDICATIONS

- Do not use on arterial bleeds, heavily bleeding wounds, and vascular fungating tumors.

APPLICATION

- Apply directly to the wound surface (pink side up) and secure in place with tape, appropriate bandage, or secondary dressing.
- Can be used under compression bandaging.

REMOVAL

- Up to 7 days.

FOAMS

New Product: Advazorb® Heel Hydrophilic Foam Dressing

Advancis Medical/DUKAL Corporation

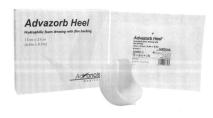

HOW SUPPLIED

Advazorb® Heel Hydrophilic Foam Dressings	6.5" × 8.5"	A6210

ACTION

- Soft and conformable, low-adherent, hydrophilic, polyurethane foam dressings with a breathable film backing.
- Ideal for use under compression bandaging with its fluid retention, low profile, and low friction film backing.
- Anatomically shaped to fi t around the heel so that the dressing is in close contact with the wound to provide an environment conducive to healing.

INDICATIONS

- Suitable for acute and chronic wounds.
- Cuts and abrasions.
- Superficial burns.
- Surgical wounds.
- Leg ulcers.
- Pressure ulcers.
- Diabetic ulcers.

CONTRAINDICATIONS

- Do not use on arterial bleeds, heavily bleeding wounds, and vascular fungating tumors.

APPLICATION

- Apply directly to the wound surface on the heel (pink side facing out) and secure in place with tape, appropriate bandage, or secondary dressing.
- Advazorb® Heel can be turned inside out and be used for wounds underarm.
- Can be used under compression bandaging.

REMOVAL

- Up to 7 days.

FOAMS

New Product: Advazorb® Lite Hydrophilic Foam Dressing

Advancis Medical/DUKAL Corporation

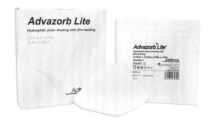

HOW SUPPLIED

Advazorb® Lite Hydrophilic Foam Dressings	3″ × 3″	A6209
Advazorb® Lite Hydrophilic Foam Dressings	4″ × 4″	A6209
Advazorb® Lite Hydrophilic Foam Dressings	5″ × 5″	A6210
Advazorb® Lite Hydrophilic Foam Dressings	6″ × 6″	A6210
Advazorb® Lite Hydrophilic Foam Dressings	4″ × 8″	A6210
Advazorb® Lite Hydrophilic Foam Dressings	8″ × 8″	A6211

ACTION

- Soft and conformable, low-adherent, hydrophilic, polyurethane foam dressings with a breathable film backing.
- Ideal for use under compression bandaging with its fluid retention, low profile, and low friction film backing.

INDICATIONS

- Suitable for acute and chronic wounds.
- Cuts and abrasions.
- Superficial burns.
- Surgical wounds.
- Leg ulcers.
- Pressure ulcers.
- Diabetic ulcers.

CONTRAINDICATIONS

- Do not use on arterial bleeds, heavily bleeding wounds, and vascular fungating tumors.

APPLICATION

- Apply directly to the wound surface (pink side up) and secure in place with tape, appropriate bandage, or secondary dressing.
- Can be used under compression bandaging.

REMOVAL

- Up to 7 days.

FOAMS

New Product: Advazorb Silfix® Hydrophilic Foam Dressing

Advancis Medical/DUKAL Corporation

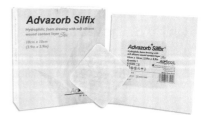

HOW SUPPLIED

Advazorb® Silflex Hydrophilic Foam Dressings	3" × 3"	A6209
Advazorb® Silflex Hydrophilic Foam Dressings	4" × 4"	A6209
Advazorb® Silflex Hydrophilic Foam Dressings	5" × 5"	A6210
Advazorb® Silflex Hydrophilic Foam Dressings	6" × 6"	A6210
Advazorb® Silflex Hydrophilic Foam Dressings	4" × 8"	A6210
Advazorb® Silflex Hydrophilic Foam Dressings	8" × 8"	A6211

ACTION

- Hydrophilic foam dressing with silicone wound contact layer.
- Wound contact layer enables the dressing to be placed onto patient while a secondary dressing is applied for retention.
- Provides gentle adherence to intact skin as the hydrophobic nature of silicone ensures that it will not adhere to a wet wound bed.

INDICATIONS

- Suitable for acute and chronic wounds.
- Cuts and abrasions.
- Superficial burns.
- Surgical wounds.
- Leg ulcers.
- Pressure ulcers.
- Diabetic ulcers.

CONTRAINDICATIONS

- Do not use on arterial bleeds, heavily bleeding wounds, or vascular fungating tumors.

APPLICATION

- Remove clear liners and apply (pink side up) to the wound ensuring the dressing covers the entire wound area and a minimum overlap of 2 cm around the edges of the wound.
- Secure in place with tape, appropriate bandage or secondary dressing.

REMOVAL

- Up to 7 days.

New Product: Advazorb Silfix® Lite Hydrophilic Foam Dressing

Advancis Medical/DUKAL Corporation

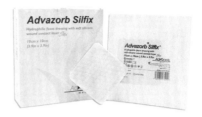

HOW SUPPLIED

Advazorb® Silflex Lite Hydrophilic Foam Dressings	3" × 3"	A6209
Advazorb® Silflex Lite Hydrophilic Foam Dressings	4" × 4"	A6209
Advazorb® Silflex Lite Hydrophilic Foam Dressings	4" × 8"	A6210
Advazorb® Silflex Lite Hydrophilic Foam Dressings	5" × 5"	A6210
Advazorb® Silflex Lite Hydrophilic Foam Dressings	6" × 6"	A6210
Advazorb® Silflex Lite Hydrophilic Foam Dressings	8" × 8"	A6211

ACTION

- Hydrophilic foam dressing with silicone wound contact layer.
- Wound contact layer enables the dressing to be placed onto patient while a secondary dressing is applied for retention.
- Provides gentle adherence to intact skin as the hydrophobic nature of silicone ensures that it won't adhere to a wet wound bed.

INDICATIONS

- Suitable for acute and chronic wounds.
- Cuts and abrasions.
- Superficial burns.
- Surgical wounds.
- Leg ulcers.
- Pressure ulcers.
- Diabetic ulcers.

CONTRAINDICATIONS

- Do not use on arterial bleeds, heavily bleeding wounds, and vascular fungating tumors.

APPLICATION

- Remove clear liners and apply (pink side up) to the wound ensuring the dressing covers the entire wound area and a minimum overlap of 2 cm around the edges of the wound.
- Secure in place with tape, appropriate bandage, or secondary dressing.

REMOVAL

- Up to 7 days.

FOAMS

AMERX® Bordered Foam Dressing

AMERX Health Care Corp.

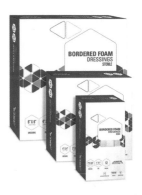

HOW SUPPLIED

Dressing	1″ × 1″	A6413
Dressing	2″ × 2″	A6212
Dressing	4″ × 4″	A6212

ACTION

AMERX Bordered Foam Dressings are breathable, non-adhesive, highly absorbent polyure-thane foam dressings to manage moderate to heavy wound exudate. The adhesive border helps secure the dressing in place and provides a barrier to outside contaminants. Soft, conformable pads are ideal for use under compression.

INDICATIONS

For use as a primary dressing over moderate to heavy exudating, chronic and acute wounds.

CONTRAINDICATIONS

- Third-degree burns or if known sensitivities to dressing components.

APPLICATION

- Dressing size should extend a minimum of 1/2″ inch beyond the wound border.
- Cleanse the wound with sterile saline solution.
- Remove the dressing from the package and remove one side of the white liner.
- Place the dressing directly over the wound and surrounding skin without tension.
- Remove the second half of the white liner.
- Carefully smooth the edge of the dressing to ensure proper contact with the surrounding skin.

REMOVAL

- If the dressing sticks, moisten with sterile saline solution prior to removal.

AMERX® Foam Dressing

AMERX Health Care Corp.

HOW SUPPLIED

Dressing	2″ × 2″	A6209
Dressing	4″ × 4″	A6209

ACTION

AMERX Foam Dressings are breathable, nonadhesive, highly absorbent polyurethane foam dressings to manage moderate to heavy wound exudate. Provides a moist wound environment to support wound healing for partial- and full-thickness wounds. Soft, conformable pads are ideal for use under compression.

INDICATIONS

For use as a primary dressing over moderate to heavy exudating, chronic and acute wounds.

CONTRAINDICATIONS

- Third-degree burns or if known sensitivities to dressing components.

APPLICATION

- Cleanse the wound with sterile saline solution and dry surrounding skin with a sterile piece of gauze.
- Place foam dressing directly over the wound.
- Dressing size should extend a minimum of one inch beyond the wound border.
- Cover foam dressing with a secondary dressing (adhesive gauze, tape or wrap).
- Smooth all edges to secure dressing in place.
- Change the dressing as indicated by the amount of drainage.

REMOVAL

- If the dressing sticks, moisten with sterile saline solution prior to removal.

FOAMS

New Product: AQUACEL™ Foam Pro Wound Dressing*

ConvaTec

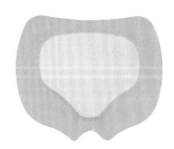

HOW SUPPLIED

Dressing	3" × 3"
Dressing	4" × 4"
Dressing	6" × 6"
Dressing, Heel	8" × 5.5"
Dressing, Sacral	8" × 7"
Dressing, Sacral	9(2/5)" × 8(2/5)"

ACTION

- Multilayered absorbent dressing conforms to the skin and wound.
- Contains a layer of polyurethane foam, a nonwoven layer of Hydrofiber® (sodium carboxymethylcellulose) and a perforated silicone adhesive wound contact layer.
- Outer film layer provides a waterproof viral and bacterial barrier which protects the wound from external contaminants, reducing the risk of infection.
- Film also helps to manage the moisture vapor transmission of the exudate absorbed by the dressing.
- Foam and Hydrofiber® materials within the dressing absorb high amounts of wound fluid and bacteria.
- Hydrofiber® layer helps maintain a moist environment in the wound (which supports the body's healing process) and aids in the removal of nonviable tissue from the wound (autolytic debridement) without damaging tissue.
- Silicone adhesive wound contact layer provides secure, skin-friendly gentle adhesion.

INDICATIONS

AQUACEL™ Foam Pro dressings may be used for the management of both chronic and acute wounds, such as leg ulcers, pressure ulcers (stage 2 to 4) and diabetic ulcers; surgical wounds (postoperative, donor sites, dermatologic); partial-thickness (second-degree) burns; traumatic or surgical wounds left to heal by secondary intention such as dehisced surgical incisions; surgical wounds that heal by primary intent, such as dermatologic and surgical incisions (e.g., orthopedic and vascular); local management of wounds that are prone to bleeding, such as wounds that have been mechanically or surgically debrided and donor sites; abrasions; lacerations; minor cuts.

- AQUACEL™ Foam Pro dressing may be included in a comprehensive protocol of care to protect against skin breakdown.

CONTRAINDICATIONS

- AQUACEL™ Foam Pro dressings should not be used on individuals who are sensitive to or who have had an allergic reaction to the dressing or its components.

APPLICATION

- Choose a dressing size to ensure that the central absorbent pad is 1 cm larger than the wound area. Remove the dressing from the sterile pack, minimizing finger contact with the adhesive surface where applicable. Remove the release liner. The dressing can be cut to shape for convenience. Hold the dressing over the wound or area of skin to be protected and line up the center of the dressing with the center of the wound or area of skin to be protected. Place the pad directly over the wound and smooth down the adhesive border. An appropriate retention bandage or tape should be used to secure the dressing in place if required or if the dressing has been cut. Discard any unused portion of the product after dressing the wound.

REMOVAL

- The dressing should be changed when clinically indicated (i.e., leakage, bleeding, increased pain, suspicion of infection). Maximum recommended wear time is up to 7 days. The wound should be cleansed at appropriate intervals. To remove the dressing, press down gently on the skin and carefully lift one corner of the dressing. Continue until all edges are free. Carefully lift away the dressing and discard according to local clinical protocols.

*See package insert for complete instructions for use.

FOAMS

New Product: AQUACEL™ Foam Wound Dressing*

ConvaTec

HOW SUPPLIED

Dressing, Adhesive	3.2″ × 3.2″
Dressing, Adhesive	4″ × 4″
Dressing, Adhesive	4″ × 8″
Dressing, Adhesive	4″ × 10″
Dressing, Adhesive	4″ × 12″
Dressing, Adhesive	5″ × 5″
Dressing, Adhesive	6″ × 6″
Dressing, Adhesive	7″ × 7″
Dressing, Heel	8″ × 5(1/2)″
Dressing, Sacral	8″ × 7″
Dressing, Sacral	9.4″ × 8.4″
Dressing, Nonadhesive	4″ × 4″
Dressing, Nonadhesive	6″ × 6″
Dressing, Nonadhesive	6″ × 8″

ACTION

AQUACEL™ Foam Dressing is the only foam that has comfort, simplicity, and the healing benefits of a Hydrofiber® interface.

INDICATIONS

AQUACEL™ Foam may be used for the management of both chronic and acute wounds, such as leg ulcers, pressure ulcers (stage 2 to 4) and diabetic ulcers; surgical wounds (post-operative, donor sites, dermatologic); partial thickness (second-degree) burns; traumatic or surgical wounds left to heal by secondary intention such as dehisced surgical incisions; surgical wounds that heal by primary intent, such as dermatologic and surgical incisions (e.g., orthopedic and vascular); local management of wounds that are prone to bleeding, such as wounds that have been mechanically or surgically debrided and donor sites; painful wounds; abrasions; lacerations; minor cuts; minor scalds and burns.

CONTRAINDICATIONS

- AQUACEL™ Foam dressings should not be used on individuals who are sensitive to or who have had an allergic reaction to the dressing or its components.

APPLICATION

- If the immediate sterile product pouch is damaged, do not use.

FOAMS

Wound site preparation and cleansing

- Before applying the dressing, cleanse the wound area with an appropriate wound cleanser and dry the surrounding skin.

Dressing preparation and application

- Choose a dressing size and shape to ensure that the central absorbent pad (area within the adhesive window) is 1 cm larger than the wound area. Remove the dressing from the sterile pack, minimizing finger contact with the wound contact surface and the adhesive surface where applicable. Remove the release liner if using the adhesive dressing.
- The dressing can be cut to shape for convenience. Hold the dressing over the wound and line up the center of the dressing with the center of the wound. Place the pad directly over the wound. For adhesive dressing, smooth down the adhesive border. An appropriate retention bandage or tape should be used to secure the dressing in place if the dressing does not have an adhesive border or if the adhesive dressing has been cut. For difficult to dress anatomical locations, such as the heel or the sacrum, the specially shaped adhesive dressings may be used. Discard any unused portion of the product after dressing the wound.

REMOVAL

- The dressing should be changed when clinically indicated (i.e., leakage, bleeding, increased pain, suspicion of infection). Maximum recommended wear time is up to 7 days. The wound should be cleansed at appropriate intervals. To remove the dressing, press down gently on the skin and carefully lift one corner of the dressing. Continue until all edges are free. Carefully lift away the dressing and discard according to local clinical protocols.

*See package insert for complete instructions for use.

FOAMS

Biatain® Non-Adhesive Foam Dressing; Biatain® Soft-Hold Foam Dressing and Biatain® Adhesive Foam Dressing

Coloplast

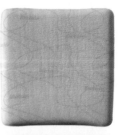

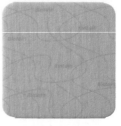

HOW SUPPLIED

Biatain Non-Adhesive Foam Dressing

Rectangle	2" × 2.75"	A6209
Square	4" × 4"	A6209
Square	6" × 6"	A6210
Square	8" × 8"	A6211

Biatain Soft-Hold Foam Dressing

Rectangle	2" × 2.75"	A6209
Square	4" × 4"	A6209
Square	6" × 6"	A6210

Biatain Adhesive Foam Dressing

Square	4" × 4"	A6212
Square	5" × 5"	A6212
Square	7" × 7"	A6213
Heel	7.5" × 8"	A6212
Sacral	9" × 9"	A6213

ACTION

Biatain® Foam Dressings are unique in their ability to manage low-to-high levels of wound exudate across a variety of wound types. 3D Polymer foam structure absorbs and locks away exudate without sticking to the wound bed. Highly permeable top film layer allows for optimal moist wound environment and protects from water and external contaminants.

INDICATIONS

Biatain Foam Dressings

- Are indicated for a wide range of exuding wounds including leg ulcers and pressure ulcers.
- May be used for second-degree burns, postoperative wounds, and skin abrasions.
- May be used on patients who are in treatment for a local or systemic infection at the discretion of a physician.
- May be used throughout the healing process to provide protection for the types of wounds indicated.

Biatain Non-Adhesive Foam Dressing

- In addition, Biatain Non-Adhesive Foam Dressings are indicated for noninfected diabetic foot ulcers.

FOAMS

Biatain Non-Adhesive and Adhesive Foam Dressings

- In addition, Biatain Non-Adhesive and Adhesive Foam Dressings are indicated for donor sites.

CONTRAINDICATIONS

- Biatain Soft-Hold Foam Dressings should not be used on donor sites.

CAUTION

- A health care professional should frequently inspect and manage infected wounds, diabetic wounds, and wounds which are solely or partially caused by arterial insufficiency in accordance with local guidelines.
- Do not use the product with oxidizing solutions, for example, hypochlorite and hydrogen peroxide solutions. Ensure that any other evaporating solution is completely dried off before dressing application.

APPLICATION

- Rinse the wound with lukewarm water or physiological saline. Gently dry the skin around the wound. The safe use of other cleansing agents in combination with Biatain Foam Dressings has not been demonstrated.
- If any film, cream, ointment or similar product is used, allow the skin to dry before applying the dressing.
- Remove the dressing aseptically from the packaging. Do not touch the plain (nonprinted) side of the foam.
- Select a dressing where the foam pad overlaps the wound edge by at least 2 cm (an overlap of 1 cm is sufficient in the case of small dressings).

Biatain Non-Adhesive Foam Dressing

- Must be applied with the plain (nonprinted) side toward the wound.
- Must be secured with a secondary bandage or compression.

Biatain Soft-Hold Foam Dressing

- Remove the protective film and apply the dressing with the plain (nonprinted) side toward the wound.
- Must be secured with a secondary bandage or compression.

Biatain Adhesive Foam Dressing

- Use the handles to avoid touching the dressing and to ensure aseptic application. Remove the protective film first and place the foam part of the dressing over the wound. Then remove the release films on the sides as part of the dressing application.

Biatain Sacral Foam Dressing

- Use the handles to ensure aseptic application. Remove the central protective film. Place the narrow end of the dressing as far down over the wound as possible and fix the dressing working up and outward. Remove the handles.

Biatain Heel Foam Dressing

- Use the handles to ensure aseptic application. Remove the central protective film. The dressing is shaped like an arrow. Fold the dressing at a 90-degree angle between the head and tail of the arrow. Hold the dressing so that the arrow is pointing away from the heel tip and fix the tail first. Then fix the head. Remove the handles one by one and fix the sides carefully so that the foam parts touch or overlap.

FOAMS

REMOVAL

- Change the dressing when clinically indicated or when visible signs of exudate approach the edge of the dressing.
- May be left in place for up to 7 days depending on the amount of exudate, dressing conditions, and type of wound.
- To remove, gently lift the corners of the dressing away from the wound.
- When removing adhesive dressings, loosen the adhesive border before lifting the dressing away from the wound.
- Biatain Sacral Foam Dressing should be removed from the top edge and down toward the anus to minimize the risk of transmitting infection.

REFERENCES

Biatain Non-Adhesive Foam Dressing

1. https://www.coloplast.us/wound/wound-/solutions/#-

Biatain Soft-Hold Foam Dressing

2. https://www.coloplast.us/wound/wound-/solutions/#-

Biatain Adhesive Foam Dressing

3. https://www.coloplast.us/wound/wound-/solutions/#-

FOAMS

Biatain® Silicone Foam Dressing; Biatain® Silicone Lite Foam Dressing

Coloplast

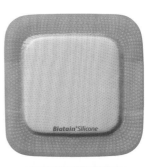

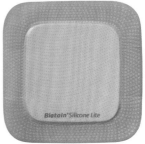

HOW SUPPLIED

Biatain Silicone Foam Dressing

Square	3″ × 3″	A6212
Square	4″ × 4″	A6212
Square	5″ × 5″	A6212
Square	6″ × 6″	A6213
Square	7″ × 7″	A6213
Post-op	4″ × 8″	A6245
Post-op	4″ × 12″	A6246
Heel	7″ × 7″	A6245
Sacral	9.8″ × 9.8″	A6213
Sacral	6″ × 7.5″	A6210
Multishape	5.5″ × 7.6″	A6212

Biatain Silicone Lite Foam Dressing

Square	2″ × 2″	A6413
Square	2″ × 5″	A6212
Square	3″ × 3″	A6212
Square	4″ × 4″	A6212
Square	5″ × 5″	A6212

FOAMS

ACTION

Biatain® Silicone Foam Dressings are unique in their ability to manage low-to-high levels of wound exudate across a variety of wound types. 3D Polymer foam structure absorbs and locks away exudate without sticking to the wound bed. Highly permeable top film layer allows for optimal moist wound environment and protects from water and external contaminants.

INDICATIONS

Biatain Silicone Foam Dressings are indicated for a wide range of exuding wounds including leg ulcers, pressure ulcers, noninfected diabetic foot ulcers, and donor sites. Biatain Silicone Lite Foam Dressings are indicated for a wide range of low exuding wounds including leg ulcers and pressure ulcers, noninfected diabetic foot ulcers, and donor sites. Both Biatain Silicone Foam Dressings and Biatain Silicone Lite Foam Dressings may be used for postoperative wounds and skin abrasions, on patients who are in treatment for local or systemic infection under the discretion of a health care professional, and throughout the healing process to provide protection for the indicated types of wounds.

CAUTION

- A health care professional should frequently inspect and manage diabetic wounds and wounds which are solely or partially caused by arterial insufficiency in accordance with local guidelines.
- Do not use the product with oxidizing solutions, for example, hypochlorite and hydrogen peroxide solutions. Ensure that any other evaporating solution is completely dried off before applying the product.

APPLICATION

- Cleanse the wound in accordance with normal procedures, for example, lukewarm water or physiological saline.
- Gently dry the skin around the wound.
- If any film, cream, ointment, or similar product is used, allow the skin to dry before applying the dressing.
- Select a dressing where the foam pad overlaps the wound edge by a minimum of 1 to 2 cm.
- Use the release liner to prevent touching the dressing and to ensure aseptic application. Remove the center protective film first and place the foam part of the dressing over the wound. Finally, remove the release liner on either side of the foam part.
- Apply the adherent side to the wound.

REMOVAL

- May be left in place for up to 7 days depending on the amount of exudate, dressing conditions, and type of wound.
- Change the dressing when clinically indicated or when visible signs of exudate approach the edge of the dressing.
- To remove the dressing, gently lift the corners of the dressing away from the wound. If is recommended to loosen the adhesive border before lifting the dressing away from the wound.

REFERENCES

Biatain Silicone Foam Dressing

1. www.biatainsiliconeus.com.

Biatain Silicone Lite Foam Dressing

2. www.biatainsiliconeus.com.

FOAMS

Bordered Foam

DermaRite Industries, LLC

HOW SUPPLIED

Island Dressing	4″ × 4″	A6212
Island Dressing	6″ × 6″	A6212
Dressing, Round Fenestrated	4″	A6212

ACTION

Bordered Foam™ is a hydrophilic foam island wound dressing with a waterproof border. Bordered Foam absorbs moderate to heavy exudate, while the waterproof backing keeps the dressing in place and protects the wound bed from contamination. Bordered Foam helps prevent periwound maceration by wicking fluids upward and away from the skin.

INDICATIONS

May be used for the management of exuding partial- or full-thickness wounds.
- Bordered Foam Round Fenestrated is indicated for partial or full thickness wounds at peritubular surgical wound sites, peritubular hypergranulation.

CONTRAINDICATIONS

- Bordered Foam should not be used on people who are sensitive or allergic to the dressing and its components.

APPLICATION

- Cleanse wound with advised liquid to remove residue according to local infection control protocol. Deep wounds should be well irrigated.
- Skin around wound should be clean and dry, use skin barrier prep as needed.
- Remove dressing from package.
- Remove backing paper from dressing.
- Apply sticky side of dressing to moist wound bed overlapping 1 to 2 inches of skin; gently smooth into place.

REMOVAL

- Dressing may be moistened to ease removal.
- Carefully remove adhesive dressings by holding the edge of the dressing and slowly pulling it parallel to the skin.
- Dispose of in accordance with local guidance.

REFERENCE

1. http://dermarite.com/product/bordered-foam/.

FOAMS

Circular Split Drain Foam

Gentell

HOW SUPPLIED

Pad	4″ Diameter	A6212

ACTION

Gentell's Circular Split Drain Foam Dressing is a pre-cut circular, bordered, absorptive dressing with a U-shaped fenestration ideal for heels, joints, and other wound sites with irregular or protruding surfaces, plus ostomy sites, catheters, and feeding tubes. This superabsorptive foam dressing reduces strike-through and prevents skin maceration by keeping the wound site dry. The hypo-allergenic, water-resistant tape allows the skin to breathe and makes application easy, which reduces nursing time.

INDICATIONS

Apply on heels, joints, and other wound sites with irregular or protruding surfaces, plus ostomy sites, catheters, and wound sites with moderate to heavy drainage.

CONTRAINDICATIONS

- None.

APPLICATION

- Irrigate the wound with Gentell Wound Cleanser and gently dry the skin surrounding the wound site.
- Ensure the dressing is large enough to provide a minimum of a one-inch margin around the edges of the wound.
- Remove paper backing from the dressing and apply directly over the surface of the wound.

REMOVAL

- Change daily or as ordered by a physician.

FOAMS

New Product: ComfortFoam

DermaRite Industries, LLC

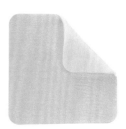

HOW SUPPLIED

Foam Wound Dressing with Soft Silicone Adhesive	2″ × 2″	A6209
Foam Wound Dressing with Soft Silicone Adhesive	3″ × 3″	A6209
Foam Wound Dressing with Soft Silicone Adhesive	4″ × 4″	A6209
Foam Wound Dressing with Soft Silicone Adhesive	4″ × 5″	A6210
Foam Wound Dressing with Soft Silicone Adhesive	4″ × 8″	A6210
Foam Wound Dressing with Soft Silicone Adhesive	6″ × 6″	A6210
Foam Wound Dressing with Soft Silicone Adhesive	6″ × 8″	A6210
Foam Wound Dressing with Soft Silicone Adhesive	8″ × 8″	A6211

ACTION

ComfortFoam® is a self-adherent silicone foam wound dressing consisting of a soft silicone contact surface, a flexible, absorbent polyurethane foam pad, and a vapor-permeable, moisture-proof outer film. The silicone adhesive sticks to surrounding skin but not to the wound bed, minimizing pain and the risk of damage to the wound and periwound areas.

INDICATIONS

For the management of moderate to heavily exuding partial or full thickness wounds, including pressure ulcers, diabetic ulcers, arterial ulcers, venous ulcers, and traumatic wounds.

CONTRAINDICATIONS

- ComfortFoam should not be used on people who are sensitive or allergic to silicone and/or any other contents of the dressing.

APPLICATION

- Cleanse wound with advised liquid to remove residue according to local infection control protocol. Deep wounds should be well irrigated.
- Skin around wound should be clean and dry, use skin barrier prep as needed.
- Remove dressing from package.
- Dressing may be cut to size prior to application.
- Remove backing paper from dressing.
- Apply sticky side of dressing to moist wound bed overlapping 1 to 2 inches of dry skin; gently smooth into place.
- Secure edges with tape if desired.

FOAMS

REMOVAL

- Dressing may be moistened to ease removal.
- Carefully remove adhesive dressings by holding the edge of the dressing and slowly pulling it parallel to the skin.
- Dispose of in accordance with local guidance.

REFERENCE

1. http://dermarite.com/product/comfortfoam-dressing/.

FOAMS

New Product: ComfortFoam Border

DermaRite Industries, LLC

HOW SUPPLIED

Bordered Foam Wound Dressing with Soft Silicone Adhesive	2" × 2"	A6413
Bordered Foam Wound Dressing with Soft Silicone Adhesive	2" × 5"	A6413
Bordered Foam Wound Dressing with Soft Silicone Adhesive	3" × 3"	A6413
Bordered Foam Wound Dressing with Soft Silicone Adhesive	4" × 4"	A6212
Bordered Foam Wound Dressing with Soft Silicone Adhesive	4" × 8"	A6212
Bordered Foam Wound Dressing with Soft Silicone Adhesive	4" × 12"	A6213
Bordered Foam Wound Dressing with Soft Silicone Adhesive	6" × 6"	A6212
Bordered Foam Wound Dressing with Soft Silicone Adhesive	6" × 8"	A6213
Bordered Foam Wound Dressing with Soft Silicone Adhesive	7" × 7"	A6213
Bordered Foam Wound Dressing with Soft Silicone Adhesive, Heel	5" × 8"	A6212
Bordered Foam Wound Dressing with Soft Silicone Adhesive, Sacral	7.2" × 7.2"	A6213
Bordered Foam Wound Dressing with Soft Silicone Adhesive, Large Sacral	9" × 9"	A6213

FOAMS

ACTION

ComfortFoam® Border is a self-adherent silicone foam island dressing consisting of a soft silicone contact surface, a flexible, absorbent polyurethane foam pad, and a vapor-permeable, moisture-proof outer film. The silicone adhesive sticks to surrounding skin but not to the wound bed, minimizing pain and the risk of damage to the wound and periwound areas.

INDICATIONS

For the management of moderate to heavily exuding partial or full thickness wounds, including pressure ulcers, diabetic ulcers, arterial ulcers, venous ulcers, and traumatic wounds.

CONTRAINDICATIONS

- ComfortFoam Border should not be used on people who are sensitive or allergic to silicone and/or any other contents of the dressing.

APPLICATION

- Cleanse wound with advised liquid to remove residue according to local infection control protocol. Deep wounds should be well irrigated.
- Skin around wound should be clean and dry, use skin barrier prep as needed.
- Remove dressing from package.
- Remove backing paper from dressing.
- Apply sticky side of dressing to moist wound bed overlapping 1 to 2 inches of dry skin; gently smooth into place.

REMOVAL

- Dressing may be moistened to ease removal.
- Carefully remove adhesive dressings by holding the edge of the dressing and slowly pulling it parallel to the skin.
- Dispose of in accordance with local guidance.

REFERENCE

1. http://dermarite.com/product/comfortfoam-border/.

FOAMS

New Product: ComfortFoam Border Lite

DermaRite Industries, LLC

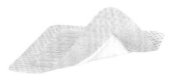

HOW SUPPLIED

Thin Bordered Foam Wound Dressing with Soft Silicone Adhesive	2″ × 2″
Thin Bordered Foam Wound Dressing with Soft Silicone Adhesive	3″ × 3″
Thin Bordered Foam Wound Dressing with Soft Silicone Adhesive	4″ × 4″

ACTION

ComfortFoam® Border Lite is a self-adherent silicone foam island dressing consisting of a soft silicone contact surface, a flexible, absorbent polyurethane foam pad, and a vapor-permeable, moisture-proof outer film. The silicone adhesive sticks to surrounding skin but not to the wound bed, minimizing pain and the risk of damage to the wound and periwound areas.

INDICATIONS

For the management of light to moderately exuding partial or full thickness wounds, including pressure ulcers, diabetic ulcers, arterial ulcers, venous ulcers, and traumatic wounds.

CONTRAINDICATIONS

- ComfortFoam Border Lite should not be used on people who are sensitive or allergic to silicone and/or any other contents of the dressing.

APPLICATION

- Cleanse wound with advised liquid to remove residue according to local infection control protocol. Deep wounds should be well irrigated.
- Skin around wound should be clean and dry, use skin barrier prep as needed.
- Remove dressing from package.
- Remove backing paper from dressing.
- Apply sticky side of dressing to moist wound bed overlapping 1 to 2 inches of dry skin; gently smooth into place.

REMOVAL

- Dressing may be moistened to ease removal.
- Carefully remove adhesive dressings by holding the edge of the dressing and slowly pulling it parallel to the skin.
- Dispose of in accordance with local guidance.

REFERENCE

1. http://dermarite.com/product/comfortfoam-border-lite/.

FOAMS

DermaFoam

DermaRite Industries, LLC

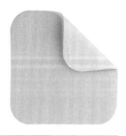

HOW SUPPLIED

Waterproof Foam Wound Dressing	2″ × 2″	A6209
Waterproof Foam Wound Dressing	4″ × 4.25″	A6210
Waterproof Foam Wound Dressing	6″ × 6″	A6210
Waterproof Foam Wound Dressing, Heel/Elbow	4.9″ × 5″	A6210
Waterproof Foam Wound Dressing, Tracheostomy	3.5″ × 3.5″	

ACTION

DermaFoam™ is a highly absorbent foam dressing that wicks wound exudate to reduce the risk for maceration in moderate to heavily draining wounds. It has a waterproof polyurethane film backing to prevent strikethrough of exudate. DermaFoam can be cut to size for irregularly shaped wounds and is nonadhesive so it is easy to remove; needs to be secured in place.

INDICATIONS

May be used as a primary dressing for the management of acute or chronic partial- or full-thickness wounds/ulcers with moderate to heavy exudate.

CONTRAINDICATIONS

- DermaFoam should not be used on people who are sensitive or allergic to the dressing and its components.

APPLICATION

- Cleanse wound with advised liquid to remove residue according to local infection control protocol. Deep wounds should be well irrigated.
- Skin around wound should be clean and dry, use skin barrier prep as needed.
- Remove dressing from package.
- Dressing may be cut to size prior to application.
- Apply foam surface of dressing to moist wound bed overlapping 1 to 2 inches of dry skin.
- Secure with tape or appropriate cover dressing that manages drainage and maintains a moist wound environment.

REMOVAL

- Dressing may be moistened to ease removal.
- Carefully remove adhesive dressings by holding the edge of the dressing and slowly pulling it parallel to the skin.
- Dispose of in accordance with local guidance.

REFERENCE

1. http://dermarite.com/product/dermafoam/.

FOAMS

DermaLevin

DermaRite Industries, LLC

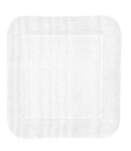

HOW SUPPLIED

Waterproof Adhesive Foam Wound Dressing	4" × 4"	A6212
Waterproof Adhesive Foam Wound Dressing	6" × 6"	A6212

ACTION

DermaLevin® is a moderately absorbent waterproof foam island dressing with a very thin hydrocolloid adhesive that protects and cushions the wound and maintains a moist wound environment. Conforms easily to awkward dressing sites.

INDICATIONS

May be used for the management of acute or chronic partial- or full-thickness wounds/ulcers with moderate exudate.

CONTRAINDICATIONS

- DermaLevin should not be used on people who are sensitive or allergic to the dressing and its components.

APPLICATION

- Cleanse wound with advised liquid to remove residue according to local infection control protocol. Deep wounds should be well irrigated.
- Skin around wound should be clean and dry, use skin barrier prep as needed.
- Warm packaged dressing in hands prior to application.
- Remove dressing from package.
- Remove backing paper from dressing.
- Apply sticky side of dressing to moist wound bed overlapping 1 to 2 inches of dry skin; gently smooth into place. Hold in place for several seconds to improve adhesion.

REMOVAL

- Dressing may be moistened to ease removal.
- Carefully remove adhesive dressings by holding the edge of the dressing and slowly pulling it parallel to the skin.
- Dispose of in accordance with local guidance.

REFERENCE

1. http://dermarite.com/product/dermalevin/.

FOAMS

New Product: Foam Lite™ ConvaTec Wound Dressing*

ConvaTec

HOW SUPPLIED

Dressing	2″ × 2″
Dressing	3.1″ × 3.1″
Dressing	4″ × 4″
Dressing	5.9″ × 5.9″
Dressing	2.1″ × 4.7″
Dressing	4″ × 8″

ACTION

Foam Lite™ is a thin, flexible foam dressing developed specifically for managing low to non-exuding wounds, such as skin abrasions, skin tears and partial-thickness burns, which do not require the absorbency of regular foam dressings.

INDICATIONS

Foam Lite™ is for the management of low to nonexuding chronic and acute wounds such as abrasions, lacerations, minor cuts and minor scalds or burns.

CONTRAINDICATIONS

- Foam Lite™ should not be used if you are sensitive to the dressing or its components, or have an allergic reaction to the dressing.

APPLICATION

- Before applying the dressing, clean the wound area with appropriate wound cleanser and dry the surrounding skin.
- Ensure that the surrounding skin is free from any oil-based products. Choose a dressing size and shape to ensure that the central pad is at least 1 cm larger than the wound area. Hold the dressing over the wound and line up the center of the dressing with the center of the wound. Smooth the dressing over the wound and ensure that the dressing is adhered all around the wound.

REMOVAL

- The dressing should be changed when clinically indicated (e.g., leakage, bleeding, increased pain, suspicion of infection). Maximum recommended wear time is up to 7 days. To remove the dressing, press down gently on the skin and carefully lift one corner of the dressing. Continue until all edges are free. Carefully lift away the dressing and discard according to local clinical protocols until all edges are free.

*See package insert for complete instructions for use.

FOAMS

HydraFoam

DermaRite Industries, LLC

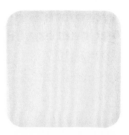

HOW SUPPLIED

Hydrophilic Foam Wound Dressing	2″ × 2″	A6209
Hydrophilic Foam Wound Dressing	4″ × 4.25″	A6210
Hydrophilic Foam Wound Dressing	6″ × 6″	A6210

ACTION

HydraFoam™ is a hydrophilic (water-loving), highly absorbent foam dressing that wicks wound exudate to reduce the risk of maceration of moderate to heavily draining wounds. HydraFoam is nonadhesive, so it is easy to remove and can be cut to size to support moist wound healing of irregularly shaped wounds. HydraFoam needs to be secured in place.

INDICATIONS

May be used as a primary dressing for the management of acute or chronic partial- or full-thickness wounds/ulcers with moderate to heavy exudate.

CONTRAINDICATIONS

- HydraFoam should not be used on people who are sensitive or allergic to the dressing and its components.

APPLICATION

- Cleanse wound with advised liquid to remove residue according to local infection control protocol. Deep wounds should be well irrigated.
- Skin around wound should be clean and dry, use skin barrier prep as needed.
- Remove dressing from package.
- Dressing may be cut to size prior to application.
- Apply foam surface of dressing to moist wound bed overlapping 1 to 2 inches of dry skin.
- Secure with tape or appropriate cover dressing that manages drainage and maintains a moist wound environment.

REMOVAL

- Dressing may be moistened to ease removal.
- Carefully remove adhesive dressings by holding the edge of the dressing and slowly pulling it parallel to the skin.
- Dispose of in accordance with local guidance.

REFERENCE

1. http://dermarite.com/product/hydrafoam/.

FOAMS

Hydrofera Blue READY™ Antibacterial Foam Dressing*

Hydrofera, LLC

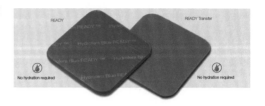

HOW SUPPLIED

Hydrofera Blue READY foam with film backing	2.5" × 2.5"	A6209
Hydrofera Blue READY foam with film backing	4" × 5"	A6210
Hydrofera Blue READY foam with film backing	8" × 8"	A6211
Hydrofera Blue READY-Transfer foam without film backing	2.5" × 2.5"	A6209
Hydrofera Blue READY-Transfer foam without film backing	4" × 5"	A6210
Hydrofera Blue READY-Transfer foam without film backing	8" × 8"	A6211

ACTION

Hydrofera Blue READY antibacterial foam dressings are sterile absorptive foam dressings made of polyurethane (PU) foam combined with two organic pigments, methylene blue and gentian violet, which provide broad-spectrum antibacterial protection.[1] Hydrofera Blue READY dressings absorb and retain exudate in the dressing.[2] Hydrofera Blue READY—Transfer dressing does not have a film backing so exudate is rapidly transferred into a secondary absorbent dressing.[3] Both are non-cytotoxic.[4]

INDICATIONS

Hydrofera Blue READY antibacterial foam dressings are intended as external dressings for use in local management of wounds such as pressure ulcers, donor sites, venous stasis ulcers, arterial ulcers, diabetic ulcers, abrasions, lacerations, superficial burns, postsurgical incisions, and other external wounds inflicted by trauma.

CONTRAINDICATIONS

- Hydrofera Blue READY antibacterial foam dressings are not indicated for third-degree burns and should not be used on individuals who are sensitive to or who have had an allergic reaction to the dressing or one of its components.

APPLICATION

- Select the appropriate dressing size to ensure the dressing will cover the entire wound.
- The dressing may be cut in order to optimize placement over wounds on heels, elbows, and so forth.
- Apply the dressing to the wound.
- Secure the dressing using a bandage or a tape over the film surface.

FOAMS

- The dressing can be applied under compression and total contact casting.
- Hydrofera Blue READY antibacterial dressings are indicated for moderate to heavily exuding wounds.

REMOVAL

- Hydrofera Blue READY antibacterial foam dressings can be left in place up to 7 days, depending on the exudate and clinical conditions of the wound.
- The dressing should be changed if it turns white.
- If the dressing has retained its color where it is in contact with the wound, the dressing may be left in place for up to 7 days.
- Do not reuse the dressing.

*See package insert for complete instructions for use.

REFERENCES

1. Instructions for Use.
2. Data on file, EN 13726-1; 2002.
3. Data on file 2017 – TR-00148.
4. Data on file 2013 – 130107-1CYT.

FOAMS

Hydrofera Blue™ Classic Antibacterial Foam Dressing*

Hydrofera, LLC

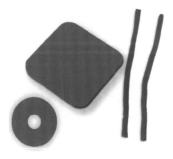

HOW SUPPLIED

Standard Dressing	2″ × 2″	A6209
Standard Dressing	4″ × 4″	A6209
Standard Dressing	6″ × 6″	A6210
Tunneling Dressing	9 mm (1.2 g)	A6215
Heavy Drainage Dressing	4″ × 4″ × 0.5″, thick	A6209
Heavy Drainage Dressing	6″ × 6″ × 0.75″, thick	A6210
Dressings with Moisture-Retentive Film	4″ × 4″	A6209
Dressings with Moisture-Retentive Film	2.25″ × 8″	A6210
Island Dressing	4″ × 4.75″ (pad size 2″ × 2.75″)	A6212
Ostomy Ring	2.5″ diameter Ostomy dressing	A6209

ACTION

Hydrofera Blue CLASSIC antibacterial foam dressing is sterile absorptive foam dressing made of polyvinyl alcohol (PVA) sponge combined with two organic pigments, methylene blue and gentian violet, which provide broad-spectrum antibacterial protection. Hydrofera Blue antibacterial foam dressings are non-cytotoxic and do not inhibit growth factors. Provide natural negative pressure, natural autolytic debridement and absorb and retain bacteria-laden exudate. Have been shown to flatten rolled wound edges, and are compatible with enzymatic debriders and HBOT. Hydrofera Blue antibacterial foam dressings have demonstrated broad-spectrum antibacterial properties, autolytic debridement, and absorbs and retains bacteria-laden exudate,[1-3] all of which assist in bioburden control and good wound bed preparation. In addition, Hydrofera Blue classic antibacterial foam dressings are noncytotoxic, may help flatten epibole[4-6] and are compatible with enzymatic debriders.[7]

INDICATIONS

To manage wounds such as pressure ulcers, donor sites, venous stasis ulcers, arterial ulcers, diabetic ulcers, abrasions, lacerations, superficial burns, postsurgical incisions, and other external wounds inflicted by trauma.

CONTRAINDICATIONS

- Contraindicated for third-degree burns.

APPLICATION

- Before initial application, debride the wound of any necrotic tissue.
- Clean the wound with normal saline or with an appropriate cleansing solution, or both.
- Open the Hydrofera Blue classic antibacterial foam dressing package, and moisten the dressing with either sterile saline or sterile water. Squeeze out excess.
- Place the dressing on or in the wound, and secure with the appropriate secondary dressing.
- Cover dressing should maintain an optimal moist wound healing environment (for example: cover with a super absorbent dressing for a highly exudating wound, OR a film/occlusive dressing for a low exudating wound).
- The dressing may be folded, layered, and cut with sterile scissors to fit the wound. NOTE: Hydrofera Blue classic dressings with moisture retentive film may not be folded or layered.

REMOVAL

- The first dressing change should occur at 24 hours.
- Examine the area of the dressing in contact with the wound bed: If the dressing has turned white or lightened in color, the dressing should be changed again at 24 hours until the dressing retains its color.
- If the dressing has retained its color where it is in contact with the wound, a new dressing can be applied and left in place for up to 72 hours.
- Do not allow the dressing to completely dry out. The dressing should be rehydrated as needed. If a Hydrofera Blue classic antibacterial foam dressing is allowed to dry out, rehydration with sterile saline or sterile water is recommended prior to removal.

*See package insert for complete instructions for use.

REFERENCES

1. Instructions for Use.
2. Applewhite AJ, Attar P, Liden B, Stevenson Q. Gentian violet and methylene blue polyvinyl alcohol foam antibacterial dressing as a viable form of autolytic debridement in the wound bed. *Surg Technol. Int* 2015;26:65–70.
3. Internal data on file.
4. Edwards K. New twist on an old favorite: gentian violet and methylene blue antibacterial foam dressings. *Adv Wound Care.* (New Rochelle). 2015. In Press.
5. Swan H, Trovela VJ. Case study review: use of an absorbent bacteriostatic dressing for multiple indications. Poster presented at Clinical Symposium on Advances in Skin and Wound Care; September 9–11, 2011; Washington DC.
6. Weir D, Blakely M. Case review of the clinical use of an antimicrobial PVA foam dressing. Poster presented at the Clinical Symposium on Advances in Skin and Wound Care; September 9–11, 2011, Washington DC.
7. Shi L, Ermis R, Kiedaisch B, Carson D. The effect of various wound dressings on the activity of debriding enzymes. *Adv Skin Wound Care.* 2010;23(10):456–462.

FOAMS

Mepiform® Soft Silicone Gel Sheeting

Mölnlycke Health Care

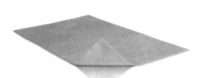

HOW SUPPLIED

Gel Sheeting	2" × 3"
Gel Sheeting	4" × 7"
Gel Sheeting	1.6" × 12"

ACTION

Mepiform® is a self-adherent soft silicone gel sheeting for scar management, featuring Safetac technology that is breathable, comfortable, and waterproof. Mepiform is thin, flexible, and discreet and can be worn during all daily activities.

INDICATIONS

To manage old and new hypertrophic and keloid scars; can be used on closed wounds, where it may prevent the formation of hypertrophic and keloid scars; may be used prophylactically for 2 to 6 months, depending on the condition of the scar.

CONTRAINDICATIONS

- None provided by the manufacturer.

APPLICATION

- Clean the scar tissue or closed wound with mild soap and water. Rinse and pat dry. Make sure the scar and surrounding skin are dry.
- If necessary, cut the dressing to the appropriate shape. No extra fixation is needed.
- Remove the release film and apply the dressing to the scar without stretching the dressing.
- Avoid the use of creams or ointments under Mepiform.

REMOVAL

- Optimally, Mepiform® should be worn 24 hours per day. It is recommended that Mepiform be removed once a day for showering or bathing and reapplied.
- Change the dressing when it begins to lose its adherent properties. Dressing wear time varies by person.

FOAMS

Mepilex® Absorbent Foam Dressing

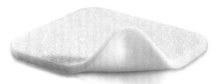

Mölnlycke Health Care

HOW SUPPLIED

Pad	4″ × 4″	A6209
Pad	4″ × 5″	A6210
Pad	4″ × 8″	A6210
Pad	6″ × 6″	A6210
Pad	8″ × 8″	A6211

ACTION

Mepilex® is a soft silicone absorbent foam dressing featuring Safetac® technology, which effectively absorbs exudate and helps maintain a moist wound environment for optimal wound healing. The Safetac® soft silicone technology layer minimizes the risk of periwound maceration and erosion and allows the dressing to be changed without causing additional pain to the patient or trauma to the wound and surrounding skin. Mepilex can be used under compression and may be cut for customization to the wound area.

INDICATIONS

To treat a wide range of exuding wounds, painful wounds, and wounds with compromised or fragile surrounding skin, including pressure ulcers and lower-extremity ulcers, such as venous and diabetic ulcers.

CONTRAINDICATIONS

- Do no use Mepilex together with oxidizing agents such as hydrogen peroxide.

APPLICATION

- Clean the wound area. Make sure the surrounding skin is dry.
- Select an appropriate dressing size. For best results, Mepilex should overlap the surrounding skin by at least 1–2 cm for smaller wounds and 5 cm for larger wounds. If necessary, cut the dressing to fit.
- Remove the release film, and apply the dressing with the adherent side toward the wound. Do not stretch the dressing.
- Secure the dressing with a bandage or other fixation when necessary.

REMOVAL

- Leave Mepilex® in place for several days, depending on the condition of the wound and the surrounding skin, or facility policy.

FOAMS

Mepilex® Border Lite Bordered Thin Foam Dressing

Mölnlycke Health Care

Mepilex® Border Lite

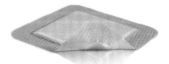

HOW SUPPLIED

Self-Adherent Soft Silicone Thin Foam Dressing	1.6″ × 2″	A6212
Self-Adherent Soft Silicone Thin Foam Dressing	2″ × 5″	A6212
Self-Adherent Soft Silicone Thin Foam Dressing	3″ × 3″	A6212
Self-Adherent Soft Silicone Thin Foam Dressing	4″ × 4″	A6212
Self-Adherent Soft Silicone Thin Foam Dressing	6″ × 6″	A6213

ACTION

Mepilex® Border Lite self-adherent soft silicone thin foam dressing is a highly conformable dressing that absorbs exudate, maintains a moist wound environment, and minimizes the risk for periwound maceration. The Safetac® technology layer allows for atraumatic removal, which prevents trauma to the wound and surrounding skin and prevents pain to the patient upon removal.

INDICATIONS

To manage a wide range of nonexuding to low-exuding wounds, painful wounds, and wounds with compromised or fragile surrounding skin, including lower-extremity wounds, pressure ulcers, and traumatic wounds such as abrasions, cuts, finger injuries, blisters, and skin tears; can also be used for protection of compromised and/or fragile skin.

CONTRAINDICATIONS

- Do not use on patients with known sensitivity to the dressing or its components.
- Do not use Mepilex® Border Lite together with oxidizing agents such as hydrogen peroxide.

APPLICATION

- Clean the wound area. Make sure the surrounding skin is dry.
- Remove the release film, and apply the dressing to the wound. Do not stretch the dressing.

REMOVAL

- Mepilex Border Lite can be left in place for several days, depending on the condition of the wound and the surrounding skin, or as indicated by accepted clinical practice. Mepilex Border Lite should be changed when exudate is present at the pad edges.

FOAMS

New Product: Mepilex® Border Post-Op

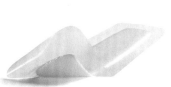

Mölnlycke Health Care

HOW SUPPLIED

Dressing	4″ × 6″	A4649
Dressing	4″ × 8″	A4649
Dressing	4″ × 10″	A4649
Dressing	4″ × 12″	A4649
Dressing	4″ × 14″	A4649

ACTION

Mepilex® Border Post-Op is a self-adherent dressing that absorbs blood exudate and minimizes the risk for maceration.

Mepilex® Border Post-Op consists of:

- A transparent film which is vapor permeable and waterproof.
- An absorbent pad in two layers: a nonwoven spreading layer and a layer with super absorbent polyacrylate fibers.
- A wound contact layer covered with a polyethylene release film.

INDICATIONS

Mepilex® Border Post-Op is a self-adhesive absorbent dressing designed for exuding wound. It is intended for acute wounds, such as surgical wounds, cuts, and abrasions.

PRECAUTIONS

- Do not use on patients with known sensitivity to the dressing or its components.
- In case of signs of clinical infection, consult a health care professional for adequate infection treatment.

APPLICATION

- Cleanse the wound in accordance to normal procedures.
- Dry the surrounding skin thoroughly.
- Open the package and remove the dressings.
- Mepilex® Border Post-Op wound pad should overlap the wound by at least 1 to 2 cm in order to protect the surrounding skin from maceration and fixate the dressing securely.
- Remove the middle release film and apply the adherent side to the wound, allowing initial fixation of the dressing. Avoid wrinkles while gently removing the release films, start with the longer part. Do not stretch the product during application.

REMOVAL

- Mepilex® Border Post-Op may be left in place for up to 7 days depending on the condition of the wound and the surrounding skin, or as indicated by accepted clinical practice.

FOAMS

Mepilex® Border Self-Adherent Bordered Foam Dressing

Mölnlycke Health Care

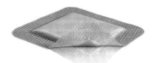

Mepilex® Border

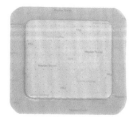

Mepilex® Border Flex

HOW SUPPLIED

Mepilex® Border	3" × 3"	A6212
Mepilex® Border	4" × 4"	A6212
Mepilex® Border	4" × 8"	A6212
Mepilex® Border	6" × 6"	A6213
Mepilex® Border	6" × 8"	A6213
Mepilex® Border	4" × 12"	A6213
Mepilex® Border Flex	3" × 3"	A6212
Mepilex® Border Flex	4" × 4"	A6212
Mepilex® Border Flex	6" × 6"	A6213
Mepilex® Border Flex	6" × 8"	A6213
Mepilex® Border Heel	8.7" × 9.1"	A6210
Mepilex® Border Sacrum	7.2" × 7.2"	A6213
Mepilex® Border Sacrum	9.2" × 9.2"	A6213

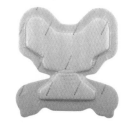

Mepilex® Border Heel

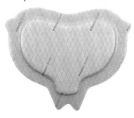

Mepilex® Border Sacrum

ACTION

Mepilex® Border self-adherent foam dressing with Safetac® technology absorbs exudate effectively, minimizes the risk of periwound skin maceration, and helps to maintain a moist environment for optimum wound healing. The Safetac® technology properties allow the dressing to be changed without causing additional trauma to the wound and surrounding skin or pain to the patient.

INDICATIONS

Designed for a wide range of exuding wounds, painful wounds, and wounds with compromised or fragile surrounding skin, including pressure ulcers, lower-extremity ulcers (such as diabetic ulcers), and traumatic wounds such as skin tears.

CONTRAINDICATIONS

- Do use on patients with known sensitivity to the dressing or its components.
- Do no use Mepilex Border together with oxidizing agents such as hydrogen peroxide.

APPLICATION

- Clean the wound area. Make sure the surrounding skin is dry.
- Remove the release film, and apply the dressing to the wound. Do not stretch the dressing.

REMOVAL

- Mepilex Border can be left in place for several days, depending on the condition of the wound and the surrounding skin, or as indicated by accepted clinical practice. Mepilex Border should be changed when exudate is present at the pad edges.

FOAMS

Mepilex® Heel Foam Heel Dressing

Mölnlycke Health Care

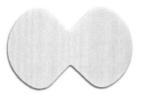

Mepilex® Heel

HOW SUPPLIED

Soft Silicone Absorbent Foam Heel Dressing	5″ × 8″

ACTION

Mepilex® Heel is a soft silicone, absorbent foam dressing featuring Safetac® technology and specifically designed for use on the heel. It is shaped to fit any heel, so there is no need for measuring or cutting. The Safetac technology provides a good seal to reduce the risk of maceration and minimizes the trauma and pain at dressing changes.

INDICATIONS

Designed for a wide range of exuding wounds, painful wounds, and wounds with compromised or fragile periwound skin, including pressure ulcers, venous ulcers, and diabetic ulcers.

CONTRAINDICATIONS

- Do not use on patients with known sensitivity to the dressing or its components.
- Do not use Mepilex® Heel together with oxidizing agents such as hydrogen peroxide.

APPLICATION

- Clean the wound area. Make sure the surrounding skin is dry.
- Remove the longer release film.
- Fix the dressing under the foot, and release the shorter release film.
- Mold the dressing around the heel, and bring edges together.
- Mepilex Heel should overlap the wound bed by at least 1″ (2.5 cm) onto the surrounding skin.

REMOVAL

- Leave Mepilex Heel in place for several days, depending on the condition of the wound and the surrounding skin, or facility policy.

FOAMS

Mepilex® Lite Thin Foam Dressing

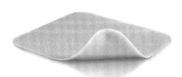

Mölnlycke Health Care

HOW SUPPLIED

Dressing	2.4" × 3.4"	A6209
Dressing	4" × 4"	A6209
Dressing	6" × 6"	A6210
Dressing	8" × 20"	A6211

ACTION

Mepilex® Lite is a highly conformable, soft silicone foam dressing that absorbs exudates and helps maintain a moist wound environment. The Safetac® technology layer seals around the wound edges, deterring exudate from leaking onto the surrounding skin, which minimizes the risk for maceration and ensures atraumatic dressing changes. Mepilex Lite can be cut to suit various wound shapes and locations.

INDICATIONS

Mepilex Lite may be used as a primary or secondary dressing for the management of a wide range of non to low exuding wounds, such as leg and foot ulcers, partial-thickness burns, radiation skin reactions, and epidermolysis bullosa (EB); Mepilex® Lite can also be used for protection of compromised and/or fragile skin and may be used under compression bandaging.

CONTRAINDICATIONS

- Do not use on patients with known sensitivity to the dressing or its components.
- Do not use Mepilex® Lite together with oxidizing agents such as hydrogen peroxide.

APPLICATION

- Clean the wound area. Make sure the surrounding skin is dry.
- Select an appropriate dressing size. For best results, Mepilex Lite should overlap the surrounding skin by at least 1–2 cm for smaller wounds and 5 cm for larger wounds. If necessary, cut the dressing to fit.
- Remove the release film, and apply the dressing with the adherent side toward the wound. Do not stretch the dressing.
- Secure the dressing with a bandage or other fixation when necessary.

REMOVAL

- Leave Mepilex Lite in place for several days, depending on the condition of the wound and the surrounding skin, or facility policy.

Mepilex® Transfer Exudate Transfer Dressing

Mölnlycke Health Care

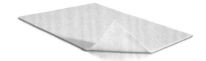

Mepilex® Transfer

HOW SUPPLIED

Pad	6″ × 8″	A6210
Pad	8″ × 20″	A6211

ACTION

Mepilex® Transfer is thin and conformable, enabling management of difficult-to-dress wounds. As the Safetac® technology layer seals around the wound margins, the foam structure allows the exudate to move vertically into a secondary absorbent pad, thus protecting the surrounding skin from excess moisture and minimizing the risk of maceration. With the Safetac® technology layer, Mepilex® Transfer ensures direct contact to the wound base and surrounding skin and helps minimize trauma and pain during dressing changes.

INDICATIONS

For a wide range of exuding wounds and difficult-to-dress wounds such as those caused by cancer, lymphedema, and Epstein–Barr virus; also used as a protective layer on minimal or low exuding wounds; covers large, awkward areas; ideal for areas with fragile skin.

CONTRAINDICATIONS

- Do not use on patients with known sensitivity to the dressing or its components.
- Do not use Mepilex® Transfer together with oxidizing agents such as hydrogen peroxide.

APPLICATION

- Clean the wound area. Make sure the surrounding skin is dry.
- Remove the release film, and apply the dressing to the wound, overlapping the surrounding skin by 1 to 2 cm for smaller wounds and 5 cm for larger wounds.
- Dressing may be used under compression.
- Secure Mepilex Transfer with a secondary dressing. Dressing choice depends on the location and exudate amount. Options include mesh net or other nonadhesive dressing holder, Mepore Film, Alldress, gauze, or Mefix.

REMOVAL

- Mepilex Transfer can be left in place for several days, depending on the condition of the wound and the surrounding skin, or as indicated by accepted clinical practice.

FOAMS

New Product: Mepilex® XT with Safetac® Technology

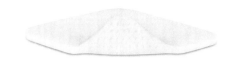

Mölnlycke Health Care

HOW SUPPLIED

Dressing	4″ × 4″	A6209
Dressing	4″ × 8″	A6210
Dressing	6″ × 6″	A6210
Dressing	8″ × 8″	A6211

ACTION

Mepilex® XT is a soft silicone wound dressing that absorbs both low and high viscous exudate. Mepilex® XT consists of:

- A soft silicone wound contact layer.
- A flexible absorbent pad of polyurethane foam.
- An outer layer film which is vapor permeable and waterproof.

INDICATIONS

Mepilex® XT is a dressing designed for a wide range of exuding acute and chronic wounds in all healing states such as leg and foot ulcers, pressure ulcers, and traumatic wounds, for example, skin tears and secondary wounds.

CONTRAINDICATIONS

- Do not use Mepilex® XT together with oxidizing agents such as hydrochloric solutions and hydrogen peroxide.
- Do no use on patients with known sensitivity to the dressing or its components.

APPLICATION

- Cleanse the wound in accordance to normal procedures.
- Dry the surrounding skin thoroughly.
- Remove the release films and apply the adherent side of the wound. Do not stretch.
- For the best results, Mepilex® XT should overlap the dry surrounding skin by at least 1 to 2 cm for the smaller sizes in order to protect the surrounding skin from maceration and excoriation and fixate the dressing securely. If required, Mepilex® XT can be cut to suit various wound shapes and locations.
- When necessary, fixate Mepilex® XT with a bandage or other fixation.
- Mepilex® XT may be left in place for several days depending on the condition of the wound and surrounding skin, or as indicated by accepted clinical practice.
- A change in dressing regimen can result in an initial increased level of exudate, which temporarily may require an increase change frequency.
- As Mepilex® XT maintains a moist wound environment, supporting debridement, there might be an initial increase in wound size. This is normal and to be expected.
- Mepilex® XT can be used under compression bandaging.

REMOVAL

- Mepilex® XT may be left in place for several days depending on the condition of the wound and surrounding skin, or as indicated by accepted clinical practice.

FOAMS

New Product: Optifoam Gentle

Medline Industries, Inc.

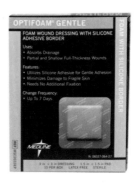

HOW SUPPLIED

Silicone Bordered Foam Island Dressing	1.6″ × 2″	A6413
Silicone Bordered Foam Island Dressing	3″ × 3″	A6212
Silicone Bordered Foam Island Dressing	4″ × 4″	A6212
Silicone Bordered Foam Island Dressing	6″ × 6″	A6213
Silicone Bordered Foam Island Dressing	7″ × 7″	A6213
Silicone Bordered Foam Island Dressing	10″ × 9″	A6213

ACTION

Optifoam Gentle Foam Island Dressing with Silicone Border is used to manage exudate in draining wounds. This hydropolymer gentle adhesive dressing is composed of a thin film backing over a hydrophilic foam island. The waterproof outer layer is coated with a medical-grade adhesive that helps maintain an optimally moist environment, which supports wound healing by encouraging autolytic debridement, which enables granulation to occur. New window-frame delivery system makes application smooth and easy. New sacral shape has anatomical shape to provide better fit and longer wear.

INDICATIONS

Partial- and full-thickness wounds with drainage.

CONTRAINDICATIONS

- Third-degree burns and lesions with active vasculitis.

APPLICATION

- Clean the wound using Skintegrity Wound Cleanser or an appropriate solution. Dry the surrounding skin to allow secure adhesion of the dressing.
- Select the appropriate size dressing to allow the foam island to cover all breached or compromised skin.
- Remove the outermost release paper, and anchor the dressing at one side.
- Smooth the dressing over the wound, and remove remaining release paper. Make sure the dressing is securely adhered without wrinkles in the adhesive border or stretching of the skin.
- Remove the paper frame, starting at the center thumb notch, following and smoothing the dressing as you lift and remove the paper frame.

REMOVAL

- The dressing may be left in place for up to 7 days or until exudate is visible and nears the edge of the dressing.
- Gently press down on the skin, and lift an edge of the dressing.
- Carefully stretch the dressing laterally to the skin to promote pain-free removal.
- Clean the wound again before applying a new dressing.

FOAMS

New Product: Optifoam Gentle Liquitrap

Medline Industries, Inc.

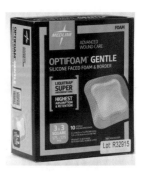

HOW SUPPLIED

Silicone Faced Foam and Border Dressing with Liquitrap Core	3" × 3"	A6212
Silicone Faced Foam and Border Dressing with Liquitrap Core	4" × 4"	A6212
Silicone Faced Foam and Border Dressing with Liquitrap Core	6" × 6"	A6213
Silicone Faced Foam and Border Dressing with Liquitrap Core	7" × 7"	A6213
Silicone Faced Foam and Border Dressing with Liquitrap Core	9" × 9"	A6213

ACTION

Optifoam Gentle Liquitrap is ideal for partial- and full-thickness wound with drainage. It has a silicone face and border that aids in gentle removal. The Liquitrap core locks in fluid, protecting the skin around the wound. The waterproof outer layer is coated with a medical-grade adhesive that helps maintain an optimally moist environment, which supports wound healing by encouraging autolytic debridement.

INDICATIONS

Partial- and full-thickness wounds with drainage.

CONTRAINDICATIONS

- Third-degree burns.

APPLICATION

- Clean the wound using Skintegrity Wound Cleanser or an appropriate solution. Dry the surrounding skin to allow secure adhesion of the dressing.
- Select the appropriate size dressing to allow the foam island to cover all breached or compromised skin.
- Remove the outermost release paper, and anchor the dressing at one side.
- Smooth the dressing over the wound, and remove remaining release paper. Make sure the dressing is securely adhered without wrinkles in the adhesive border or stretching of the skin.
- Remove the paper frame, starting at the center thumb notch, following and smoothing the dressing as you lift and remove the paper frame.

REMOVAL

- The dressing may be left in place for up to 7 days or until exudate is visible and nears the edge of the dressing.
- Gently press down on the skin, and lift an edge of the dressing.
- Carefully stretch the dressing laterally to the skin to promote pain-free removal.
- Clean the wound again before applying a new dressing.

FOAMS

New Product: Optifoam Gentle Lite

Medline Industries, Inc.

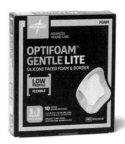

HOW SUPPLIED

Silicone Faced Foam and Border Dressing	1.6″ × 2″	A6413
Silicone Faced Foam and Border Dressing	3″ × 3″	A6212
Silicone Faced Foam and Border Dressing	4″ × 4″	A6212
Silicone Faced Foam and Border Dressing	6″ × 6″	A6213

ACTION

Optifoam Gentle Lite is ideal for partial- and full-thickness wound with minimal drainage. It has a silicone face and border that aids in gentle removal. The foam core locks in fluid, protecting the skin around the wound. The waterproof outer layer is coated with a medical-grade adhesive that helps maintain an optimally moist environment, which supports wound healing by encouraging autolytic debridement.

INDICATIONS

Partial- and full-thickness wounds with minimal drainage.

CONTRAINDICATIONS

• Third-degree burns.

APPLICATION

• Clean the wound using Skintegrity Wound Cleanser or an appropriate solution. Dry the surrounding skin to allow secure adhesion of the dressing.
• Select the appropriate size dressing to allow the foam island to cover all breached or compromised skin.
• Remove the outermost release paper, and anchor the dressing at one side.
• Smooth the dressing over the wound, and remove remaining release paper. Make sure the dressing is securely adhered without wrinkles in the adhesive border or stretching of the skin.
• Remove the paper frame, starting at the center thumb notch, following and smoothing the dressing as you lift and remove the paper frame.

REMOVAL

• The dressing may be left in place for up to 7 days or until exudate is visible and nears the edge of the dressing.
• Gently press down on the skin, and lift an edge of the dressing.
• Carefully stretch the dressing laterally to the skin to promote pain-free removal.
• Clean the wound again before applying a new dressing.

FOAMS

New Product: Optifoam Gentle Lite Non-Bordered

Medline Industries, Inc.

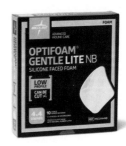

HOW SUPPLIED

Lite Non-Bordered Silicone Faced Foam Dressing	4″ × 4″	A6209
Lite Non-Bordered Silicone Faced Foam Dressing	6″ × 6″	A6210

ACTION

Optifoam Gentle Lite Non-Bordered is ideal for partial- and full-thickness wound with minimal drainage. It has a silicone face that aids in gentle removal. The foam core locks in fluid, protecting the skin around the wound.

INDICATIONS

Partial- and full-thickness wounds with minimal drainage.

CONTRAINDICATIONS

- Third-degree burns.

APPLICATION

- Clean the wound using Skintegrity Wound Cleanser or an appropriate solution. Dry the surrounding skin.
- Select the appropriate size dressing to allow the foam to cover all breached or compromised skin. May be cut to accommodate bony prominences or smaller wound sizes or fenestrated to accommodate a gastrostomy tube or other leaking drain tubes.
- Apply the dressing, and secure it with elastic net, gauze roll, or tape.

REMOVAL

- The dressing may be left in place for up to 7 days or until exudate is visible and nears the edge of the dressing.
- Gently remove the dressing.
- Clean the wound again before applying a new dressing.

FOAMS

New Product: Optifoam Gentle NB

Medline Industries, Inc.

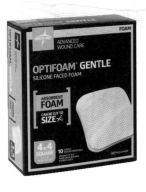

HOW SUPPLIED

Non-Bordered Silicone Faced Foam Dressing	4″ × 4″	A6209
Non-Bordered Silicone Faced Foam Dressing	6″ × 6″	A6210
Non-Bordered Silicone Faced Foam Dressing	8″ × 8″	A6211

ACTION

Optifoam Gentle Non-Bordered is ideal for partial- and full-thickness wound with drainage. It has a silicone face that aids in gentle removal. The foam core locks in fluid, protecting the skin around the wound. Can be cut to size.

INDICATIONS

Partial- and full-thickness wounds with minimal drainage.

CONTRAINDICATIONS

- Third-degree burns.

APPLICATION

- Clean the wound using Skintegrity Wound Cleanser or an appropriate solution. Dry the surrounding skin.
- Select the appropriate size dressing to allow the foam to cover all breached or compromised skin.
- May be cut to accommodate bony prominences or smaller wound sizes or fenestrated to accommodate a gastrostomy tube or other leaking drain tubes.
- Apply the dressing, and secure it with elastic net, gauze roll, or tape.

REMOVAL

- The dressing may be left in place for up to 7 days or until exudate is visible and nears the edge of the dressing.
- Gently remove the dressing.
- Clean the wound again before applying a new dressing.

New Product: Optifoam Gentle SA

Medline Industries, Inc.

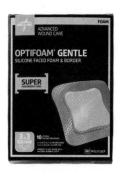

HOW SUPPLIED

Silicone Faced Foam and Border Dressing with Superabsorbent Core	3" × 3"	A6212
Silicone Faced Foam and Border Dressing with Superabsorbent Core	4" × 4"	A6212
Silicone Faced Foam and Border Dressing with Superabsorbent Core	6" × 6"	A6213
Silicone Faced Foam and Border Dressing with Superabsorbent Core	7" × 7"	A6213
Silicone Faced Foam and Border Dressing with Superabsorbent Core	9" × 9"	A6213

ACTION

Optifoam Gentle SA is ideal for partial- and full-thickness wound with drainage. It has a silicone face and border that aids in gentle removal. The foam core locks in fluid, protecting the skin around the wound. The waterproof outer layer is coated with a medical-grade adhesive that helps maintain an optimally moist environment, which supports wound healing by encouraging autolytic debridement.

INDICATIONS

Partial- and full-thickness wounds with drainage.

CONTRAINDICATIONS

- Third-degree burns.

APPLICATION

- Clean the wound using Skintegrity Wound Cleanser or an appropriate solution. Dry the surrounding skin to allow secure adhesion of the dressing.
- Select the appropriate size dressing to allow the foam island to cover all breached or compromised skin.
- Remove the outermost release paper, and anchor the dressing at one side.
- Smooth the dressing over the wound, and remove remaining release paper. Make sure the dressing is securely adhered without wrinkles in the adhesive border or stretching of the skin.
- Remove the paper frame, starting at the center thumb notch, following and smoothing the dressing as you lift and remove the paper frame.

REMOVAL

- The dressing may be left in place for up to 7 days or until exudate is visible and nears the edge of the dressing.
- Gently press down on the skin, and lift an edge of the dressing.
- Carefully stretch the dressing laterally to the skin to promote pain-free removal.
- Clean the wound again before applying a new dressing.

FOAMS

New Product: Optifoam Heel

Medline Industries, Inc.

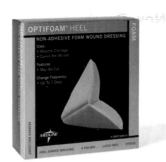

HOW SUPPLIED

Non-Adhesive Heel Shaped Foam Wound Dressing	A6210

ACTION

Optifoam Heel is a highly comfortable and absorbent polyurethane foam dressing that absorbs moderate to heavy drainage. Optifoam Heel helps create an ideal healing environment and the waterproof outer layer protects the wound and keeps bacteria out.

INDICATIONS

Pressure injuries, partial- and full-thickness wounds and diabetic foot ulcers.

CONTRAINDICATIONS

- Third-degree burns and lesions with active vasculitis.

APPLICATION

- Clean the wound using Skintegrity Wound Cleanser or an appropriate solution. Dry the surrounding skin.
- Select the appropriate size dressing to allow the foam to cover all breached or compromised skin.
- Apply the dressing, and secure with tape or gauze.

REMOVAL

- The dressing may be left in place for up to 7 days or until exudate is visible and nears the edge of the dressing.
- Clean the wound again before applying a new dressing.

FOAMS

New Product: Optifoam Thin

Medline Industries, Inc.

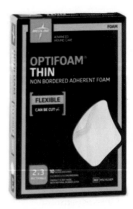

HOW SUPPLIED

Thin Adhesive Faced Dressing	2″ × 3″	N/A
Thin Adhesive Faced Dressing	4″ × 4″	N/A

ACTION

Optifoam Thin is a highly comfortable polyurethane foam adhesive dressing. It is ideal for in the management of lightly draining wounds and skin tears. It has a self-adhesive face. The foam core locks in fluid, protecting the skin around the wound. Optifoam Thin has a waterproof backing and can be cut to size.

INDICATIONS

Skin tears, abrasions, superficial pressure injuries.

CONTRAINDICATIONS

- Third-degree burns.

APPLICATION

- Clean the wound using Skintegrity Wound Cleanser or an appropriate solution. Dry the surrounding skin.
- Select the appropriate size dressing to allow the foam to cover all breached or compromised skin.
- May be cut to accommodate bony prominences or smaller wound sizes or fenestrated to accommodate a gastrostomy tube or other leaking drain tubes.
- Apply the dressing, and secure if needed.

REMOVAL

- The dressing may be left in place for up to 7 days or until exudate is visible and nears the edge of the dressing.
- Gently press down on the skin, and lift an edge of the dressing.
- Carefully stretch the dressing laterally to the skin to promote pain-free removal.
- Clean the wound again before applying a new dressing.

POLYDERM Hydrophilic Polyurethane Foam Dressing

DeRoyal

HOW SUPPLIED

Foam Pad	2 1/4″ × 2 1/4″	A6209
Foam Pad	3 3/4″ × 3 3/4″	A6212

ACTION

POLYDERM is a nonadherent, highly absorbent, lint-free foam dressing for the management of heavily exuding wounds.

INDICATIONS

For use as a primary or secondary dressing to manage pressure ulcers (stages 2 to 4), partial- and full-thickness wounds, donor sites, second-degree burns, lacerations, cuts, abrasions, and draining wounds; may also be used for red, yellow, and black wounds and for exuding wounds.

CONTRAINDICATIONS

- None provided by the manufacturer.

APPLICATION

- Clean the wound site with normal saline solution.
- Center the foam over the wound.
- Secure the dressing.

REMOVAL

- Remove any secondary dressing.
- Gently lift the foam dressing from the wound.

FOAMS

POLYDERM PLUS Barrier Foam Dressing

DeRoyal

HOW SUPPLIED

Foam Pad with Border	2 1/4" × 2 1/4" foam with 4" × 4" border	A6212
Foam Pad with Border	3 3/4" × 3 3/4" foam with 6" × 6" border	A6212

ACTION

POLYDERM PLUS is a nonadherent, highly absorbent, semiocclusive, lint-free foam dressing with a nonwoven tape border. It maintains a moist wound environment conducive to healing and resists external contaminants and blood or drainage strike-through.

INDICATIONS

For use as a primary or secondary dressing to manage pressure ulcers (stages 2 to 4), partial- and full-thickness wounds, donor sites, tunneling wounds, infected and noninfected wounds, and draining wounds; may also be used for red, yellow, or black wounds and for exuding wounds.

CONTRAINDICATIONS

- None provided by the manufacturer.

APPLICATION

- Clean the wound with normal saline solution.
- Peel back the release liner from the dressing's center to expose the foam.
- Center the foam over the wound, and press into place.

REMOVAL

- Gently lift the edges of the border, and then peel off the dressing.

FOAMS

New Product: PolyMem® and PolyMem® MAX® Film Adhesive Dressings*

Ferris Mfg. Corp.

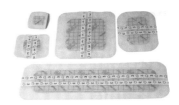

HOW SUPPLIED

Film Adhesive PMD Dot	1″ × 1″ pad with 2″ × 2″ adhesive	A6212
Film Adhesive PMD Island	2″ × 3″ pad with 3.5″ × 4.5″ adhesive, New Product	A6212
Film Adhesive Extra-absorbent PMD Island	1.25″ × 1.5″ extra-absorbent pad with 2.75″ × 3″ adhesive, New Product	A6212
Film Adhesive Extra-absorbent PMD Island	3.5″ × 3.5″ extra-absorbent pad with 5.25″ × 5.25″ adhesive, New Product	A6212
Film Adhesive Extra-absorbent PMD Island	2″ × 10″ extra-absorbent pad with 3.5″ × 11.75″ adhesive, New Product	A6213

FOAMS

ACTION

PolyMem (standard and MAX) with Film Adhesive Border Dressings are multifunctional,[1–4] interactive[5] bordered polymeric membrane dressings (PMDs) that are breathable yet tough, protective,[3,6] and water-resistant.[7] These polymeric membrane dressings are designed to continuously cleanse,[6,8] balance moisture,[3,5,9–11] limit inflammation,[1,12–14] reduce odor,[3,5,6,15] and wound pain[4,6,16–18] and protect wounds[3,6] while partnering with the body to promote quick healing.[9–11,16,19–22] Many new wound products are being developed to include small aspects of PolyMem dressings' many benefits, but none are able to furnish the integrated solutions PolyMem products have reliably provided for nearly three decades.[6]

Activated by moisture, PolyMem products gradually release a nontoxic surfactant cleanser and glycerin to loosen bonds between the wound bed and adherent substances that may impair healing.[1,5,23–25] Glycerin pulls nutrient-filled, enzyme-rich fluid from the body into the wound bed, enhancing healing and autolytic debridement while floating the contaminants.[3,5,11,26,27] The PolyMem membrane pulls in the undesirable substances along with the fluid, which are locked into the porous superabsorbent structure.[1,6,28,29] The wound contaminants are atraumatically removed and discarded when the PolyMem dressing is changed, eliminating the need for routine rinsing at dressing changes.[10,24,28,29]

The glycerin and surfactant in PolyMem products help moisturize dry areas of wounds while pulling fluid from the body into the wound bed and redistributing it.[3,5,9–11] Simultaneously, excess fluid from overly wet areas is absorbed into the dressing and is locked into a gel.[3,5,28,30] The "intelligent" backing allows excess fluid to evaporate while retaining the fluid needed to keep dry wounds moist.[31] Other available dressings have only portions of this complete moisture balancing system.[6]

All occlusive dressings provide some pain relief. However, PolyMem products are the only drug-free dressings with evidence showing that they also relieve pain by altering the response of the pain-sensing nerves (nociceptors).[9,12–14,25,32,33] PolyMem products' alteration of the nociceptor response occurs even on intact skin, and has been shown in clinical studies to decrease the excess inflammation that leads to excess swelling and often slows healing.[6,9,12–14,27,33]

PolyMem dressings are non-adherent while conforming to the wound bed.[5,10,11,26,28,32,34,35] They are flexible and comfortable to wear.[1,6,26,34–36]

INDICATIONS

Indicated for virtually all wounds at every stage of healing,[1,3,11,24,28] including closed tissue injuries,[13,33,37,38] multifunctional PolyMem dressings meet or exceed every criterion wound experts identify for an *Ideal Dressing*.[7,29,39] PolyMem dressings are safe for use over structures like tendon, bone, and exposed vessels because they can donate moisture.[1,5,11,26,27] PolyMem is suitable for use even when wounds are infected, provided that the infection is otherwise appropriately addressed.[1,5,6,21,40] PolyMem is especially suitable for chronic, trauma, and burn wounds because it helps subdue excess inflammation and is a pain relieving dressing.[2,6,9,12,16,21,30,41,42]

- PolyMem (standard and MAX) Film Adhesive Border Dressings are designed with unsurpassed versatility, accommodating dry to heavily exudating wounds. The breathable, water resistant, adhesive-coated thin-film backing, when applied without tension, provides exceptional comfort for patients.[7]

CONTRAINDICATIONS

- None.

APPLICATION

- Initially, irrigate or debride the wound bed as indicated or prescribed. Rinse with water or saline. Additional topical products are not necessary or recommended for use with PolyMem. Simply pat the periwound dry, leaving the wound bed slightly moist.
- Fill any deep cavities lightly with PolyMem WIC (with or without silver) or WIC Silver Rope, allowing for about 30% expansion.
- Select a PolyMem (standard and MAX) Film Adhesive Border Dressing with a membrane pad that is large enough to cover the open wound **AND** all of the surrounding inflamed (reddened, raw, tender, warm, itchy, or swollen) skin. Apply dressing, carefully ensuring that the adhesive borders are not under tension. Smooth into place. See Instructions for Use for details.

How to know when to change PolyMem dressings

- Do NOT change PolyMem on a calendar schedule, especially in the first week of use; anticipate changes in exudate levels, which may dramatically increase initially.
- PolyMem is an indicator dressing: the backing will become a darker color when the membrane becomes saturated. Change the dressing when the darker color reaches any of the wound edges.

REMOVAL

- Simply, gently remove the PolyMem (standard or MAX) Film Adhesive Border Dressing and any wound filler and replace it with an appropriate new PolyMem configuration. In most cases, when using PolyMem, there is no need to rinse the wound.
- PolyMem is designed to continuously cleanse the wound and does not leave residue that needs to be removed. Excessive cleaning may injure regenerating tissue and delay wound healing.

FOAMS

Guidelines for optimal use

(See *Instructions for Use* provided in each box and **PolyMem.com for detailed information.**)

Independent wound experts have created a robust evidence base for PolyMem dressings by documenting their success in using PolyMem over the past 25+ years. Ferris has developed these guidelines based upon their documented experiences.

- Using PolyMem is simple. However, using PolyMem optimally (knowing which dressing configuration to use, and how) is an art.[6,19] PolyMem use saves time, giving wound specialists more time to address the whole patient, improving healing by optimizing offloading, compression therapy, circulation, nutrition, medications, and so forth.[4,9,16,19,26,30,32,38,43,44]
- PolyMem dressings should be changed when indicated, rather than on a schedule. Changing PolyMem more frequently than necessary on a healthy, granulating wound bed may slow healing. Tracing the approximate wound borders on the outer film of the PolyMem dressing makes it easy to see when a change is needed without "peeking" at the wound.[39]
- PolyMem is an interactive dressing. PolyMem often recruits LARGE amounts of wound fluid, containing debris and metabolic wastes, for the first few days of use, which may prompt frequent dressing changes.[1,24,43] When the wound is clean and granulating, reduced exudate may allow PolyMem to be left in place for up to 7 days.[6]
- On first application, irrigate or debride the wound to remove causes of delayed healing that are easy to address; then allow PolyMem to remove the remainder of the contaminants atraumatically. The PolyMem membrane may become discolored or malodorous, but the wound bed itself will become cleaner and healthier.
- Experienced users gain the confidence to avoid routine rinsing at dressing changes.[3,4,6,44,45] Simply applying a PolyMem dressing **IS** wound cleansing.[6,19] Because rinsing cools the wound bed, washes away valuable nutrients, and can damage fragile new tissue, it is best to rinse only if loose contaminants are visible or the dressing has become dislodged prior to the dressing change, allowing the wound to become dirty and dry.[46]
- Patients with large surface area third degree burns must be carefully supervised by a burn specialist, especially when any absorptive dressing is used, including PolyMem.
- Healing wounds quickly is the most cost-saving choice. PolyMem is proven to help close wounds quickly.

*See package insert for complete information.

FOAMS

REFERENCES

PDFs of many of the footnoted references are available at www.polymem.com/clinicalguide/

1. Benskin LL. PolyMem Wic Silver Rope: A multifunctional dressing for decreasing pain, swelling, and inflammation. *Adv Wound Care (New Rochelle)*. 2012;1(1):44–47.
2. Dawson, Lewis C, Boch R. Total Joint Replacement Surgical Site Infections Eliminated by Using Multifunctional Dressing. 900 Cases Report over 4 years. May 2010.
3. Cutting KF, Vowden P, Wiegand C. Wound inflammation and the role of a multifunctional polymeric dressing. *Wounds International Journal*. 2015;6(2):41–46.
4. White L. Optimal Management for Upper Extremity Wounds with a Multifunctional Polymeric Membrane Dressing. September 2015.
5. Denyer J, White R, Ousey K, et al. PolyMem dressings Made Easy. *Wounds International*. May 2015. http://www.woundsinternational.com/made-easys/view/polymem-dressings-made-easy. Accessed May 7, 2016.
6. Benskin LL. Polymeric Membrane Dressings for topical wound management of patients with infected wounds in a challenging environment: A protocol with 3 case examples. *Ostomy Wound Management*. 2016;62(6):42–50. (OWM website adds evidence summaries, Tables 1 & 2)
7. Benskin L. PolyMem The Ideal Dressing. August 2015.
8. Blackman JD, Senseng D, Quinn L, et al. Clinical evaluation of a semipermeable polymeric membrane dressing for the treatment of chronic diabetic foot ulcers. *Diabetes Care*. 1994;17(4):322–325.
9. Weissman O, Hundeshagen G, Harats M, et al. Custom-fit polymeric membrane dressing masks in the treatment of second degree facial burns. *Burns*. 2013;39(6):1316–1320.

10. Scott A. Polymeric membrane dressings for radiotherapy-induced skin damage. *Br J Nurs.* 2014; 23(10):S24, S26–S31.

11. Dabiri G, Damstetter E, Phillips T. Choosing a wound dressing based on common wound characteristics. *Adv Wound Care (New Rochelle).* 2016;5(1):32–41.

12. Kim YJ, Lee SW, Hong SH, et al. The effects of PolyMem(R) on the wound healing. *J Korean Soc Plast Reconstr Surg.* 1999;26(6):1165–1172.

13. Hayden JK, Cole BJ. The effectiveness of a pain wrap compared to a standard dressing on the reduction of postoperative morbidity following routine knee arthroscopy: a prospective randomized single-blind study. *Orthopedics.* 2003;26(1):59–63; discussion 63.

14. Beitz AJ, Newman A, Kahn AR, et al. A polymeric membrane dressing with antinociceptive properties: analysis with a rodent model of stab wound secondary hyperalgesia. *J Pain.* 2004;5(1):38–47.

15. Agathangelou C. Treating Fungating Breast Cancer Wounds with Polymeric Membrane Dressings, an Innovation in Fungating Wound Management. May 2015.

16. Haik J, Weissman O, Demetrius S, Tamir J. Polymeric Membrane Dressings* for Skin Graft Donor Sites: 6 Years Experience on 1200 Cases. April 2011.

17. Man D, Aleksinko P. Use of Polymeric Membrane Dressings After Occlusive Deep Facial and Neck Chemical Peel Improves Outcomes. April 2010.

18. Man D, Aleksinko P. Intra-Operative Use Followed with Post-Op Application of Polymeric Membrane Dressings Reduces Post-Op Pain, Edema and Bruising After Full Face Lift Surgery. April 2010.

19. Denyer J. Six Years' Experience Of PolyMem Dressings Used On Children With Epidermolysis Bullosa (EB). September 2015.

20. Scott A. Involving patients in the monitoring of radiotherapy-induced skin reactions. *Journal of Community Nursing.* 2013;27(5):16–22.

21. Aaltonen M. Developing a Protocol For Burns in a Private Out-Patient Wound Clinic. May 2015.

22. Curtin C. The new diabetic foot ulcer standard of care: Instant total contact cast plus polymeric membrane dressings. November 2012.

23. Rodeheaver GT, Kurtz L, Kircher BJ, et al. Pluronic F-68: a promising new skin wound cleanser. *Ann Emerg Med.* 1980;9(11):572–576.

24. Denyer JE, Pillay E. Best practice guidelines for skin and wound care in epidermolysis bullosa—International Consensus. 2012. http://www.woundsinternational.com/other-resources/view/best-practice-guidelines-for-skin-and-wound-care-in-epidermolysis-bullosa. Accessed March 30, 2015.

25. Davies SL, White RJ. Defining a holistic pain-relieving approach to wound care via a drug free polymeric membrane dressing. *J Wound Care.* 2011;20(5):250, 252, 254 passim.

26. Rafter L, Oforka E. Standard versus polymeric membrane finger dressing and outcomes following pain diaries. *Wounds UK.* 2014;10(2):40–49.

27. Cahn A, Kleinman Y. A novel approach to the treatment of diabetic foot abscesses—a case series. *J Wound Care.* 2014;23(8):394, 396–399.

28. Fowler E, Papen JC. Clinical evaluation of a polymeric membrane dressing in the treatment of dermal ulcers. *Ostomy Wound Manage.* 1991;35:35–38, 40–44.

29. Yastrub DJ. Relationship between type of treatment and degree of wound healing among institutionalized geriatric patients with stage II pressure ulcers. *Care Manag J.* 2004;5(4):213–218.

30. Stoddart J. Circumferential Wrap Technique with Polymeric Membrane Dressings after Arthroscopic ACL Reconstruction Reduces Blistering, Inflammation and Bruising; Rapid Recovery and Improved Patient Satisfaction: 80 Prospective Patient Series. May 2013.

31. Fulton JA, Blasiole KN, Cottingham T, et al. Wound dressing absorption: A comparative study. *Adv Skin Wound Care.* 2012;25(7):315–320.

32. Bolhuis J. Evidence-based skin tear protocol. *Long-Term Living: For the Continuing Care Professional.* 2008;57(6):48–52.

33. Kahn AR, Sessions RW, Apasova EV. A superficial cutaneous dressing inhibits pain, inflammation and swelling in deep tissues. *Pain Medicine.* 2000;1(2):187–187.

34. Bauer J, Diem A, Ploder M. Efficiency and Safety of Using a Polymeric Membrane Wound Dressing in Patients with Epidermolysis Bullosa after a Release Operation. May 2013.

35. Bauer J, Brandtner G. Chirurgische Korrektur der Handfehlbildungen bei Epidermolysis bullosa dystrophicans. *Arzt+Kind.* 2013.

36. Rafter L, Oforka E. Trauma-free fingertip dressing changes. *Wounds UK.* 2013;9(1):96–100.

37. Hegarty F, Wong M. Polymeric membrane dressing for radiotherapy-induced skin reactions. *Br J Nurs.* 2014;23 Suppl 20:S38–S46.

38. Wilson D. Application of Polymeric Membrane Dressings to Stage I Pressure Ulcers Speeds Resolution, Reduces Ulcer Site Discomfort and Reduces Staff Time Devoted to Management of Ulcers. April 2010.

39. Carr RD, Lalagos DE. Clinical evaluation of a polymeric membrane dressing in the treatment of pressure ulcers. *Decubitus.* 1990;3(3):38–42.

40. Denyer JE. Wound management for children with epidermolysis bullosa. *Dermatologic Clinics.* 2010; 28(2):257–264.

41. Rahman S, Shokri A. Total Knee Arthroplasty (TKA) Infections Eliminated and Rehabilitation Improved Using Polymeric Membrane Dressing Circumferential Wrap Technique: 120 Patients at 12-month Follow-up. May 2013.

42. Edwards J, Mason S. An evaluation of the use of PolyMem Silver in burn management. *Journal of Community Nursing.* 2010;24(6):16–19.

43. Denyer J. Managing pain in children with epidermolysis bullosa. *Nurs Times.* 2012;108(29):21–23.

44. Vanwalleghem G. A New Protocol for the Treatment of Pilonidal Cysts. May 2011.

45. Agathangelou C. Patients with Chronic Wound Pain Stop Hurting, Why? May 2011.

46. McGuiness W, Vella E, Harrison D. Influence of dressing changes on wound temperature. *J Wound Care.* 2004;13(9):383–385.

FOAMS

PolyMem® Cloth Adhesive Dressings*

Ferris Mfg. Corp.

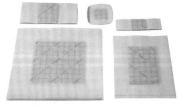

HOW SUPPLIED

Cloth Adhesive PMD Dot	1″ × 1″ pad with 2″ × 2″ adhesive	A6212
Cloth Adhesive PMD Island	2″ × 3″ pad with 4″ × 5″ adhesive	A6212
Cloth Adhesive PMD Island	3.5″ × 3.5″ pad with 6″ × 6″ adhesive	A6212
Cloth Adhesive PMD Strip	1″ × 1″ pad with 1″ × 3″ adhesive	A6212
Cloth Adhesive PMD Strip	2″ × 1.5″ pad with 2″ × 4″ adhesive	A6212

ACTION

PolyMem Cloth Adhesive dressings are multifunctional,[1–4] interactive[5] polymeric membrane dressings (PMDs) with a comfortable cloth border.[6,7] These polymeric membrane dressings are designed to control inflammation,[1,8–10] pain,[4,7,11–13] and odor[3,5,7,14] and to protect wounds[3,7] while partnering with the body to promote quick healing.[11,15–21] Many new wound products are being developed to include small aspects of PolyMem dressings' many benefits, but none are able to furnish the integrated solutions PolyMem products have reliably provided for nearly three decades.[7]

Activated by moisture, PolyMem products gradually release a nontoxic surfactant cleanser and glycerin to loosen bonds between the wound bed and adherent substances that may impair healing.[1,5,22–24] Glycerin pulls nutrient-filled, enzyme-rich fluid from the body into the wound bed, enhancing healing and autolytic debridement while floating the contaminants.[3,5,21,25,26] The PolyMem membrane pulls in the undesirable substances along with the fluid, which are locked into the porous superabsorbent structure.[1,7,27,28] The wound contaminants are atraumatically removed and discarded when the PolyMem dressing is changed, eliminating the need for routine rinsing at dressing changes.[18,23,27,28]

The glycerin and surfactant in PolyMem products help moisturize dry areas of wounds while pulling fluid from the body into the wound bed and redistributing it.[3,5,15,18,21] Simultaneously, excess fluid from overly wet areas is absorbed into the dressing and is locked into a gel.[3,5,27,29] The "intelligent" backing allows excess fluid to evaporate while retaining the fluid needed to keep dry wounds moist.[30] Other available dressings have only portions of this complete moisture balancing system.[7]

All occlusive dressings provide some pain relief. However, PolyMem products are the only drug-free dressings with evidence showing that they also relieve pain by altering the response of the pain-sensing nerves (nociceptors).[8–10,15,24,32] PolyMem products' alteration of the nociceptor response occurs even on intact skin, and has been shown in clinical studies to decrease the excess inflammation that leads to excess swelling and often slows healing.[7–10,15,26,32]

PolyMem dressings are nonadherent while conforming to the wound bed.[5,18,21,25,27,31,33,34] They are flexible and comfortable to wear.[1,7,25,33–35]

INDICATIONS

Indicated for virtually all wounds at every stage of healing,[1,3,21,23,27] including closed tissue injuries,[9,32,36,37] multifunctional PolyMem dressings meet or exceed every criterion wound experts identify for an *Ideal Dressing*.[6,28,38] PolyMem dressings are safe for use over structures like tendon, bone, and exposed vessels because they can donate moisture.[1,5,21,25,26] PolyMem is suitable for use even when wounds are infected, provided that the infection is

FOAMS

otherwise appropriately addressed.[1,5,7,19,39] PolyMem is especially suitable for chronic, trauma, and burn wounds because it helps subdue excess inflammation and is a pain-relieving dressing.[2,7,8,11,15,19,29,40,41]

- PolyMem Cloth Adhesive Border Dressings are especially suited for closed tissue injuries and wounds in active patients and those who are sensitive to urethane adhesive borders. The breathable, adhesive-coated cloth backing provides exceptional comfort for patients, particularly in warm environments.[6,7]

CONTRAINDICATIONS

- None.

APPLICATION

- Initially, irrigate or debride the wound bed as indicated or prescribed. Rinse with water or saline. Additional topical products are not necessary or recommended for use with PolyMem. Simply pat the periwound dry, leaving the wound bed slightly moist.
- Fill any deep cavities lightly with PolyMem WIC (with or without silver) or WIC Silver Rope, allowing for about 30% expansion. Apply the PolyMem dressing with the moisture-barrier film (printed side) out.
- Select a PolyMem Cloth Adhesive Dressing with a membrane pad that is large enough to cover the open wound **AND** all of the surrounding inflamed (reddened, raw, tender, warm, itchy, or swollen) skin. Apply adhesive without tension.

How to know when to change PolyMem dressings

- Do NOT change PolyMem on a calendar schedule, especially in the first week of use; anticipate changes in exudate levels, which may dramatically increase initially.
- PolyMem is an indicator dressing: The backing will become a darker color when the membrane becomes saturated. Change the dressing when the darker color reaches any of the wound edges.

REMOVAL

- Simply, gently remove the PolyMem Cloth Adhesive Dressing and any wound filler and replace them with an appropriate new PolyMem configuration. In most cases, when using PolyMem, there is no need to rinse the wound.
- PolyMem is designed to continuously cleanse the wound and does not leave residue that needs to be removed. Excessive cleaning may injure regenerating tissue and delay wound healing.

Guidelines for optimal use

(See *Instructions for Use* provided in each box and **PolyMem.com for detailed information**.)

Independent wound experts have created a robust evidence base for PolyMem dressings by documenting their success in using PolyMem over the past 25+ years. Ferris has developed these guidelines based upon their documented experiences.

- Using PolyMem is simple. However, using PolyMem optimally (knowing which dressing configuration to use, and how) is an art.[7,16] PolyMem use saves time, giving wound specialists more time to address the whole patient, improving healing by optimizing offloading, compression, circulation, nutrition, medications, and so forth.[4,11,15,16,25,29,31,37,42,43]
- PolyMem dressings should be changed when indicated, rather than on a schedule. Changing PolyMem more frequently than necessary on a healthy, granulating wound bed may slow healing. Tracing the approximate wound borders on the outer film of the PolyMem dressing makes it easy to see when a change is needed without "peaking" at the wound.[38]

FOAMS

- PolyMem is an interactive dressing. PolyMem often recruits LARGE amounts of wound fluid, containing debris and metabolic wastes, for the first few days of use, which may prompt frequent dressing changes.[1,23,42] When the wound is clean and granulating, reduced exudate may allow PolyMem to be left in place for up to 7 days.[7]
- On first application, irrigate or debride the wound to remove causes of delayed healing that are easy to address; then allow PolyMem to remove the remainder of the contaminants atraumatically. The PolyMem membrane may become discolored or malodorous, but the wound bed itself will become cleaner and healthier.
- Experienced users gain the confidence to avoid routine rinsing at dressing changes.[3,4,7,43,44] Simply applying a PolyMem dressing **IS** wound cleansing.[7,16] Because rinsing cools the wound bed, washes away valuable nutrients, and can damage fragile new tissue, it is best to rinse only if loose contaminants are visible or the dressing became dislodged prior to the dressing change, allowing the wound to become dirty and dry.[45]
- Patients with large surface area, third-degree burns must be carefully supervised by a burn specialist, especially when any absorptive dressing is used, including PolyMem.
- Healing wounds quickly is the most cost-saving choice. PolyMem is proven to help close wounds quickly.

*See package insert for complete information.

REFERENCES

PDFs of many of the footnoted references are available at www.polymem.com/clinicalguide/

1. Benskin LL. PolyMem Wic Silver Rope: A multifunctional dressing for decreasing pain, swelling, and inflammation. *Adv Wound Care (New Rochelle)*. 2012;1(1):44–47.
2. Dawson, Lewis C, Boch R. Total Joint Replacement Surgical Site Infections Eliminated by Using Multifunctional Dressing. 900 Cases Report over 4 years. May 2010.
3. Cutting KF, Vowden P, Wiegand C. Wound inflammation and the role of a multifunctional polymeric dressing. *Wounds International Journal*. 2015;6(2):41–46.
4. White L. Optimal Management for Upper Extremity Wounds with a Multifunctional Polymeric Membrane Dressing. September 2015.
5. Denyer J, White R, Ousey K, et al. PolyMem dressings Made Easy. *Wounds International*. May 2015. http://www.woundsinternational.com/made-easys/view/polymem-dressings-made-easy. Accessed May 7, 2016.
6. Benskin L. PolyMem The Ideal Dressing. August 2015.
7. Benskin LL. Polymeric membrane dressings for topical wound management of patients with infected wounds in a challenging environment: A protocol with 3 case examples. *Ostomy Wound Manage*. 2016;62(6):42–50. (OWM website adds evidence summaries, Tables 1 & 2)
8. Kim YJ, Lee SW, Hong SH, et al. The effects of PolyMem(R) on the wound healing. *J Korean Soc Plast Reconstr Surg*. 1999;26(6):1165–1172.
9. Hayden JK, Cole BJ. The effectiveness of a pain wrap compared to a standard dressing on the reduction of postoperative morbidity following routine knee arthroscopy: a prospective randomized single-blind study. *Orthopedics*. 2003;26(1):59–63; discussion 63.
10. Beitz AJ, Newman A, Kahn AR, et al. A polymeric membrane dressing with antinociceptive properties: analysis with a rodent model of stab wound secondary hyperalgesia. *J Pain*. 2004;5(1):38–47.
11. Haik J, Weissman O, Demetrius S, et al. Polymeric Membrane Dressings* for Skin Graft Donor Sites: 6 Years Experience on 1200 Cases. April 2011.
12. Man D, Aleksinko P. Use of Polymeric Membrane Dressings After Occlusive Deep Facial and Neck Chemical Peel Improves Outcomes. April 2010.
13. Man D, Aleksinko P. Intra-Operative Use Followed with Post-Op Application of Polymeric Membrane Dressings Reduces Post-Op Pain, Edema and Bruising After Full Face Lift Surgery. April 2010.
14. Agathangelou C. Treating Fungating Breast Cancer Wounds with Polymeric Membrane Dressings, an Innovation in Fungating Wound Management. May 2015.
15. Weissman O, Hundeshagen G, Harats M, et al. Custom-fit polymeric membrane dressing masks in the treatment of second degree facial burns. *Burns*. 2013;39(6):1316–1320.
16. Denyer J. Six Years' Experience Of PolyMem Dressings Used On Children With Epidermolysis Bullosa (EB). September 2015.

17. Scott A. Involving patients in the monitoring of radiotherapy-induced skin reactions. *Journal of Community Nursing*. 2013;27(5):16–22.

18. Scott A. Polymeric membrane dressings for radiotherapy-induced skin damage. *Br J Nurs*. 2014; 23(10):S24, S26–S31.

19. Aaltonen M. Developing a Protocol For Burns in a Private Out-Patient Wound Clinic. May 2015.

20. Curtin C. The new diabetic foot ulcer standard of care: Instant total contact cast plus polymeric membrane dressings. November 2012.

21. Dabiri G, Damstetter E, Phillips T. Choosing a wound dressing based on common wound characteristics. *Adv Wound Care (New Rochelle)*. 2016;5(1):32–41.

22. Rodeheaver GT, Kurtz L, Kircher BJ, et al. Pluronic F-68: a promising new skin wound cleanser. *Ann Emerg Med*. 1980;9(11):572–576.

23. Denyer JE, Pillay E. Best practice guidelines for skin and wound care in epidermolysis bullosa— International Consensus. 2012. http://www.woundsinternational.com/other-resources/view/best-practice-guidelines-for-skin-and-wound-care-in-epidermolysis-bullosa. Accessed March 30, 2015.

24. Davies SL, White RJ. Defining a holistic pain-relieving approach to wound care via a drug free polymeric membrane dressing. *J Wound Care*. 2011;20(5):250, 252, 254 passim.

25. Rafter L, Oforka E. Standard versus polymeric membrane finger dressing and outcomes following pain diaries. *Wounds UK*. 2014;10(2):40–49.

26. Cahn A, Kleinman Y. A novel approach to the treatment of diabetic foot abscesses—a case series. *J Wound Care*. 2014;23(8):394, 396–399.

27. Fowler E, Papen JC. Clinical evaluation of a polymeric membrane dressing in the treatment of dermal ulcers. *Ostomy Wound Manage*. 1991;35:35–38, 40–44.

28. Yastrub DJ. Relationship between type of treatment and degree of wound healing among institutionalized geriatric patients with stage II pressure ulcers. *Care Manag J*. 2004;5(4):213–218.

29. Stoddart J. Circumferential Wrap Technique with Polymeric Membrane Dressings after Arthroscopic ACL Reconstruction Reduces Blistering, Inflammation and Bruising; Rapid Recovery and Improved Patient Satisfaction: 80 Prospective Patient Series. May 2013.

30. Fulton JA, Blasiole KN, Cottingham T, et al. Wound dressing absorption: A comparative study. *Adv Skin Wound Care*. 2012;25(7):315–320.

31. Bolhuis J. Evidence-based skin tear protocol. *Long-Term Living: For the Continuing Care Professional*. 2008;57(6):48–52.

32. Kahn AR, Sessions RW, Apasova EV. A superficial cutaneous dressing inhibits pain, inflammation and swelling in deep tissues. *Pain Medicine*. 2000;1(2):187.

33. Bauer J, Diem A, Ploder M. Efficiency and Safety of Using a Polymeric Membrane Wound Dressing in Patients with Epidermolysis Bullosa after a Release Operation. May 2013.

34. Bauer J, Brandtner G. Chirurgische Korrektur der Handfehlbildungen bei Epidermolysis bullosa dystrophicans. *Arzt+Kind*. 2013.

35. Rafter L, Oforka E. Trauma-free fingertip dressing changes. *Wounds UK*. 2013;9(1):96–100.

36. Hegarty F, Wong M. Polymeric membrane dressing for radiotherapy-induced skin reactions. *Br J Nurs*. 2014;23 Suppl 20:S38–S46.

37. Wilson D. Application of Polymeric Membrane Dressings to Stage I Pressure Ulcers Speeds Resolution, Reduces Ulcer Site Discomfort and Reduces Staff Time Devoted to Management of Ulcers. April 2010.

38. Carr RD, Lalagos DE. Clinical evaluation of a polymeric membrane dressing in the treatment of pressure ulcers. *Decubitus*. 1990;3(3):38–42.

39. Denyer JE. Wound management for children with epidermolysis bullosa. *Dermatologic Clinics*. 2010;28(2):257–264.

40. Rahman S, Shokri A. Total Knee Arthroplasty (TKA) Infections Eliminated and Rehabilitation Improved Using Polymeric Membrane Dressing Circumferential Wrap Technique: 120 Patients at 12-month Follow-up. May 2013.

41. Edwards J, Mason S. An evaluation of the use of PolyMem Silver in burn management. *Journal of Community Nursing*. 2010;24(6):16–19.

42. Denyer J. Managing pain in children with epidermolysis bullosa. *Nurs Times*. 2012;108(29):21–23.

43. Vanwalleghem G. A New Protocol for the Treatment of Pilonidal Cysts. May 2011.

44. Agathangelou C. Patients with Chronic Wound Pain Stop Hurting, Why? May 2011.

45. McGuiness W, Vella E, Harrison D. Influence of dressing changes on wound temperature. *J Wound Care*. 2004;13(9):383–385.

FOAMS

PolyMem® Dressing*

Ferris Mfg. Corp.

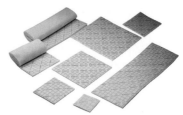

HOW SUPPLIED

Nonadhesive PMD Pad	1.8″ × 1.8″, New Size	A6209
Nonadhesive PMD Pad	3″ × 3″	A6209
Nonadhesive PMD Pad	4″ × 4″	A6209
Nonadhesive PMD Pad	5″ × 5″	A6210
Nonadhesive PMD Pad	6.5″ × 7.5″	A6210
Nonadhesive PMD Pad	4″ × 12.5″	A6210
Nonadhesive PMD Roll	4″ × 24″	A6211
Nonadhesive PMD Roll	8″ × 24″	A6211

ACTION

PolyMem is a multifunctional,[1-4] interactive[5] polymeric membrane dressing (PMD) designed for handling exudate[3,6-9] while providing protection from contamination,[3,9] continuously cleansing,[9,10] balancing moisture,[3,5,6,11,12] helping to subdue and focus inflammation,[1,13-15] and reducing odor[3,5,9,16] and wound pain.[4,9,17-19] Many new wound products are being developed to include small aspects of PolyMem dressings' many benefits, but none are able to furnish the integrated solutions PolyMem products have reliably provided for nearly three decades.[9]

Activated by moisture, PolyMem products gradually release a nontoxic surfactant cleanser and glycerin to loosen bonds between the wound bed and adherent substances that may impair healing.[1,5,20-22] Glycerin pulls nutrient-filled, enzyme-rich fluid from the body into the wound bed, enhancing healing and autolytic debridement while floating the contaminants.[3,5,6,23,24] The PolyMem membrane pulls in the undesirable substances along with the fluid, which are locked into the porous superabsorbent structure.[1,9,25,26] The wound contaminants are atraumatically removed and discarded when the PolyMem dressing is changed, eliminating the need for routine rinsing at dressing changes.[12,21,25,26]

The glycerin and surfactant in PolyMem products help moisturize dry areas of wounds while pulling fluid from the body into the wound bed and redistributing it.[3,5,6,11,12] Simultaneously, excess fluid from overly wet areas is absorbed into the dressing and is locked into a gel.[3,5,25,27] The "intelligent" backing allows excess fluid to evaporate while retaining the fluid needed to keep dry wounds moist.[28] Other available dressings have only portions of this complete moisture balancing system.[9]

All occlusive dressings provide some pain relief. However, PolyMem products are the only drug-free dressings with evidence showing that they also relieve pain by altering the response of the pain-sensing nerves (nociceptors).[11,13-15,22,29,30] PolyMem products' alteration of the nociceptor response occurs even on intact skin, and has been shown in clinical studies to decrease the excess inflammation that leads to excess swelling and often slows healing.[9,11,13-15,24,30]

PolyMem dressings are nonadherent while conforming to the wound bed.[5,6,12,23,25,29,31,32] They are flexible and comfortable to wear.[1,9,23,31-33]

INDICATIONS

Indicated for virtually all wounds at every stage of healing,[1,3,6,21,25] including closed tissue injuries,[14,30,34,35] multifunctional PolyMem dressings meet or exceed every criterion wound

experts identify for an *ideal dressing*.[26,36,37] PolyMem dressings are safe for use over structures like tendon, bone, and exposed vessels because they can donate moisture.[1,5,6,23,24] PolyMem is suitable for use even when wounds are infected, provided that the infection is otherwise appropriately addressed.[1,5,9,38,39] PolyMem is especially suitable for chronic, trauma, and burn wounds because it helps subdue excess inflammation and is a pain-relieving dressing.[2,8,9,11,13,17,27,39,40]

- Standard PolyMem dressings are the optimal choice for closed tissue injuries and low to moderately exudating wounds, particularly when cutting dressings to size and taping is the preferred method of application. See PolyMem Cutting Guides[41–43] for examples.

CONTRAINDICATIONS

- None.

APPLICATION

- Initially, irrigate or debride the wound bed as indicated or prescribed. Rinse with water or saline. Additional topical products are not necessary or recommended for use with PolyMem. Simply pat the periwound dry, leaving the wound bed slightly moist.
- Select a PolyMem dressing with a membrane pad that is large enough to cover the open wound **AND** all of the surrounding inflamed (reddened, raw, tender, warm, itchy, or swollen) skin. Fill any deep cavities lightly with PolyMem WIC (with or without silver) or WIC Silver Rope, allowing for about 30% expansion. Apply the PolyMem dressing with the moisture-barrier film (printed side) out.
- Secure PolyMem appropriately. Apply adhesives without tension.

How to know when to change PolyMem dressings

- Do NOT change PolyMem on a calendar schedule, especially in the first week of use; anticipate changes in exudate levels, which may dramatically increase initially.
- PolyMem is an indicator dressing: the backing will become a darker color when the membrane becomes saturated. Change the dressing when the darker color reaches any of the wound edges.

REMOVAL

- Simply, gently remove the PolyMem dressing and replace it with an appropriate new PolyMem configuration. In most cases, when using PolyMem, there is no need to rinse the wound.
- PolyMem is designed to continuously cleanse the wound and does not leave a residue that needs to be removed. Excessive cleaning may injure regenerating tissue and delay wound healing.

Guidelines for optimal use

(See *Instructions for Use* provided in each box and **PolyMem.com for detailed information.**)
Independent wound experts have created a robust evidence base for PolyMem dressings by documenting their success in using PolyMem over the past 25+ years. Ferris has developed these guidelines based upon their documented experiences.

- Using PolyMem is simple. However, using PolyMem optimally (knowing which dressing configuration to use, and how) is an art.[9,44] PolyMem use saves time, giving wound specialists more time to address the whole patient, improving healing by optimizing offloading, compression, circulation, nutrition, medications, etc.[4,11,17,23,27,29,35,44–46]
- PolyMem dressings should be changed when indicated, rather than on a schedule. Changing PolyMem more frequently than necessary on a healthy, granulating wound bed may slow healing. Tracing the approximate wound borders on the outer film of the

FOAMS

PolyMem dressing makes it easy to see when a change is needed without "peeking" at the wound.[36]

- PolyMem is an interactive dressing. PolyMem often recruits LARGE amounts of wound fluid, containing debris and metabolic wastes, for the first few days of use, which may prompt frequent dressing changes.[1,21,45] When the wound is clean and granulating, reduced exudate may allow PolyMem to be left in place for up to 7 days.[9]

- On first application, irrigate or debride the wound to remove causes of delayed healing that are easy to address; then allow PolyMem to remove the remainder of the contaminants atraumatically. The PolyMem membrane may become discolored or malodorous, but the wound bed itself will become cleaner and healthier.

- Experienced users gain the confidence to avoid routine rinsing at dressing changes.[3,4,9,46,47] Simply applying a PolyMem dressing **IS** wound cleansing.[9,44] Because rinsing cools the wound bed, washes away valuable nutrients, and can damage fragile new tissue, it is best to rinse only if loose contaminants are visible or the dressing has become dislodged prior to the dressing change, allowing the wound to become dirty and dry.[48]

- Patients with large surface area third-degree burns must be carefully supervised by a burn specialist, especially when any absorptive dressing is used, including PolyMem.

- Healing wounds quickly is the most cost-saving choice. PolyMem is proven to help close wounds quickly.

*See package insert for complete information.

REFERENCES

PDFs of many of the footnoted references are available at www.polymem.com/clinicalguide/

1. Benskin LLL. PolyMem wic silver rope: A multifunctional dressing for decreasing pain, swelling, and inflammation. *Adv Wound Care.* 2012;1(1):44–47.
2. Dawson LC, Boch R. Total Joint Replacement Surgical Site Infections Eliminated by Using Multifunctional Dressing. 900 Cases Report Over 4 Years. May 2010.
3. Cutting KF, Vowden P, Wiegand C. Wound inflammation and the role of a multifunctional polymeric dressing. *Int Wound J.* 2015;6(2):41–46.
4. White L. Optimal Management for Upper Extremity Wounds With a Multifunctional Polymeric Membrane Dressing. September 2015.
5. Denyer J, White R, Ousey K, et al. PolyMem Dressings Made Easy. *Wounds International.* May 2015. http://www.woundsinternational.com/made-easys/view/polymem-dressings-made-easy. Accessed May 7, 2016.
6. Dabiri G, Damstetter E, Phillips T. Choosing a wound dressing based on common wound characteristics. *Adv Wound Care.* 2016;5(1):32–41.
7. Langemo DK, Black J. National pressure ulcer advisory panel. Pressure ulcers in individuals receiving palliative care: a National Pressure Ulcer Advisory Panel white paper. *Adv Skin Wound Care.* 2010;23(2):59–72.
8. Edwards J, Mason S. An evaluation of the use of PolyMem Silver in burn management. *J Commun Nurs.* 2010;24(6):16–19.
9. Benskin LL. Polymeric membrane dressings for topical wound management of patients with infected wounds in a challenging environment: A protocol with 3 case examples. *Ostomy Wound Manage.* 2016;62(6):42–50. (OWM website adds evidence summaries, Tables 1 & 2)
10. Blackman JD, Senseng D, Quinn L, et al. Clinical evaluation of a semipermeable polymeric membrane dressing for the treatment of chronic diabetic foot ulcers. *Diab Care.* 1994;17(4):322–325.
11. Weissman O, Hundeshagen G, Harats M, et al. Custom-fit polymeric membrane dressing masks in the treatment of second degree facial burns. *Burns.* 2013;39(6):1316–1320.
12. Scott A. Polymeric membrane dressings for radiotherapy-induced skin damage. *Br J Nurs.* 2014; 23(10):S24, S26–S31.
13. Kim YJ, Lee SW, Hong SH, et al. The effects of PolyMem(R) on the wound healing. *J Korean Soc Plast Reconstruct Surg.* 1999;26(6):1165–1172.
14. Hayden JK, Cole BJ. The effectiveness of a pain wrap compared to a standard dressing on the reduction of postoperative morbidity following routine knee arthroscopy: a prospective randomized single-blind study. *Orthopedics.* 2003;26(1):59–63; discussion 63.

FOAMS

15. Beitz AJ, Newman A, Kahn AR, et al. A polymeric membrane dressing with antinociceptive properties: analysis with a rodent model of stab wound secondary hyperalgesia. *J Pain.* 2004;5(1):38–47.
16. Agathangelou C. Treating Fungating Breast Cancer Wounds with Polymeric Membrane Dressings, an Innovation in Fungating Wound Management. May 2015.
17. Haik J, Weissman O, Demetrius S, et al. Polymeric Membrane Dressings* for Skin Graft Donor Sites: 6 Years Experience on 1200 Cases. April 2011.
18. Man D, Aleksinko P. Use of Polymeric Membrane Dressings After Occlusive Deep Facial and Neck Chemical Peel Improves Outcomes. April 2010.
19. Man D, Aleksinko P. Intra-Operative Use Followed with Post-Op Application of Polymeric Membrane Dressings Reduces Post-Op Pain, Edema and Bruising After Full Face Lift Surgery. April 2010.
20. Rodeheaver GT, Kurtz L, Kircher BJ, et al. Pluronic F-68: a promising new skin wound cleanser. *Ann Emerg Med.* 1980;9(11):572–576.
21. Denyer JE, Pillay E, Clapham J. Best Practice Guidelines for Skin and Wound Care in Epidermolysis Bullosa—International Consensus. 2017. https://www.woundsinternational.com/resources/details/best-practice-guidelines-skin-and-wound-care-in-epidermolysis-bullosa. Accessed November 20, 2018.
22. Davies SL, White RJ. Defining a holistic pain-relieving approach to wound care via a drug free polymeric membrane dressing. *J Wound Care.* 2011;20(5):250, 252, 254 passim.
23. Rafter L, Oforka E. Standard versus polymeric membrane finger dressing and outcomes following pain diaries. *Wounds UK.* 2014;10(2):40–49.
24. Cahn A, Kleinman Y. A novel approach to the treatment of diabetic foot abscesses—a case series. *J Wound Care.* 2014;23(8):394, 396–399.
25. Fowler E, Papen JC. Clinical evaluation of a polymeric membrane dressing in the treatment of dermal ulcers. *Ostomy Wound Manage.* 1991;35:35–38, 40–44.
26. Yastrub DJ. Relationship between type of treatment and degree of wound healing among institutionalized geriatric patients with stage II pressure ulcers. *Care Manag J.* 2004;5(4):213–218.
27. Stoddart J. Circumferential Wrap Technique with Polymeric Membrane Dressings after Arthroscopic ACL Reconstruction Reduces Blistering, Inflammation and Bruising; Rapid Recovery and Improved Patient Satisfaction: 80 Prospective Patient Series. May 2013.
28. Fulton JA, Blasiole KN, Cottingham T, et al. Wound dressing absorption: A comparative study. *Adv Skin & Wound Care.* 2012;25(7):315–320.
29. Bolhuis J. Evidence-based skin tear protocol. *Long-Term Living.* 2008;57(6):48–52.
30. Kahn AR, Sessions RW, Apasova EV. A superficial cutaneous dressing inhibits pain, inflammation and swelling in deep tissues. *Pain Med.* 2000;1(2):187–187.
31. Bauer J, Diem A, Ploder M. Efficiency and Safety of Using a Polymeric Membrane Wound Dressing in Patients with Epidermolysis Bullosa after a Release Operation. May 2013.
32. Bauer J, Brandtner G. Chirurgische Korrektur der Handfehlbildungen bei Epidermolysis bullosa dystrophicans. *Arzt+Kind.* 2013.
33. Rafter L, Oforka E. Trauma-free fingertip dressing changes. *Wounds UK.* 2013;9(1):96–100.
34. Hegarty F, Wong M. Polymeric membrane dressing for radiotherapy-induced skin reactions. *Br J Nurs.* 2014;23 Suppl 20:S38–S46.
35. Wilson D. Application of Polymeric Membrane Dressings to Stage I Pressure Ulcers Speeds Resolution, Reduces Ulcer Site Discomfort and Reduces Staff Time Devoted to Management of Ulcers. April 2010.
36. Carr RD, Lalagos DE. Clinical evaluation of a polymeric membrane dressing in the treatment of pressure ulcers. *Decubitus.* 1990;3(3):38–42.
37. Benskin L. PolyMem The Ideal Dressing. August 2015.
38. Denyer JE. Wound management for children with epidermolysis bullosa. *Dermatol Clin.* 2010; 28(2):257–264.
39. Aaltonen M. Developing a Protocol For Burns in a Private Out-Patient Wound Clinic. May 2015.
40. Rahman S, Shokri A. Total Knee Arthroplasty (TKA) Infections Eliminated and Rehabilitation Improved Using Polymeric Membrane Dressing Circumferential Wrap Technique: 120 Patients at 12-month Follow-up. May 2013.
41. Hegarty F, Scott A, Wong M, et al. PolyMem Cutting guide for dressing radiotherapy induced skin reactions. 2015.
42. Bostock S. Improving management of radiotherapy-induced skin reactions: a radiographer's perspective. *Wounds UK.* 2016;12(3). http://www.wounds-uk.com/journal-articles/improving-management-of-radiotherapy-induced-skin-reactions-a-radiographers-perspective. Accessed June 26, 2017.

FOAMS

43. Denyer J, Winblad R. PolyMem Dressings in the Management of Epidermolysis Bullosa. 2014. https://pages.cld.bz/data/tyEnNjo/common/downloads/publication.pdf.

44. Denyer J. Six Years' Experience Of PolyMem Dressings Used On Children With Epidermolysis Bullosa (EB). September 2015.

45. Denyer J. Managing pain in children with epidermolysis bullosa. *Nurs Times*. 2012;108(29):21–23.

46. Vanwalleghem G. A New Protocol for the Treatment of Pilonidal Cysts. May 2011.

47. Agathangelou C. Patients with Chronic Wound Pain Stop Hurting, Why? May 2011.

48. McGuiness W, Vella E, Harrison D. Influence of dressing changes on wound temperature. *J Wound Care*. 2004;13(9):383–385.

New Product: PolyMem® Finger/Toe Dressings*

Ferris Mfg. Corp.

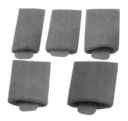

HOW SUPPLIED

#1 (Small) Finger/Toe PMD	1.8″ × 2.2″, New Size	A6209
#2 (Medium) Finger/Toe PMD	2.2″ × 2.6″, New Size	A6209
#3 (Large) Finger/Toe PMD	2.6″ × 3.0″, New Size	A6209
#4 (Extra Large) Finger/Toe PMD	3.0″ × 3.4″, New Size	A6209
#5 (XXL) Finger/Toe PMD	3.4″ × 3.8″, New Size	A6210

ACTION

PolyMem Finger/Toe Dressings are multifunctional[1–4] polymeric membrane dressings (PMDs) designed to easily roll onto appendages or nearby joints, making dressing changes simple, atraumatic, and quick.[3,5,6] PolyMem helps diminish pain[3,7,8,8,9] and edema,[4,10–12] and promotes healing by continuously cleansing wounds,[9,13,14] balancing moisture,[2,15–18] helping to subdue and focus inflammation.[4,10–12] Many new wound products are being developed to include small aspects of PolyMem dressings' many benefits, but none are able to furnish the integrated solutions PolyMem products have reliably provided for nearly three decades.[9]

Activated by moisture, PolyMem products gradually release a nontoxic surfactant cleanser and glycerin to loosen bonds between the wound bed and adherent substances that may impair healing.[4,15,19–21] Glycerin pulls nutrient-filled, enzyme-rich fluid from the body into the wound bed, enhancing healing and autolytic debridement while floating the contaminants.[2,5,15,18,22] The PolyMem membrane pulls in the undesirable substances along with the fluid, which are locked into the porous superabsorbent structure.[4,9,23,24] The wound contaminants are atraumatically removed and discarded when the PolyMem dressing is changed, eliminating the need for routine rinsing at dressing changes.[17,20,23,24]

The glycerin and surfactant in PolyMem products help moisturize dry areas of wounds while pulling fluid from the body into the wound bed and redistributing it.[2,15–18] Simultaneously, excess fluid from overly wet areas is absorbed into the dressing and is locked into a gel.[2,15,23,25] The "intelligent" backing allows excess fluid to evaporate while retaining the fluid needed to keep dry wounds moist.[26] Other available dressings have only portions of this complete moisture balancing system.[9]

All occlusive dressings provide some pain relief. However, PolyMem products are the only drug-free dressings with evidence showing that they also relieve pain by altering the response of the pain-sensing nerves (nociceptors).[10–12,16,21,27,28] PolyMem products' alteration of the nociceptor response occurs even on intact skin, and has been shown in clinical studies to decrease the excess inflammation that leads to excess swelling and often slows healing.[9–12,16,22,28]

PolyMem dressings are non-adherent while conforming to the wound bed.[5,15,17,18,23,27,29,30] They are flexible and comfortable to wear.[4–6,9,29,30]

INDICATIONS

Indicated for virtually all wounds at every stage of healing,[2,4,18,20,23] including closed tissue injuries,[11,28,31,32] multifunctional PolyMem dressings meet or exceed every criterion wound experts identify for an *Ideal Dressing*.[24,33,34] PolyMem dressings are safe for use over structures like tendon, bone, and exposed vessels because they can donate moisture.[4,5,15,18,22] PolyMem is suitable for use even when wounds are infected, provided that the infection is otherwise appropriately addressed.[4,9,15,35,36] PolyMem is especially suitable for chronic, trauma, and burn wounds because it helps subdue excess inflammation and is a pain relieving dressing.[1,7,9,10,16,25,36–38]

- PolyMem Finger/Toe dressings are especially suited for wounds and closed tissue injuries on appendages and adjacent joints.[3,5,6] They can also be opened along one seam to fit ears and can form sleeves for neonates and infants.[39,40]

CONTRAINDICATIONS

- None.

APPLICATION

- Initially, irrigate or debride the wound bed as indicated or prescribed. Rinse with water or saline. Additional topical products are not necessary or recommended for use with PolyMem. Simply pat the periwound dry, leaving the wound bed slightly moist.
- Select a PolyMem Finger/Toe dressing the appropriate diameter for the appendage. Trim excess length. Fill large voids lightly with PolyMem WIC (standard or silver). Insert tip of finger or toe into the rolled end of the dressing. Roll the PolyMem dressing onto the appendage with the moisture-barrier film (printed side) out.
- For joints, the dressing may be cut to form a ring or sleeve, and it may be split along seams with the ends secured with tape. See website and Instructions for Use for detailed application instructions.

How to know when to change PolyMem dressings

- Do NOT change PolyMem on a calendar schedule, especially in the first week of use; anticipate changes in exudate levels, which may dramatically increase initially.
- PolyMem is an indicator dressing: the backing will become a darker color when the membrane becomes saturated. Change the dressing when the darker color reaches any of the wound edges.

REMOVAL

- Simply, gently remove the PolyMem Finger/Toe dressing and replace it with an appropriate new PolyMem configuration. In most cases, when using PolyMem, there is no need to rinse the wound.
- PolyMem is designed to continuously cleanse the wound and does not leave residue that needs to be removed. Excessive cleaning may injure regenerating tissue and delay wound healing.

Guidelines for optimal use

(See *Instructions for Use* provided in each box and **PolyMem.com for detailed information**.)

Independent wound experts have created a robust evidence base for PolyMem dressings by documenting their success in using PolyMem over the past 25+ years. Ferris has developed these guidelines based upon their documented experiences.

- Using PolyMem is simple. However, using PolyMem optimally (knowing which dressing configuration to use, and how) is an art.[9,41] PolyMem use saves time, giving wound specialists more time to address the whole patient, improving healing by optimizing offloading, compression, circulation, nutrition, medications, and so forth.[3,5,7,16,25,27,32,41–43]
- PolyMem dressings should be changed when indicated, rather than on a schedule. Changing PolyMem more frequently than necessary on a healthy, granulating wound bed may slow healing. Tracing the approximate wound borders on the outer film of the PolyMem dressing makes it easy to see when a change is needed without "peeking" at the wound.[33]

- PolyMem is an interactive dressing. PolyMem often recruits LARGE amounts of wound fluid, containing debris and metabolic wastes, for the first few days of use, which may prompt frequent dressing changes.[4,20,42] When the wound is clean and granulating, reduced exudate may allow PolyMem to be left in place for up to 7 days.[9]
- On first application, irrigate or debride the wound to remove causes of delayed healing that are easy to address; then allow PolyMem to remove the remainder of the contaminants atraumatically. The PolyMem membrane may become discolored or malodorous, but the wound bed itself will become cleaner and healthier.
- Experienced users gain the confidence to avoid routine rinsing at dressing changes.[2,3,9,43,44] Simply applying a PolyMem dressing **IS** wound cleansing.[9,41] Because rinsing cools the wound bed, washes away valuable nutrients, and can damage fragile new tissue, it is best to rinse only if loose contaminants are visible or the dressing has become dislodged prior to the dressing change, allowing the wound to become dirty and dry.[45]
- Patients with large surface area third degree burns must be carefully supervised by a burn specialist, especially when any absorptive dressing is used, including PolyMem.
- Healing wounds quickly is the most cost-saving choice. PolyMem is proven to help close wounds quickly.

*See package insert for complete information.

REFERENCES

PDFs of many of the footnoted references are available at www.polymem.com/clinicalguide/

1. Dawson, Lewis C, Boch R. Total Joint Replacement Surgical Site Infections Eliminated by Using Multifunctional Dressing. 900 Cases Report over 4 years. May 2010.
2. Cutting KF, Vowden P, Wiegand C. Wound inflammation and the role of a multifunctional polymeric dressing. *Wounds International Journal.* 2015;6(2):41–46.
3. White L. Optimal Management for Upper Extremity Wounds with a Multifunctional Polymeric Membrane Dressing. September 2015.
4. Benskin LL. PolyMem Wic Silver Rope: A multifunctional dressing for decreasing pain, swelling, and inflammation. *Adv Wound Care* (New Rochelle). 2012;1(1):44–47.
5. Rafter L, Oforka E. Standard versus polymeric membrane finger dressing and outcomes following pain diaries. *Wounds UK.* 2014;10(2):40–49.
6. Rafter L, Oforka E. Trauma-free fingertip dressing changes. *Wounds UK.* 2013;9(1):96–100.
7. Haik J, Weissman O, Demetrius S, et al. Polymeric Membrane Dressings* for Skin Graft Donor Sites: 6 Years Experience on 1200 Cases. April 2011.
8. Man D, Aleksinko P. Intra-Operative Use Followed with Post-Op Application of Polymeric Membrane Dressings Reduces Post-Op Pain, Edema and Bruising After Full Face Lift Surgery. April 2010.
9. Benskin LL. Polymeric Membrane Dressings for topical wound management of patients with infected wounds in a challenging environment: A protocol with 3 case examples. *Ostomy Wound Management.* 2016;62(6):42–50. (OWM website adds evidence summaries, Tables 1 & 2)
10. Kim YJ, Lee SW, Hong SH, et al. The effects of polyMem(R) on the wound healing. *J Korean Soc Plast Reconstr Surg.* 1999;26(6):1165–1172.
11. Hayden JK, Cole BJ. The effectiveness of a pain wrap compared to a standard dressing on the reduction of postoperative morbidity following routine knee arthroscopy: a prospective randomized single-blind study. *Orthopedics.* 2003;26(1):59–63; discussion 63.
12. Beitz AJ, Newman A, Kahn AR, et al. A polymeric membrane dressing with antinociceptive properties: analysis with a rodent model of stab wound secondary hyperalgesia. *J Pain.* 2004;5(1):38–47.
13. Blackman JD, Senseng D, Quinn L, et al. Clinical evaluation of a semipermeable polymeric membrane dressing for the treatment of chronic diabetic foot ulcers. *Diabetes Care.* 1994;17(4):322–325.
14. Langemo DK, Black J; National Pressure Ulcer Advisory Panel. Pressure ulcers in individuals receiving palliative care: a National Pressure Ulcer Advisory Panel white paper. *Adv Skin Wound Care.* 2010;23(2):59–72.
15. Denyer J, White R, Ousey K, et al. PolyMem dressings Made Easy. *Wounds International.* May 2015. http://www.woundsinternational.com/made-easys/view/polymem-dressings-made-easy. Accessed May 7, 2016.
16. Weissman O, Hundeshagen G, Harats M, et al. Custom-fit polymeric membrane dressing masks in the treatment of second degree facial burns. *Burns.* 2013;39(6):1316–1320.

FOAMS

17. Scott A. Polymeric membrane dressings for radiotherapy-induced skin damage. *Br J Nurs.* 2014; 23(10):S24, S26–S31.
18. Dabiri G, Damstetter E, Phillips T. Choosing a wound dressing based on common wound characteristics. *Adv Wound Care* (New Rochelle). 2016;5(1):32–41.
19. Rodeheaver GT, Kurtz L, Kircher BJ, et al. Pluronic F-68: a promising new skin wound cleanser. *Ann Emerg Med.* 1980;9(11):572–576.
20. Denyer JE, Pillay E. Best practice guidelines for skin and wound care in epidermolysis bullosa—International Consensus. 2012. http://www.woundsinternational.com/other-resources/view/best-practice-guidelines-for-skin-and-wound-care-in-epidermolysis-bullosa. Accessed March 30, 2015.
21. Davies SL, White RJ. Defining a holistic pain-relieving approach to wound care via a drug free polymeric membrane dressing. *J Wound Care.* 2011;20(5):250, 252, 254 passim.
22. Cahn A, Kleinman Y. A novel approach to the treatment of diabetic foot abscesses—a case series. *J Wound Care.* 2014;23(8):394, 396–399.
23. Fowler E, Papen JC. Clinical evaluation of a polymeric membrane dressing in the treatment of dermal ulcers. *Ostomy Wound Manage.* 1991;35:35–38, 40–44.
24. Yastrub DJ. Relationship between type of treatment and degree of wound healing among institutionalized geriatric patients with stage II pressure ulcers. *Care Manag J.* 2004;5(4):213–218.
25. Stoddart J. Circumferential Wrap Technique with Polymeric Membrane Dressings after Arthroscopic ACL Reconstruction Reduces Blistering, Inflammation and Bruising; Rapid Recovery and Improved Patient Satisfaction: 80 Prospective Patient Series. May 2013.
26. Fulton JA, Blasiole KN, Cottingham T, et al. Wound dressing absorption: A comparative study. *Adv Skin Wound Care.* 2012;25(7):315–320.
27. Bolhuis J. Evidence-based skin tear protocol. *Long-Term Living: For the Continuing Care Professional.* 2008;57(6):48–52.
28. Kahn AR, Sessions RW, Apasova EV. A superficial cutaneous dressing inhibits pain, inflammation and swelling in deep tissues. *Pain Medicine.* 2000;1(2):187.
29. Bauer J, Diem A, Ploder M. Efficiency and Safety of Using a Polymeric Membrane Wound Dressing in Patients with Epidermolysis Bullosa after a Release Operation. May 2013.
30. Bauer J, Brandtner G. Chirurgische Korrektur der Handfehlbildungen bei Epidermolysis bullosa dystrophicans. *Arzt+Kind.* 2013.
31. Hegarty F, Wong M. Polymeric membrane dressing for radiotherapy-induced skin reactions. *Br J Nurs.* 2014;23 Suppl 20:S38–S46.
32. Wilson D. Application of Polymeric Membrane Dressings to Stage I Pressure Ulcers Speeds Resolution, Reduces Ulcer Site Discomfort and Reduces Staff Time Devoted to Management of Ulcers. April 2010.
33. Carr RD, Lalagos DE. Clinical evaluation of a polymeric membrane dressing in the treatment of pressure ulcers. *Decubitus.* 1990;3(3):38–42.
34. Benskin L. PolyMem The Ideal Dressing. August 2015.
35. Denyer JE. Wound management for children with epidermolysis bullosa. *Dermatologic Clinics.* 2010; 28(2):257–264.
36. Aaltonen M. Developing a Protocol For Burns in a Private Out-Patient Wound Clinic. May 2015.
37. Rahman S, Shokri A. Total Knee Arthroplasty (TKA) Infections Eliminated and Rehabilitation Improved Using Polymeric Membrane Dressing Circumferential Wrap Technique: 120 Patients at 12-month Follow-up. May 2013.
38. Edwards J, Mason S. An evaluation of the use of PolyMem Silver in burn management. *Journal of Community Nursing.* 2010;24(6):16–19.
39. Hegarty F, Scott A, Wong M, et al. PolyMem Cutting guide for dressing radiotherapy induced skin reactions. 2015.
40. Denyer J, Winblad R. PolyMem Dressings in the Management of Epidermolysis Bullosa. 2014. https://pages.cld.bz/data/tyEnNjo/common/downloads/publication.pdf.
41. Denyer J. Six Years' Experience Of PolyMem Dressings Used On Children With Epidermolysis Bullosa (EB). September 2015.
42. Denyer J. Managing pain in children with epidermolysis bullosa. *Nurs Times.* 2012;108(29):21–23.
43. Vanwalleghem G. A New Protocol for the Treatment of Pilonidal Cysts. May 2011.
44. Agathangelou C. Patients with Chronic Wound Pain Stop Hurting, Why? May 2011.
45. McGuiness W, Vella E, Harrison D. Influence of dressing changes on wound temperature. *J Wound Care.* 2004;13(9):383–385.

New Product: Polymem® MAX® Dressing*

Ferris Mfg. Corp.

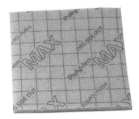

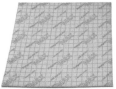

HOW SUPPLIED

Extra-absorbent Non-adhesive PMD Pad	3″ × 3″, New Size	A6209
Extra-absorbent Non-adhesive PMD Pad	4.5″ × 4.5″	A6210
Extra-absorbent Non-adhesive PMD Pad	8″ × 8″	A6211

ACTION

PolyMem MAX is an extra-absorbent multifunctional,[1–4] interactive[5] polymeric membrane dressing (PMD) designed for handling high levels of exudate[3,6–9] while providing protection from contamination,[3,6] continuously cleansing,[6,10] balancing moisture,[3,5,7,11,12] helping to subdue and focus inflammation,[1,13–15] and reducing odor[3,5,6,16] and wound pain.[4,9,17–19] Many new wound products are being developed to include small aspects of PolyMem dressings' many benefits, but none are able to furnish the integrated solutions PolyMem products have reliably provided for nearly three decades.[9]

Activated by moisture, PolyMem products gradually release a nontoxic surfactant cleanser and glycerin to loosen bonds between the wound bed and adherent substances that may impair healing.[1,5,20–22] Glycerin pulls nutrient-filled, enzyme-rich fluid from the body into the wound bed, enhancing healing and autolytic debridement while floating the contaminants.[3,5,6,23,24] The PolyMem membrane pulls in the undesirable substances along with the fluid, which are locked into the porous superabsorbent structure.[1,9,25,26] The wound contaminants are atraumatically removed and discarded when the PolyMem dressing is changed, eliminating the need for routine rinsing at dressing changes.[12,21,25,26]

The glycerin and surfactant in PolyMem products help moisturize dry areas of wounds while pulling fluid from the body into the wound bed and redistributing it.[3,5,6,11,12] Simultaneously, excess fluid from overly wet areas is absorbed into the dressing and is locked into a gel.[3,5,25,27] The "intelligent" backing allows excess fluid to evaporate while retaining the fluid needed to keep dry wounds moist.[28] Other available dressings have only portions of this complete moisture balancing system.[9]

All occlusive dressings provide some pain relief. However, PolyMem products are the only drug-free dressings with evidence showing that they also relieve pain by altering the response of the pain-sensing nerves (nociceptors).[11,13–15,22,29,30] PolyMem products' alteration of the nociceptor response occurs even on intact skin, and has been shown in clinical studies to decrease the excess inflammation that leads to excess swelling and often slows healing.[9,11,13–15,24,30]

PolyMem dressings are non-adherent while conforming to the wound bed.[5,6,12,23,25,29,31,32] They are flexible and comfortable to wear.[1,9,23,31–33]

INDICATIONS

Indicated for virtually all wounds at every stage of healing,[1,3,6,21,25] including closed tissue injuries,[14,30,34,35] multifunctional PolyMem dressings meet or exceed every criterion wound

experts identify for an *Ideal Dressing*.[26,36,37] PolyMem dressings are safe for use over structures like tendon, bone, and exposed vessels because they can donate moisture.[1,5,6,23,24] PolyMem is suitable for use even when wounds are infected, provided that the infection is otherwise appropriately addressed.[1,5,9,38,39] PolyMem is especially suitable for chronic, trauma, and burn wounds because it helps subdue excess inflammation and is a pain relieving dressing.[2,8,9,11,13,17,27,39,40]

- PolyMem MAX dressings are especially suited for moderately to heavily exudating wounds.[6,17,28,41] They are 60% more absorbent and have a higher MVTR (they permit faster evaporation) than standard thickness PolyMem dressings.

CONTRAINDICATIONS

- None.

APPLICATION

- Initially, irrigate or debride the wound bed as indicated or prescribed. Rinse with water or saline. Additional topical products are not necessary or recommended for use with PolyMem. Simply pat the periwound dry, leaving the wound bed slightly moist.
- Select a PolyMem MAX dressing with a membrane pad that is large enough to cover the open wound **AND** all of the surrounding inflamed (reddened, raw, tender, warm, itchy, or swollen) skin. Fill any deep cavities lightly with PolyMem WIC (with or without silver) or WIC Silver Rope, allowing for about 30% expansion. Apply the PolyMem dressing with the moisture-barrier film (printed side) out.
- Secure PolyMem appropriately. Apply adhesives without tension.

How to know when to change PolyMem dressings

- Do NOT change PolyMem on a calendar schedule, especially in the first week of use; anticipate changes in exudate levels, which may dramatically increase initially.
- PolyMem is an indicator dressing: the backing will become a darker color when the membrane becomes saturated. Change the dressing when the darker color reaches any of the wound edges.

REMOVAL

- Simply, gently remove the PolyMem MAX dressing and replace it with an appropriate new PolyMem configuration. In most cases, when using PolyMem, there is no need to rinse the wound.
- PolyMem is designed to continuously cleanse the wound and does not leave residue that needs to be removed. Excessive cleaning may injure regenerating tissue and delay wound healing.

Guidelines for optimal use

(See *Instructions for Use* provided in each box and **PolyMem.com for detailed information**.)

Independent wound experts have created a robust evidence base for PolyMem dressings by documenting their success in using PolyMem over the past 25+ years. Ferris has developed these guidelines based upon their documented experiences.

- Using PolyMem is simple. However, using PolyMem optimally (knowing which dressing configuration to use, and how) is an art.[9,42] PolyMem use saves time, giving wound specialists more time to address the whole patient, improving healing by optimizing offloading, compression, circulation, nutrition, medications, etc.[4,11,17,23,27,29,35,42–44]
- PolyMem dressings should be changed when indicated, rather than on a schedule. Changing PolyMem more frequently than necessary on a healthy, granulating wound bed may slow healing. Tracing the approximate wound borders on the outer film of the PolyMem dressing makes it easy to see when a change is needed without "peeking" at the wound.[36]

- PolyMem is an interactive dressing. PolyMem often recruits LARGE amounts of wound fluid, containing debris and metabolic wastes, for the first few days of use, which may prompt frequent dressing changes.[1,21,43] When the wound is clean and granulating, reduced exudate may allow PolyMem to be left in place for up to 7 days.[9]
- On first application, irrigate or debride the wound to remove causes of delayed healing that are easy to address; then allow PolyMem to remove the remainder of the contaminants atraumatically. The PolyMem membrane may become discolored or malodorous, but the wound bed itself will become cleaner and healthier.
- Experienced users gain the confidence to avoid routine rinsing at dressing changes.[3,4,9,44,45] Simply applying a PolyMem dressing **IS** wound cleansing.[9,42] Because rinsing cools the wound bed, washes away valuable nutrients, and can damage fragile new tissue, it is best to rinse only if loose contaminants are visible or the dressing has become dislodged prior to the dressing change, allowing the wound to become dirty and dry.[46]
- Patients with large surface area third degree burns must be carefully supervised by a burn specialist, especially when any absorptive dressing is used, including PolyMem.
- Healing wounds quickly is the most cost-saving choice. PolyMem is proven to help close wounds quickly.

*See package insert for complete information.

REFERENCES

PDFs of many of the footnoted references are available at www.polymem.com/clinicalguide/

1. Benskin LL. PolyMem Wic Silver Rope: A multifunctional dressing for decreasing pain, swelling, and inflammation. *Adv Wound Care* (New Rochelle). 2012;1(1):44–47.
2. Dawson, Lewis C, Boch R. Total Joint Replacement Surgical Site Infections Eliminated by Using Multifunctional Dressing. 900 Cases Report over 4 years. May 2010.
3. Cutting KF, Vowden P, Wiegand C. Wound inflammation and the role of a multifunctional polymeric dressing. *Wounds International Journal*. 2015;6(2):41–46.
4. White L. Optimal Management for Upper Extremity Wounds with a Multifunctional Polymeric Membrane Dressing. September 2015.
5. Denyer J, White R, Ousey K, et al. PolyMem dressings Made Easy. *Wounds International*. May 2015. http://www.woundsinternational.com/made-easys/view/polymem-dressings-made-easy. Accessed May 7, 2016.
6. Dabiri G, Damstetter E, Phillips T. Choosing a wound dressing based on common wound characteristics. *Adv Wound Care* (New Rochelle). 2016;5(1):32–41.
7. Langemo DK, Black J; National Pressure Ulcer Advisory Panel. Pressure ulcers in individuals receiving palliative care: a National Pressure Ulcer Advisory Panel white paper. *Adv Skin Wound Care*. 2010;23(2):59–72.
8. Edwards J, Mason S. An evaluation of the use of PolyMem Silver in burn management. *Journal of Community Nursing*. 2010;24(6):16–19.
9. Benskin LL. Polymeric Membrane Dressings for topical wound management of patients with infected wounds in a challenging environment: A protocol with 3 case examples. *Ostomy Wound Management*. 2016;62(6):42–50. (OWM website adds evidence summaries, Tables 1 & 2)
10. Blackman JD, Senseng D, Quinn L, et al. Clinical evaluation of a semipermeable polymeric membrane dressing for the treatment of chronic diabetic foot ulcers. *Diabetes Care*. 1994;17(4):322–325.
11. Weissman O, Hundeshagen G, Harats M, et al. Custom-fit polymeric membrane dressing masks in the treatment of second degree facial burns. *Burns*. 2013;39(6):1316–1320.
12. Scott A. Polymeric membrane dressings for radiotherapy-induced skin damage. *Br J Nurs*. 2014; 23(10):S24, S26–S31.
13. Kim YJ, Lee SW, Hong SH, et al. The effects of PolyMem(R) on the wound healing. *J Korean Soc Plast Reconstr Surg*. 1999;26(6):1165–1172.
14. Hayden JK, Cole BJ. The effectiveness of a pain wrap compared to a standard dressing on the reduction of postoperative morbidity following routine knee arthroscopy: a prospective randomized single-blind study. *Orthopedics*. 2003;26(1):59–63; discussion 63.
15. Beitz AJ, Newman A, Kahn AR, et al. A polymeric membrane dressing with antinociceptive properties: analysis with a rodent model of stab wound secondary hyperalgesia. *J Pain*. 2004;5(1):38–47.
16. Agathangelou C. Treating Fungating Breast Cancer Wounds with Polymeric Membrane Dressings, an Innovation in Fungating Wound Management. May 2015.

FOAMS

17. Haik J, Weissman O, Demetrius S, et al. Polymeric Membrane Dressings® for Skin Graft Donor Sites: 6 Years Experience on 1200 Cases. April 2011.
18. Man D, Aleksinko P. Use of Polymeric Membrane Dressings After Occlusive Deep Facial and Neck Chemical Peel Improves Outcomes. April 2010.
19. Man D, Aleksinko P. Intra-Operative Use Followed with Post-Op Application of Polymeric Membrane Dressings Reduces Post-Op Pain, Edema and Bruising After Full Face Lift Surgery. April 2010.
20. Rodeheaver GT, Kurtz L, Kircher BJ, et al. Pluronic F-68: a promising new skin wound cleanser. *Ann Emerg Med*. 1980;9(11):572–576.
21. Denyer JE, Pillay E. Best practice guidelines for skin and wound care in epidermolysis bullosa— International Consensus. 2012. http://www.woundsinternational.com/other-resources/view/best-practice-guidelines-for-skin-and-wound-care-in-epidermolysis-bullosa. Accessed March 30, 2015.
22. Davies SL, White RJ. Defining a holistic pain-relieving approach to wound care via a drug free polymeric membrane dressing. *J Wound Care*. 2011;20(5):250, 252, 254 passim.
23. Rafter L, Oforka E. Standard versus polymeric membrane finger dressing and outcomes following pain diaries. *Wounds UK*. 2014;10(2):40–49.
24. Cahn A, Kleinman Y. A novel approach to the treatment of diabetic foot abscesses—a case series. *J Wound Care*. 2014;23(8):394, 396–399.
25. Fowler E, Papen JC. Clinical evaluation of a polymeric membrane dressing in the treatment of dermal ulcers. *Ostomy Wound Manage*. 1991;35:35-38, 40–44.
26. Yastrub DJ. Relationship between type of treatment and degree of wound healing among institutionalized geriatric patients with stage II pressure ulcers. *Care Manag J*. 2004;5(4):213–218.
27. Stoddart J. Circumferential Wrap Technique with Polymeric Membrane Dressings after Arthroscopic ACL Reconstruction Reduces Blistering, Inflammation and Bruising; Rapid Recovery and Improved Patient Satisfaction: 80 Prospective Patient Series. May 2013.
28. Fulton JA, Blasiole KN, Cottingham T, et al. Wound dressing absorption: A comparative study. *Adv Skin Wound Care*. 2012;25(7):315–320.
29. Bolhuis J. Evidence-based skin tear protocol. *Long-Term Living: For the Continuing Care Professional*. 2008;57(6):48-52.
30. Kahn AR, Sessions RW, Apasova EV. A superficial cutaneous dressing inhibits pain, inflammation and swelling in deep tissues. *Pain Medicine*. 2000;1(2):187–187.
31. Bauer J, Diem A, Ploder M. Efficiency and Safety of Using a Polymeric Membrane Wound Dressing in Patients with Epidermolysis Bullosa after a Release Operation. May 2013.
32. Bauer J, Brandtner G. Chirurgische Korrektur der Handfehlbildungen bei Epidermolysis bullosa dystrophicans. *Arzt+Kind*. 2013.
33. Rafter L, Oforka E. Trauma-free fingertip dressing changes. *Wounds UK*. 2013;9(1):96–100.
34. Hegarty F, Wong M. Polymeric membrane dressing for radiotherapy-induced skin reactions. *Br J Nurs*. 2014;23 Suppl 20:S38–S46.
35. Wilson D. Application of Polymeric Membrane Dressings to Stage I Pressure Ulcers Speeds Resolution, Reduces Ulcer Site Discomfort and Reduces Staff Time Devoted to Management of Ulcers. April 2010.
36. Carr RD, Lalagos DE. Clinical evaluation of a polymeric membrane dressing in the treatment of pressure ulcers. *Decubitus*. 1990;3(3):38–42.
37. Benskin L. PolyMem The Ideal Dressing. August 2015.
38. Denyer JE. Wound management for children with epidermolysis bullosa. *Dermatologic Clinics*. 2010; 28(2):257–264.
39. Aaltonen M. Developing a Protocol For Burns in a Private Out-Patient Wound Clinic. May 2015.
40. Rahman S, Shokri A. Total Knee Arthroplasty (TKA) Infections Eliminated and Rehabilitation Improved Using Polymeric Membrane Dressing Circumferential Wrap Technique: 120 Patients at 12-month Follow-up. May 2013.
41. Benskin L. Crush injury treated with extra-thick polymeric membrane dressings until complete wound closure. June 2008.
42. Denyer J. Six Years' Experience Of PolyMem Dressings Used On Children With Epidermolysis Bullosa (EB). September 2015.
43. Denyer J. Managing pain in children with epidermolysis bullosa. *Nurs Times*. 2012;108(29):21–23.
44. Vanwalleghem G. A New Protocol for the Treatment of Pilonidal Cysts. May 2011.
45. Agathangelou C. Patients with Chronic Wound Pain Stop Hurting, Why? May 2011.
46. McGuiness W, Vella E, Harrison D. Influence of dressing changes on wound temperature. *J Wound Care*. 2004;13(9):383–385.

New Product: Polymem® WIC® Wound Filler*

Ferris Mfg. Corp.

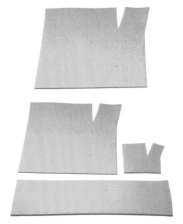

HOW SUPPLIED

PMD Wound Filler	3″ × 3″ 4 g	A6215
PMD Wound Filler	3″ × 12″ 16 g	A6215
PMD Wound Filler	8″ × 8″ 28 g, New Size	A6215

ACTION

PolyMem WIC is a multifunctional,[1–4] interactive[5] primary polymeric membrane dressing (PMD) designed to gently expand to fill cavities, and to wick excess fluid into outer (secondary) dressings or compression wraps,[6–8] while limiting inflammation,[1,9–11] decreasing persistent and procedural wound pain,[4,8,12–14] balancing moisture,[3,5,15–17] and continuously cleansing wounds.[8,18] Many new wound products are being developed to include small aspects of PolyMem dressings' many benefits, but none are able to furnish the integrated solutions PolyMem products have reliably provided for nearly three decades.[8]

Activated by moisture, PolyMem products gradually release a nontoxic surfactant cleanser and glycerin to loosen bonds between the wound bed and adherent substances that may impair healing.[1,5,19–21] Glycerin pulls nutrient-filled, enzyme-rich fluid from the body into the wound bed, enhancing healing and autolytic debridement while floating the contaminants.[3,5,17,22,23] The PolyMem membrane pulls in the undesirable substances along with the fluid, which are locked into the porous superabsorbent structure.[1,8,24,25] The wound contaminants are atraumatically removed and discarded when the PolyMem dressing is changed, eliminating the need for routine rinsing at dressing changes.[16,20,24,25]

The glycerin and surfactant in PolyMem products help moisturize dry areas of wounds while pulling fluid from the body into the wound bed and redistributing it.[3,5,15–17] Simultaneously, excess fluid from overly wet areas is absorbed into the dressing and is locked into a gel.[3,5,24,26] The "intelligent" backing allows excess fluid to evaporate while retaining the fluid needed to keep dry wounds moist.[27] Other available dressings have only portions of this complete moisture balancing system.[8]

All occlusive dressings provide some pain relief. However, PolyMem products are the only drug-free dressings with evidence showing that they also relieve pain by altering the response of the pain-sensing nerves (nociceptors).[9–11,15,21,28,29] PolyMem products' alteration of the nociceptor response occurs even on intact skin, and has been shown in clinical studies to decrease the excess inflammation that leads to excess swelling and often slows healing.[8–11,15,23,29]

PolyMem dressings are non-adherent while conforming to the wound bed.[5,16,17,22,24,28,30,31] They are flexible and comfortable to wear.[1,8,22,30–32]

INDICATIONS

Indicated for virtually all wounds at every stage of healing,[1,3,17,20,24] including closed tissue injuries,[10,29,33,34] multifunctional PolyMem dressings meet or exceed every criterion wound experts identify for an *Ideal Dressing*.[7,25,35] PolyMem dressings are safe for use over structures like tendon, bone, and exposed vessels because they can donate moisture.[1,5,17,22,23] PolyMem is suitable for use even when wounds are infected, provided that the infection is otherwise appropriately addressed.[1,5,8,36,37] PolyMem is especially suitable for chronic, trauma, and burn wounds because it helps subdue excess inflammation and is a pain relieving dressing.[2,8,9,12,15,26,37–39]

- PolyMem WIC wound filler is indicated to lightly fill dead space in dry to heavily exudating wounds.[40–43] It is also useful for providing extra absorption under PolyMem secondary dressings and to provide PolyMem's unique benefits under absorptive compression wraps.[6,8]

CONTRAINDICATIONS

- None.

APPLICATION

- Initially, irrigate or debride the wound bed as indicated or prescribed. Rinse with water or saline. Additional topical products are not necessary or recommended for use with PolyMem. Simply pat the periwound dry, leaving the wound bed slightly moist.
- For cavity wounds, cut or tear PolyMem WIC wound filler so that it lightly fills the cavity, allowing for about 30% expansion as the dressing becomes saturated. Lay PolyMem WIC flat when used under secondary dressings or absorptive compression wraps.
- Cover PolyMem WIC with a PolyMem dressing with a membrane pad that is large enough to cover the wound filler **AND** all of the surrounding inflamed (reddened, raw, tender, warm, itchy, or swollen) skin, with the moisture-barrier film (printed side) out. Secure the secondary (outer) dressing appropriately (see website for securement hints). Apply adhesives without tension.

How to know when to change PolyMem dressings

- Do NOT change PolyMem on a calendar schedule, especially in the first week of use; anticipate changes in exudate levels, which may dramatically increase initially.
- PolyMem is an indicator dressing: the backing will become a darker color when the membrane becomes saturated. Change the dressing when the darker color reaches any of the wound edges.

REMOVAL

- Simply, gently remove the PolyMem WIC wound filler and replace it with an appropriate new PolyMem configuration. In most cases, when using PolyMem, there is no need to rinse the wound.
- PolyMem is designed to continuously cleanse the wound and does not leave residue that needs to be removed. Excessive cleaning may injure regenerating tissue and delay wound healing.

Guidelines for optimal use

(See *Instructions for Use* provided in each box and **PolyMem.com for detailed information.**)

Independent wound experts have created a robust evidence base for PolyMem dressings by documenting their success in using PolyMem over the past 25+ years. Ferris has developed these guidelines based upon their documented experiences.

- Using PolyMem is simple. However, using PolyMem optimally (knowing which dressing configuration to use, and how) is an art.[8,44] PolyMem use saves time, giving wound specialists more time to address the whole patient, improving healing by optimizing offloading, compression, circulation, nutrition, medications, and so forth.[4,12,15,22,26,28,34,44–46]
- PolyMem dressings should be changed when indicated, rather than on a schedule. Changing PolyMem more frequently than necessary on a healthy, granulating wound bed may slow healing. Tracing the approximate wound borders on the outer film of the

PolyMem dressing makes it easy to see when a change is needed without "peeking" at the wound.[35]

- PolyMem is an interactive dressing. PolyMem often recruits LARGE amounts of wound fluid, containing debris and metabolic wastes, for the first few days of use, which may prompt frequent dressing changes.[1,20,45] When the wound is clean and granulating, reduced exudate may allow PolyMem to be left in place for up to 7 days.[8]
- On first application, irrigate or debride the wound to remove causes of delayed healing that are easy to address; then allow PolyMem to remove the remainder of the contaminants atraumatically. The PolyMem membrane may become discolored or malodorous, but the wound bed itself will become cleaner and healthier.
- Experienced users gain the confidence to avoid routine rinsing at dressing changes.[3,4,8,46,47] Simply applying a PolyMem dressing **IS** wound cleansing.[8,44] Because rinsing cools the wound bed, washes away valuable nutrients, and can damage fragile new tissue, it is best to rinse only if loose contaminants are visible or the dressing has become dislodged prior to the dressing change, allowing the wound to become dirty and dry.[48]
- Patients with large surface area third degree burns must be carefully supervised by a burn specialist, especially when any absorptive dressing is used, including PolyMem.
- Healing wounds quickly is the most cost-saving choice. PolyMem is proven to help close wounds quickly.

*See package insert for complete information.

REFERENCES

PDFs of many of the footnoted references are available at www.polymem.com/clinicalguide/

1. Benskin LL. PolyMem Wic Silver Rope: A multifunctional dressing for decreasing pain, swelling, and inflammation. *Adv Wound Care (New Rochelle)*. 2012;1(1):44–47.
2. Dawson, Lewis C, Boch R. Total Joint Replacement Surgical Site Infections Eliminated by Using Multifunctional Dressing. 900 Cases Report over 4 years. May 2010.
3. Cutting KF, Vowden P, Wiegand C. Wound inflammation and the role of a multifunctional polymeric dressing. *Wounds International Journal*. 2015;6(2):41–46.
4. White L. Optimal Management for Upper Extremity Wounds with a Multifunctional Polymeric Membrane Dressing. September 2015.
5. Denyer J, White R, Ousey K, et al. PolyMem dressings Made Easy. *Wounds International*. May 2015. http://www.woundsinternational.com/made-easys/view/polymem-dressings-made-easy. Accessed May 7, 2016.
6. Harrison JE. Chronic Venous Ulcer Closing Steadily with Complete Elimination of Wound Pain Using Standard or Silver Polymeric Membrane Wound Filler Under Compression. June 2008.
7. Benskin L. PolyMem The Ideal Dressing. August 2015.
8. Benskin LL. Polymeric Membrane Dressings for topical wound management of patients with infected wounds in a challenging environment: A protocol with 3 case examples. *Ostomy Wound Management*. 2016;62(6):42–50. (OWM website adds evidence summaries, Tables 1 & 2)
9. Kim YJ, Lee SW, Hong SH, et al. The Effects of PolyMem(R) on the Wound Healing. *J Korean Soc Plast Reconstr Surg*. 1999;26(6):1165–1172.
10. Hayden JK, Cole BJ. The effectiveness of a pain wrap compared to a standard dressing on the reduction of postoperative morbidity following routine knee arthroscopy: a prospective randomized single-blind study. *Orthopedics*. 2003;26(1):59–63; discussion 63.
11. Beitz AJ, Newman A, Kahn AR, et al. A polymeric membrane dressing with antinociceptive properties: analysis with a rodent model of stab wound secondary hyperalgesia. *J Pain*. 2004;5(1):38–47.
12. Haik J, Weissman O, Demetrius S, et al. Polymeric Membrane Dressings* for Skin Graft Donor Sites: 6 Years Experience on 1200 Cases. April 2011.
13. Man D, Aleksinko P. Use of Polymeric Membrane Dressings After Occlusive Deep Facial and Neck Chemical Peel Improves Outcomes. April 2010.
14. Man D, Aleksinko P. Intra-Operative Use Followed with Post-Op Application of Polymeric Membrane Dressings Reduces Post-Op Pain, Edema and Bruising After Full Face Lift Surgery. April 2010.
15. Weissman O, Hundeshagen G, Harats M, et al. Custom-fit polymeric membrane dressing masks in the treatment of second degree facial burns. *Burns*. 2013;39(6):1316–1320.

FOAMS

16. Scott A. Polymeric membrane dressings for radiotherapy-induced skin damage. *Br J Nurs*. 2014; 23(10):S24, S26–S31.

17. Dabiri G, Damstetter E, Phillips T. Choosing a Wound Dressing Based on Common Wound Characteristics. *Adv Wound Care (New Rochelle)*. 2016;5(1):32–41.

18. Blackman JD, Senseng D, Quinn L, et al. Clinical evaluation of a semipermeable polymeric membrane dressing for the treatment of chronic diabetic foot ulcers. *Diabetes Care*. 1994;17(4): 322–325.

19. Rodeheaver GT, Kurtz L, Kircher BJ, et al. Pluronic F-68: a promising new skin wound cleanser. *Ann Emerg Med*. 1980;9(11):572–576.

20. Denyer JE, Pillay E. Best practice guidelines for skin and wound care in epidermolysis bullosa— International Consensus. 2012. http://www.woundsinternational.com/other-resources/view/best-practice-guidelines-for-skin-and-wound-care-in-epidermolysis-bullosa. Accessed March 30, 2015.

21. Davies SL, White RJ. Defining a holistic pain-relieving approach to wound care via a drug free polymeric membrane dressing. *J Wound Care*. 2011;20(5):250, 252, 254 passim.

22. Rafter L, Oforka E. Standard versus polymeric membrane finger dressing and outcomes following pain diaries. *Wounds UK*. 2014;10(2):40–49.

23. Cahn A, Kleinman Y. A novel approach to the treatment of diabetic foot abscesses—a case series. *J Wound Care*. 2014;23(8):394, 396–399.

24. Fowler E, Papen JC. Clinical evaluation of a polymeric membrane dressing in the treatment of dermal ulcers. *Ostomy Wound Manage*. 1991;35:35–38, 40–44.

25. Yastrub DJ. Relationship between type of treatment and degree of wound healing among institutionalized geriatric patients with stage II pressure ulcers. *Care Manag J*. 2004;5(4):213–218.

26. Stoddart J. Circumferential Wrap Technique with Polymeric Membrane Dressings after Arthroscopic ACL Reconstruction Reduces Blistering, Inflammation and Bruising; Rapid Recovery and Improved Patient Satisfaction: 80 Prospective Patient Series. May 2013.

27. Fulton JA, Blasiole KN, Cottingham T, et al. Wound Dressing Absorption: A Comparative Study. *Adv Skin Wound Care*. 2012;25(7):315–320.

28. Bolhuis J. Evidence-based skin tear protocol. *Long-Term Living: For the Continuing Care Professional*. 2008;57(6):48–52.

29. Kahn AR, Sessions RW, Apasova EV. A superficial cutaneous dressing inhibits pain, inflammation and swelling in deep tissues. *Pain Medicine*. 2000;1(2):187–187.

30. Bauer J, Diem A, Ploder M. Efficiency and Safety of Using a Polymeric Membrane Wound Dressing in Patients with Epidermolysis Bullosa after a Release Operation. May 2013.

31. Bauer J, Brandtner G. Chirurgische Korrektur der Handfehlbildungen bei Epidermolysis bullosa dystrophicans. *Arzt+Kind*. 2013.

32. Rafter L, Oforka E. Trauma-free fingertip dressing changes. *Wounds UK*. 2013;9(1):96–100.

33. Hegarty F, Wong M. Polymeric membrane dressing for radiotherapy-induced skin reactions. *Br J Nurs*. 2014;23 Suppl 20:S38–S46.

34. Wilson D. Application of Polymeric Membrane Dressings to Stage I Pressure Ulcers Speeds Resolution, Reduces Ulcer Site Discomfort and Reduces Staff Time Devoted to Management of Ulcers. April 2010.

35. Carr RD, Lalagos DE. Clinical evaluation of a polymeric membrane dressing in the treatment of pressure ulcers. *Decubitus*. 1990;3(3):38–42.

36. Denyer JE. Wound Management for Children with Epidermolysis Bullosa. *Dermatologic Clinics*. 2010;28(2):257–264.

37. Aaltonen M. Developing a Protocol For Burns in a Private Out-Patient Wound Clinic. May 2015.

38. Rahman S, Shokri A. Total Knee Arthroplasty (TKA) Infections Eliminated and Rehabilitation Improved Using Polymeric Membrane Dressing Circumferential Wrap Technique: 120 Patients at 12-month Follow-up. May 2013.

39. Edwards J, Mason S. An evaluation of the use of PolyMem Silver in burn management. *Journal of Community Nursing*. 2010;24(6):16–19.

40. Benskin L. Deep Ulceration Treated with Polymeric Membrane Dressings Until Complete Wound Closure. June 2008.

41. Benskin L. Diabetic foot salvaged, wounds closed in only two months using polymeric membrane cavity filler® and polymeric membrane dressings. June 2007.

42. Barnes L. The Use of Polymeric Membrane Dressings for Management of a Full-Thickness/Tunneling Dehisced Surgical Abdominal Wound. June 2006.

43. Benskin L. Extensive tunneling lower leg wounds with exposed tendons closed quickly using various polymeric membrane dressing configurations. October 2008.

44. Denyer J. Six Years' Experience Of PolyMem Dressings Used On Children With Epidermolysis Bullosa (EB). September 2015.

45. Denyer J. Managing pain in children with epidermolysis bullosa. *Nurs Times*. 2012;108(29):21–23.

46. Vanwalleghem G. A New Protocol for the Treatment of Pilonidal Cysts. May 2011.

47. Agathangelou C. Patients with Chronic Wound Pain Stop Hurting, Why? May 2011.

48. McGuiness W, Vella E, Harrison D. Influence of dressing changes on wound temperature. *J Wound Care*. 2004;13(9):383–385.

FOAMS

Shapes® by PolyMem® Oval and Sacral Dressings*

Ferris Mfg. Corp.

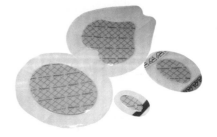

HOW SUPPLIED

#3 Oval-Shaped PMD	1" × 2" pad with 2" × 3" adhesive	A6212
#5 Oval-Shaped PMD	2" × 3" pad with 3.5" × 5" adhesive	A6212
#8 Oval-Shaped PMD	4" × 5.7" pad with 6.5" × 8.2" adhesive	A6213
Sacral (Heart-Shaped) PMD	4.5" × 4.7" pad with 7.2" × 7.8" adhesive	A6212

ACTION

Shapes by PolyMem Oval and Sacral Dressings are wound-shaped water-resistant[1] multi-functional,[2–5] interactive[6] polymeric membrane dressings (PMDs) with a thin-film adhesive border.[7] These polymeric membrane dressings are designed to decrease pain,[5,8–11] odor,[4,6,11,12] and inflammation[2,13–15] and protect wounds[4,11] while promoting quick healing.[1] Many new wound products are being developed to include small aspects of PolyMem dressings' many benefits, but none are able to furnish the integrated solutions PolyMem products have reliably provided for nearly three decades.[11]

Activated by moisture, PolyMem products gradually release a nontoxic surfactant cleanser and glycerin to loosen bonds between the wound bed and adherent substances that may impair healing.[2,6,16–18] Glycerin pulls nutrient-filled, enzyme-rich fluid from the body into the wound bed, enhancing healing and autolytic debridement while floating the contaminants.[4,6,19–21] The PolyMem membrane pulls in the undesirable substances along with the fluid, which are locked into the porous superabsorbent structure.[2,11,22,23] The wound contaminants are atraumatically removed and discarded when the PolyMem dressing is changed, eliminating the need for routine rinsing at dressing changes.[17,22–24]

The glycerin and surfactant in PolyMem products help moisturize dry areas of wounds while pulling fluid from the body into the wound bed and redistributing it.[4,6,21,24,25] Simultaneously, excess fluid from overly wet areas is absorbed into the dressing and is locked into a gel.[4,6,22,26] The "intelligent" backing allows excess fluid to evaporate while retaining the fluid needed to keep dry wounds moist.[27] Other available dressings have only portions of this complete moisture balancing system.[11]

All occlusive dressings provide some pain relief. However, PolyMem products are the only drug-free dressings with evidence showing that they also relieve pain by altering the response of the pain-sensing nerves (nociceptors).[1,13–15,18,25,28] PolyMem products' alteration of the nociceptor response occurs even on intact skin, and has been shown in clinical studies to decrease the excess inflammation that leads to excess swelling and often slows healing.[11,13–15,20,25,28]

PolyMem dressings are non-adherent while conforming to the wound bed.[1,6,19,21,22,24,29,30] They are flexible and comfortable to wear.[2,11,19,29–31]

INDICATIONS

Indicated for virtually all wounds at every stage of healing,[2,4,17,21,22] including closed tissue injuries,[14,28,32,33] multifunctional PolyMem dressings meet or exceed every criterion wound

experts identify for an *Ideal Dressing*.[23,34,35] PolyMem dressings are safe for use over structures like tendon, bone, and exposed vessels because they can donate moisture.[2,6,19–21] PolyMem is suitable for use even when wounds are infected, provided that the infection is otherwise appropriately addressed.[2,6,11,36,37] PolyMem is especially suitable for chronic, trauma, and burn wounds because it helps subdue excess inflammation and is a pain relieving dressing.[3,8,11,13,25,26,37–39]

- Shapes by PolyMem dressings are especially suited to offer a secure fit for contoured areas of the body where the dressing needs to bend and conform.[1,7,40]

CONTRAINDICATIONS

- None.

APPLICATION

- Initially, irrigate or debride the wound bed as indicated or prescribed. Rinse with water or saline. Additional topical products are not necessary or recommended for use with PolyMem. Simply pat the periwound dry, leaving the wound bed slightly moist.
- Fill any deep cavities lightly with PolyMem WIC (standard or silver) or WIC Silver Rope, allowing for expansion. Apply the Shapes by PolyMem dressing with the membrane pad covering the open wound **AND** all of the surrounding inflamed (reddened, raw, tender, warm, itchy, or swollen) skin.
- Apply the adhesive borders without tension. Smooth into place. See Instructions for Use for details.

How to know when to change PolyMem dressings

- Do NOT change PolyMem on a calendar schedule, especially in the first week of use; anticipate changes in exudate levels, which may dramatically increase initially.
- PolyMem is an indicator dressing: the backing will become a darker color when the membrane becomes saturated. Change the dressing when the darker color reaches any of the wound edges.

REMOVAL

- Simply, gently remove the Shapes by PolyMem dressing and any wound filler and replace with an appropriate new PolyMem configuration. In most cases, when using PolyMem, there is no need to rinse the wound.
- PolyMem is designed to continuously cleanse the wound and does not leave residue that needs to be removed. Excessive cleaning may injure regenerating tissue and delay wound healing.

Guidelines for optimal use

(See *Instructions for Use* provided in each box and **PolyMem.com for detailed information**.)

Independent wound experts have created a robust evidence base for PolyMem dressings by documenting their success in using PolyMem over the past 25+ years. Ferris has developed these guidelines based upon their documented experiences.

- Using PolyMem is simple. However, using PolyMem optimally (knowing which dressing configuration to use, and how) is an art.[11,41] PolyMem use saves time, giving wound specialists more time to address the whole patient, improving healing by optimizing offloading, compression, circulation, nutrition, medications, and so forth.[1,5,8,19,25,26,33,41–43]
- PolyMem dressings should be changed when indicated, rather than on a schedule. Changing PolyMem more frequently than necessary on a healthy, granulating wound bed may slow healing. Tracing the approximate wound borders on the outer film of the PolyMem dressing makes it easy to see when a change is needed without "peeking" at the wound.[34]

FOAMS

- PolyMem is an interactive dressing. PolyMem often recruits LARGE amounts of wound fluid, containing debris and metabolic wastes, for the first few days of use, which may prompt frequent dressing changes.[2,17,42] When the wound is clean and granulating, reduced exudate may allow PolyMem to be left in place for up to 7 days.[11]
- On first application, irrigate or debride the wound to remove causes of delayed healing that are easy to address; then allow PolyMem to remove the remainder of the contaminants atraumatically. The PolyMem membrane may become discolored or malodorous, but the wound bed itself will become cleaner and healthier.
- Experienced users gain the confidence to avoid routine rinsing at dressing changes.[4,5,11,43,44] Simply applying a PolyMem dressing **IS** wound cleansing.[11,41] Because rinsing cools the wound bed, washes away valuable nutrients, and can damage fragile new tissue, it is best to rinse only if loose contaminants are visible or the dressing has become dislodged prior to the dressing change, allowing the wound to become dirty and dry.[45]
- Patients with large surface area third degree burns must be carefully supervised by a burn specialist, especially when any absorptive dressing is used, including PolyMem.
- Healing wounds quickly is the most cost-saving choice. PolyMem is proven to help close wounds quickly.

*See package insert for complete information.

REFERENCES

PDFs of many of the footnoted references are available at www.polymem.com/clinicalguide/

1. Bolhuis J. Evidence-based skin tear protocol. *Long-Term Living: For the Continuing Care Professional.* 2008;57(6):48–52.
2. Benskin LLL. PolyMem Wic Silver Rope: A multifunctional dressing for decreasing pain, swelling, and inflammation. *Adv Wound Care (New Rochelle).* 2012;1(1):44–47.
3. Dawson, Lewis C, Boch R. Total Joint Replacement Surgical Site Infections Eliminated by Using Multifunctional Dressing. 900 Cases Report over 4 years. May 2010.
4. Cutting KF, Vowden P, Wiegand C. Wound inflammation and the role of a multifunctional polymeric dressing. *Wounds International Journal.* 2015;6(2):41–46.
5. White L. Optimal Management for Upper Extremity Wounds with a Multifunctional Polymeric Membrane Dressing. September 2015.
6. Denyer J, White R, Ousey K, et al. PolyMem dressings Made Easy. *Wounds International.* May 2015. http://www.woundsinternational.com/made-easys/view/polymem-dressings-made-easy. Accessed May 7, 2016.
7. Yastrub D. Heel Ulcer in Hospice Patient Closed Quickly Using Polymeric Membrane Dressings. June 2008.
8. Haik J, Weissman O, Demetrius S, et al. Polymeric Membrane Dressings® for Skin Graft Donor Sites: 6 Years Experience on 1200 Cases. April 2011.
9. Man D, Aleksinko P. Use of Polymeric Membrane Dressings After Occlusive Deep Facial and Neck Chemical Peel Improves Outcomes. April 2010.
10. Man D, Aleksinko P. Intra-Operative Use Followed with Post-Op Application of Polymeric Membrane Dressings Reduces Post-Op Pain, Edema and Bruising After Full Face Lift Surgery. April 2010.
11. Benskin LL. Polymeric Membrane Dressings for topical wound management of patients with infected wounds in a challenging environment: A protocol with 3 case examples. *Ostomy Wound Management.* 2016;62(6):42–50. (OWM website adds evidence summaries, Tables 1 & 2)
12. Agathangelou C. Treating Fungating Breast Cancer Wounds with Polymeric Membrane Dressings, an Innovation in Fungating Wound Management. May 2015.
13. Kim YJ, Lee SW, Hong SH, et al. The effects of PolyMem(R) on the wound healing. *J Korean Soc Plast Reconstr Surg.* 1999;26(6):1165–1172.
14. Hayden JK, Cole BJ. The effectiveness of a pain wrap compared to a standard dressing on the reduction of postoperative morbidity following routine knee arthroscopy: a prospective randomized single-blind study. *Orthopedics.* 2003;26(1):59–63; discussion 63.
15. Beitz AJ, Newman A, Kahn AR, et al. A polymeric membrane dressing with antinociceptive properties: analysis with a rodent model of stab wound secondary hyperalgesia. *J Pain.* 2004;5(1):38–47.

16. Rodeheaver GT, Kurtz L, Kircher BJ, et al. Pluronic F-68: a promising new skin wound cleanser. *Ann Emerg Med.* 1980;9(11):572-576.

17. Denyer JE, Pillay E. Best practice guidelines for skin and wound care in epidermolysis bullosa— International Consensus. 2012. http://www.woundsinternational.com/other-resources/view/best-practice-guidelines-for-skin-and-wound-care-in-epidermolysis-bullosa. Accessed March 30, 2015.

18. Davies SL, White RJ. Defining a holistic pain-relieving approach to wound care via a drug free polymeric membrane dressing. *J Wound Care.* 2011;20(5):250, 252, 254 passim.

19. Rafter L, Oforka E. Standard versus polymeric membrane finger dressing and outcomes following pain diaries. *Wounds UK.* 2014;10(2):40–49.

20. Cahn A, Kleinman Y. A novel approach to the treatment of diabetic foot abscesses—a case series. *J Wound Care.* 2014;23(8):394, 396–399.

21. Dabiri G, Damstetter E, Phillips T. Choosing a wound dressing based on common wound characteristics. *Adv Wound Care (New Rochelle).* 2016;5(1):32–41.

22. Fowler E, Papen JC. Clinical evaluation of a polymeric membrane dressing in the treatment of dermal ulcers. *Ostomy Wound Manage.* 1991;35:35–38, 40–44.

23. Yastrub DJ. Relationship between type of treatment and degree of wound healing among institutionalized geriatric patients with stage II pressure ulcers. *Care Manag J.* 2004;5(4):213–218.

24. Scott A. Polymeric membrane dressings for radiotherapy-induced skin damage. *Br J Nurs.* 2014; 23(10):S24, S26–S31.

25. Weissman O, Hundeshagen G, Harats M, et al. Custom-fit polymeric membrane dressing masks in the treatment of second degree facial burns. *Burns.* 2013;39(6):1316–1320.

26. Stoddart J. Circumferential Wrap Technique with Polymeric Membrane Dressings after Arthroscopic ACL Reconstruction Reduces Blistering, Inflammation and Bruising; Rapid Recovery and Improved Patient Satisfaction: 80 Prospective Patient Series. May 2013.

27. Fulton JA, Blasiole KN, Cottingham T, et al. Wound dressing absorption: A comparative study. *Adv Skin Wound Care.* 2012;25(7):315–320.

28. Kahn AR, Sessions RW, Apasova EV. A superficial cutaneous dressing inhibits pain, inflammation and swelling in deep tissues. *Pain Medicine.* 2000;1(2):187–187.

29. Bauer J, Diem A, Ploder M. Efficiency and Safety of Using a Polymeric Membrane Wound Dressing in Patients with Epidermolysis Bullosa after a Release Operation. May 2013.

30. Bauer J, Brandtner G. Chirurgische Korrektur der Handfehlbildungen bei Epidermolysis bullosa dystrophicans. *Arzt+Kind.* 2013.

31. Rafter L, Oforka E. Trauma-free fingertip dressing changes. *Wounds UK.* 2013;9(1):96–100.

32. Hegarty F, Wong M. Polymeric membrane dressing for radiotherapy-induced skin reactions. *Br J Nurs.* 2014;23 Suppl 20:S38–S46.

33. Wilson D. Application of Polymeric Membrane Dressings to Stage I Pressure Ulcers Speeds Resolution, Reduces Ulcer Site Discomfort and Reduces Staff Time Devoted to Management of Ulcers. April 2010.

34. Carr RD, Lalagos DE. Clinical evaluation of a polymeric membrane dressing in the treatment of pressure ulcers. *Decubitus.* 1990;3(3):38–42.

35. Benskin L. PolyMem The Ideal Dressing. August 2015.

36. Denyer JE. Wound management for children with epidermolysis bullosa. *Dermatologic Clinics.* 2010;28(2):257–264.

37. Aaltonen M. Developing a Protocol For Burns in a Private Out-Patient Wound Clinic. May 2015.

38. Rahman S, Shokri A. Total Knee Arthroplasty (TKA) Infections Eliminated and Rehabilitation Improved Using Polymeric Membrane Dressing Circumferential Wrap Technique: 120 Patients at 12-month Follow-up. May 2013.

39. Edwards J, Mason S. An evaluation of the use of PolyMem Silver in burn management. *Journal of Community Nursing.* 2010;24(6):16–19.

40. Wilson D. Skin tear healing improved through the use of polymeric membrane dressings. June 2008.

41. Denyer J. Six Years' Experience Of PolyMem Dressings Used On Children With Epidermolysis Bullosa (EB). September 2015.

42. Denyer J. Managing pain in children with epidermolysis bullosa. *Nurs Times.* 2012;108(29):21–23.

43. Vanwalleghem G. A New Protocol for the Treatment of Pilonidal Cysts. May 2011.

44. Agathangelou C. Patients with Chronic Wound Pain Stop Hurting, Why? May 2011.

45. McGuiness W, Vella E, Harrison D. Influence of dressing changes on wound temperature. *J Wound Care.* 2004;13(9):383–385.

Shapes® by PolyMem® Tube Dressing*

Ferris Mfg. Corp.

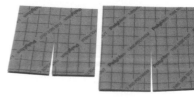

HOW SUPPLIED

| Small PMD Designed for Tube Sites | 2.75" × 2.75" | A6209 |
| Large PMD Designed for Tube Sites | 3.5" × 3.5" | A6209 |

ACTION

Shapes by PolyMem Tube Dressings are multifunctional,[1–4] interactive[5] polymeric membrane dressings (PMDs) precut to fit tube sites of any diameter.[6–8] These polymeric membrane dressings are designed to protect tube sites from pressure[6–8] and contamination[3,9] while helping decrease inflammation,[1,10–12] balancing moisture,[3,5,13–15] and continuously cleansing[9,16] to help prevent[7] and resolve[6,8] tube site complications. Many new wound products are being developed to include small aspects of PolyMem dressings' many benefits, but none are able to furnish the integrated solutions PolyMem products have reliably provided for nearly three decades.[9]

Activated by moisture, PolyMem products gradually release a nontoxic surfactant cleanser and glycerin to loosen bonds between the wound bed and adherent substances that may impair healing.[1,5,17–19] Glycerin pulls nutrient-filled, enzyme-rich fluid from the body into the wound bed, enhancing healing and autolytic debridement while floating the contaminants.[3,5,15,20,21] The PolyMem membrane pulls in the undesirable substances along with the fluid, which are locked into the porous superabsorbent structure.[1,9,22,23] The wound contaminants are atraumatically removed and discarded when the PolyMem dressing is changed, eliminating the need for routine rinsing at dressing changes.[14,18,22,23]

The glycerin and surfactant in PolyMem products help moisturize dry areas of wounds while pulling fluid from the body into the wound bed and redistributing it.[3,5,13–15] Simultaneously, excess fluid from overly wet areas is absorbed into the dressing and is locked into a gel.[3,5,22,24] The "intelligent" backing allows excess fluid to evaporate while retaining the fluid needed to keep dry wounds moist.[25] Other available dressings have only portions of this complete moisture balancing system.[9]

All occlusive dressings provide some pain relief. However, PolyMem products are the only drug-free dressings with evidence showing that they also relieve pain by altering the response of the pain-sensing nerves (nociceptors).[10–13,19,26,27] PolyMem products' alteration of the nociceptor response occurs even on intact skin, and has been shown in clinical studies to decrease the excess inflammation that leads to excess swelling and often slows healing.[9–13,21,27]

PolyMem dressings are nonadherent while conforming to the wound bed.[5,14,15,20,22,26,28,29] They are flexible and comfortable to wear.[1,9,20,28–30]

INDICATIONS

Indicated for virtually all wounds at every stage of healing,[1,3,15,18,22] including closed tissue injuries,[11,27,31,32] multifunctional PolyMem dressings meet or exceed every criterion wound experts identify for an *Ideal Dressing*.[23,33,34] PolyMem dressings are safe for use over structures like tendon, bone, and exposed vessels because they can donate moisture.[1,5,15,20,21] PolyMem is suitable for use even when wounds are infected, provided that the infection is otherwise appropriately addressed.[1,5,9,35,36] PolyMem is especially suitable for chronic, trauma, and burn wounds because it helps subdue excess inflammation and is a pain relieving dressing.[2,9,10,13,24,36–39]

FOAMS

- Shapes by PolyMem Tube dressings are especially designed to enhance patient comfort and help clinicians easily apply the dressing to tube sites.[6-8] Unlike other dressings used on tube sites, PolyMem dressings do not shed fibers.[34]

CONTRAINDICATIONS

- None.

APPLICATION

- Initially, prepare the tube site as indicated or prescribed. Rinse with water or saline. Pat entire area dry. Additional topical products are not necessary or recommended for use with PolyMem.
- Gently slide the Shapes by PolyMem Tube dressing into place so that it fits neatly and easily around the tube with the film (printed) side out and the membrane pad covering the open wound **AND** all of the surrounding inflamed (reddened, raw, tender, warm, itchy, or swollen) skin.
- Apply tape sparingly, only as needed. Smooth into place. See Instructions for Use for details.

How to know when to change PolyMem dressings

- Change when secretions or moisture saturate the dressing.
- PolyMem is an indicator dressing: the backing will become a darker color when the membrane becomes saturated. Change the dressing when the darker color is visible through the dressing backing.

REMOVAL

- Simply, gently remove the Shapes by PolyMem Tube dressing and replace it with an appropriate new PolyMem configuration.
- PolyMem is designed to continuously cleanse the tube site and does not leave residue that needs to be removed. Any visible mucous or loosened debris can be removed with a sterile cotton-tipped applicator. Excessive cleaning may injure the fragile tissue surrounding the tube site. Do not routinely cleanse or rinse at dressing changes.

Guidelines for optimal use

(See *Instructions for Use* provided in each box and **PolyMem.com for detailed information**.)

Independent wound experts have created a robust evidence base for PolyMem dressings by documenting their success in using PolyMem over the past 25+ years. Ferris has developed these guidelines based upon their documented experiences.

- Using PolyMem is simple. However, using PolyMem optimally (knowing which dressing configuration to use, and how) is an art.[9,40] PolyMem use saves time, giving wound specialists more time to address the whole patient, improving healing by optimizing offloading, compression, circulation, nutrition, medications, and so forth.[4,13,20,24,26,32,38,40–42]
- PolyMem dressings should be changed when indicated, rather than on a schedule. Changing PolyMem more frequently than necessary on a healthy, granulating wound bed may slow healing. Tracing the approximate wound borders on the outer film of the PolyMem dressing makes it easy to see when a change is needed without "peeking" at the wound.[33]
- PolyMem is an interactive dressing. PolyMem often recruits LARGE amounts of wound fluid, containing debris and metabolic wastes, for the first few days of use, which may prompt frequent dressing changes.[1,18,41] When the wound is clean and granulating, reduced exudate may allow PolyMem to be left in place for up to 7 days.[9]
- On first application, irrigate or debride the wound to remove causes of delayed healing that are easy to address; then allow PolyMem to remove the remainder of the contaminants

FOAMS

atraumatically. The PolyMem membrane may become discolored or malodorous, but the wound bed itself will become cleaner and healthier.

- Experienced users gain the confidence to avoid routine rinsing at dressing changes.[3,4,9,42,43] Simply applying a PolyMem dressing IS wound cleansing.[9,40] Because rinsing cools the wound bed, washes away valuable nutrients, and can damage fragile new tissue, it is best to rinse only if loose contaminants are visible or the dressing has become dislodged prior to the dressing change, allowing the wound to become dirty and dry.[44]
- Patients with large surface area third degree burns must be carefully supervised by a burn specialist, especially when any absorptive dressing is used, including PolyMem.
- Healing wounds quickly is the most cost-saving choice. PolyMem is proven to help close wounds quickly.

*See package insert for complete information.

REFERENCES

PDFs of many of the footnoted references are available at www.polymem.com/clinicalguide/

1. Benskin LL. PolyMem Wic Silver Rope: A multifunctional dressing for decreasing pain, swelling, and inflammation. *Adv Wound Care (New Rochelle).* 2012;1(1):44–47.
2. Dawson, Lewis C, Boch R. Total Joint Replacement Surgical Site Infections Eliminated by Using Multifunctional Dressing. 900 Cases Report over 4 years. May 2010.
3. Cutting KF, Vowden P, Wiegand C. Wound inflammation and the role of a multifunctional polymeric dressing. *Wounds International Journal.* 2015;6(2):41–46.
4. White L. Optimal Management for Upper Extremity Wounds with a Multifunctional Polymeric Membrane Dressing. September 2015.
5. Denyer J, White R, Ousey K, et al. PolyMem dressings made easy. *Wounds International.* May 2015. http://www.woundsinternational.com/made-easys/view/polymem-dressings-made-easy. Accessed May 7, 2016.
6. Lonie G. Polymeric Membrane Tube Site Dressings Improve Tracheostomy Site Management While Increasing Patient Comfort. March 2010.
7. O'Toole TR, Jacobs N, Hondorp B, et al. Prevention of tracheostomy-related hospital-acquired pressure ulcers. *Otolaryngol Head Neck Surg.* 2017;156(4):642–651.
8. Agathangelou C. Using Polymeric Membrane Dressings to Solve Problematic Skin Damage From Gastronomy Leakage on Elderly Patients. May 2013.
9. Benskin LL. Polymeric Membrane Dressings for topical wound management of patients with infected wounds in a challenging environment: A protocol with 3 case examples. *Ostomy Wound Management.* 2016;62(6):42–50. (OWM website adds evidence summaries, Tables 1 & 2)
10. Kim YJ, Lee SW, Hong SH, et al. The effects of PolyMem(R) on the wound healing. *J Korean Soc Plast Reconstr Surg.* 1999;26(6):1165–1172.
11. Hayden JK, Cole BJ. The effectiveness of a pain wrap compared to a standard dressing on the reduction of postoperative morbidity following routine knee arthroscopy: a prospective randomized single-blind study. *Orthopedics.* 2003;26(1):59–63; discussion 63.
12. Beitz AJ, Newman A, Kahn AR, et al. A polymeric membrane dressing with antinociceptive properties: analysis with a rodent model of stab wound secondary hyperalgesia. *J Pain.* 2004;5(1):38–47.
13. Weissman O, Hundeshagen G, Harats M, et al. Custom-fit polymeric membrane dressing masks in the treatment of second degree facial burns. *Burns.* 2013;39(6):1316–1320.
14. Scott A. Polymeric membrane dressings for radiotherapy-induced skin damage. *Br J Nurs.* 2014; 23(10):S24, S26–S31.
15. Dabiri G, Damstetter E, Phillips T. Choosing a wound dressing based on common wound characteristics. *Adv Wound Care (New Rochelle).* 2016;5(1):32–41.
16. Blackman JD, Senseng D, Quinn L, et al. Clinical evaluation of a semipermeable polymeric membrane dressing for the treatment of chronic diabetic foot ulcers. *Diabetes Care.* 1994;17(4):322–325.
17. Rodeheaver GT, Kurtz L, Kircher BJ, et al. Pluronic F-68: a promising new skin wound cleanser. *Ann Emerg Med.* 1980;9(11):572–576.
18. Denyer JE, Pillay E. Best practice guidelines for skin and wound care in epidermolysis bullosa— International Consensus. 2012. http://www.woundsinternational.com/other-resources/view/best-practice-guidelines-for-skin-and-wound-care-in-epidermolysis-bullosa. Accessed March 30, 2015.

19. Davies SL, White RJ. Defining a holistic pain-relieving approach to wound care via a drug free polymeric membrane dressing. *J Wound Care.* 2011;20(5):250, 252, 254 passim.

20. Rafter L, Oforka E. Standard versus polymeric membrane finger dressing and outcomes following pain diaries. *Wounds UK.* 2014;10(2):40–49.

21. Cahn A, Kleinman Y. A novel approach to the treatment of diabetic foot abscesses—a case series. *J Wound Care.* 2014;23(8):394, 396–399.

22. Fowler E, Papen JC. Clinical evaluation of a polymeric membrane dressing in the treatment of dermal ulcers. *Ostomy Wound Manage.* 1991;35:35–38, 40–44.

23. Yastrub DJ. Relationship between type of treatment and degree of wound healing among institutionalized geriatric patients with stage II pressure ulcers. *Care Manag J.* 2004;5(4):213–218.

24. Stoddart J. Circumferential Wrap Technique with Polymeric Membrane Dressings after Arthroscopic ACL Reconstruction Reduces Blistering, Inflammation and Bruising; Rapid Recovery and Improved Patient Satisfaction: 80 Prospective Patient Series. May 2013.

25. Fulton JA, Blasiole KN, Cottingham T, et al. Wound dressing absorption: A comparative study. *Adv Skin Wound Care.* 2012;25(7):315–320.

26. Bolhuis J. Evidence-based skin tear protocol. *Long-Term Living: For the Continuing Care Professional.* 2008;57(6):48–52.

27. Kahn AR, Sessions RW, Apasova EV. A superficial cutaneous dressing inhibits pain, inflammation and swelling in deep tissues. *Pain Medicine.* 2000;1(2):187–187.

28. Bauer J, Diem A, Ploder M. Efficiency and Safety of Using a Polymeric Membrane Wound Dressing in Patients with Epidermolysis Bullosa after a Release Operation. May 2013.

29. Bauer J, Brandtner G. Chirurgische Korrektur der Handfehlbildungen bei Epidermolysis bullosa dystrophicans. *Arzt+Kind.* 2013.

30. Rafter L, Oforka E. Trauma-free fingertip dressing changes. *Wounds UK.* 2013;9(1):96-100.

31. Hegarty F, Wong M. Polymeric membrane dressing for radiotherapy-induced skin reactions. *Br J Nurs.* 2014;23 Suppl 20:S38–S46.

32. Wilson D. Application of Polymeric Membrane Dressings to Stage I Pressure Ulcers Speeds Resolution, Reduces Ulcer Site Discomfort and Reduces Staff Time Devoted to Management of Ulcers. April 2010.

33. Carr RD, Lalagos DE. Clinical evaluation of a polymeric membrane dressing in the treatment of pressure ulcers. *Decubitus.* 1990;3(3):38–42.

34. Benskin L. PolyMem The Ideal Dressing. August 2015.

35. Denyer JE. Wound management for children with epidermolysis bullosa. *Dermatologic Clinics.* 2010;28(2):257–264.

36. Aaltonen M. Developing a Protocol For Burns in a Private Out-Patient Wound Clinic. May 2015.

37. Rahman S, Shokri A. Total Knee Arthroplasty (TKA) Infections Eliminated and Rehabilitation Improved Using Polymeric Membrane Dressing Circumferential Wrap Technique: 120 Patients at 12-month Follow-up. May 2013.

38. Haik J, Weissman O, Demetrius S, et al. Polymeric Membrane Dressings* for Skin Graft Donor Sites: 6 Years Experience on 1200 Cases. April 2011.

39. Edwards J, Mason S. An evaluation of the use of PolyMem Silver in burn management. *Journal of Community Nursing.* 2010;24(6):16–19.

40. Denyer J. Six Years' Experience Of PolyMem Dressings Used On Children With Epidermolysis Bullosa (EB). September 2015.

41. Denyer J. Managing pain in children with epidermolysis bullosa. *Nurs Times.* 2012;108(29):21–23.

42. Vanwallghem G. A New Protocol for the Treatment of Pilonidal Cysts. May 2011.

43. Agathangelou C. Patients with Chronic Wound Pain Stop Hurting, Why? May 2011.

44. McGuiness W, Vella E, Harrison D. Influence of dressing changes on wound temperature. *J Wound Care.* 2004;13(9):383–385.

FOAMS

Silicone Foam Bordered

Gentell

HOW SUPPLIED

Foam	4″ × 4″	A6212
Foam	6″ × 6″	A6213

ACTION

Gentell Silicone Foam Bordered Dressing is a primary or secondary multi-layered dressing with an absorbent foam to minimize maceration and a silicone contact layer for gentle adherence.

INDICATIONS

Gentell Silicone Foam Bordered Dressing is a primary or secondary wound dressing for chronic and acute, partial and full-thickness wounds including superficial wounds and second-degree burns.

CONTRAINDICATIONS

- None.

APPLICATION

- Irrigate the wound with Gentell Wound Cleanser and gently dry the skin surrounding the wound site.
- Remove and discard "Silicone"-labeled backing.
- Apply Gentell Silicone Foam Dressing by centering pad over wound.

REMOVAL

- Change daily or as ordered by a physician.

TIELLE™ Hydropolymer Adhesive Dressing with LIQUALOCK™ Technology*

Systagenix, An ACELITY™ Company

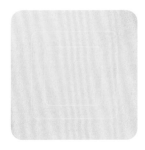

HOW SUPPLIED

TIELLE™ Hydropolymer Adhesive Dressing with LIQUALOCK™ Technology	2 3/4" × 3 1/2"	A6212
TIELLE™ Hydropolymer Adhesive Dressing with LIQUALOCK™ Technology	4 1/4" × 4 1/4"	A6212
TIELLE™ Hydropolymer Adhesive Dressing with LIQUALOCK™ Technology	5 7/8" × 7 7/8"	A6213
TIELLE™ Hydropolymer Adhesive Dressing with LIQUALOCK™ Technology	7" × 7"	A6213

ACTION

The TIELLE™ Dressing Family has a unique design compared with ordinary foams: It contains LIQUALOCK™ Technology, which cleverly retains exudates while also letting moisture vapor pass through the dressing, helping to provide an optimal moist wound healing environment.

INDICATIONS

TIELLE™ Hydropolymer Adhesive Dressing with LIQUALOCK™ Technology in indicated for the management of low to moderately exuding wounds and should be used under health care professional direction for the following indications: pressure ulcers, lower-extremity ulcers, venous, arterial, and mixed etiology ulcers, diabetic ulcers, and donor sites.

CONTRAINDICATIONS

- Not for use on third-degree burns.
- Not for use on lesions with active vasculitis.
- Should not be used when visible signs of infection are present; however, under proper medical treatment that addresses the cause, the dressing may be used.

APPLICATION

- Prepare the wound per your standard wound care protocol. TIELLE™ Adhesive Dressings may be used when visible signs of infection are present in the wound area only when proper medical treatment addresses the underlying cause.
- Choose the appropriate TIELLE™ Adhesive Dressings.
- The size selected should allow the absorbent island to overlap the wound edge by approximately 1 cm.
- Peel open the package and remove the dressing.
- Partially peel back side backing papers. Ensure skin surrounding the wound is dry.
- Position absorbent island centrally over wound site and smooth in place. One at a time, peel away side backing papers while smoothing adhesive border onto intact skin.

FOAMS

- For additional water repellency, after the application of TIELLE™ Adhesive Dressing, petroleum jelly or other petroleum-based products can be applied to the edges of the dressing and surrounding skin.

REMOVAL

- On removal lift one corner and carefully peel back. On fragile or friable skin, water or saline may be used to break the adhesive seal.

*See package insert for complete information.

FOAMS

UrgoTul™ Absorb Border with TLC™ Technology*

Urgo Medical

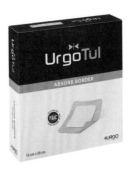

HOW SUPPLIED

Dressing, Pad	4″ × 4″ with 2.5″ × 2.5″	A6212
Dressing, Pad	6″ × 6″ with 4″ × 4″	A6212
Dressing, Pad	6″ × 8″ with 4″ × 6″	A6213
Dressing, Pad	8″ × 8″ Sacral with 5″ × 5.5″	A6213

ACTION

TLC Technology foam dressings are an absorbent foam dressing comprised of a layer of lipido-colloid matrix that gels in the presence of exudate, thus providing a moist wound interface for virtually pain-free dressing changes and reduced trauma to delicate tissue. An absorbent layer combined with the lipido-colloid matrix that includes a polyurethane foam and a superabsorbent layer that allows containment of exudate and protects the periwound skin from maceration. The silicone-border backing provides a vapor permeable, waterproof, and bacterial barrier.

INDICATIONS

Indicated for moderate to heavily exuding acute wounds (such as burns, dermabrasions/skin tears, traumatic wounds, postoperative wounds . . .) and chronic wounds (such as leg ulcers, pressure ulcers, diabetic foot ulcers). The sacrum version is recommended for exuding wounds location in the sacral area (sacral pressure ulcers . . .).

CONTRAINDICATIONS

- UrgoTul Absorb Border should not be used on individuals who are sensitive to or who have had an allergic reaction to the dressing or one of its components.

APPLICATION

- Cleanse the wound in accordance to established procedures.
- Carefully dry the periwound tissue.
- Select the appropriate dressing size to ensure the central pad will cover the entire wound.
- Remove one of the protective tabs and apply the dressing to the skin, positioning the central pad directly over the wound.
- Smooth down the dressing over the wound and remove the second protective tab, making sure that the dressing sticks properly. Do not pull or attempt to stretch the dressing during placement in order to eliminate periwound tissue shear.
- The dressing can be applied under compression.
- Do not use the dressing under compression bandages/wraps and total contact casting if the wound shows signs of infection.

REMOVAL

- UrgoTul Absorb Border with TLC Technology can be left in place for up to 7 days, depending on the exudate level and clinical condition of the wound. Duration of use is determined by the health care provider and depends on wound types and conditions.

*See package insert for complete instructions for use.

FOAMS

Waterproof Foam Non-Bordered

Gentell

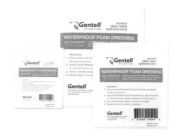

HOW SUPPLIED

Foam	2″ × 2″	A6209
Foam	4″ × 4″	A6209
Foam	5″ × 5″	A6210
Foam	8″ × 8″	A6211

ACTION

Gentell Waterproof Non-Bordered Foam Dressing is a primary wound dressing for chronic and acute, moderate-to-heavy exuding, partial to full-thickness wounds including superficial wounds and second-degree burns. Waterproof Non-Bordered Foam can also be used as a secondary wound dressing.

INDICATIONS

Use Gentell Waterproof Non-Bordered Foam as a cover dressing for primary or secondary treatments.

CONTRAINDICATIONS

- None.

APPLICATION

- Irrigate the wound with Gentell Wound Cleanser and gently dry the skin surrounding the wound site.
- Select appropriate size Gentell Waterproof Non-Bordered Foam Dressing based on the dimensions of the wound.
- Remove the dressing from the package and apply directly over the surface of the wound.

REMOVAL

- Change daily or as ordered by a physician.

FOAMS

3M™ Tegaderm™ Foam Adhesive Dressing

3M™ Health Care

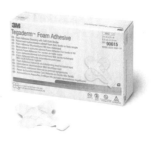

HOW SUPPLIED

Mini Wrap	2 3/4″ × 2 3/4″ (1″ × 1″ pad)	A6212

ACTION

3M™ Tegaderm™ Foam Adhesive Dressing mini wrap is constructed of a conformable, absorbent, polyurethane foam pad with a highly breathable, non-waterproof film backing reinforced with soft cloth tape, making it a perfect choice for toes, feet, noses, elbows, and chins. The unique single-spoke design allows for one-handed application for difficult-to-dress wounds. The border tabs are perforated Tegaderm film reinforced with soft cloth tape to allow high exchange of both moisture and oxygen.

INDICATIONS

3M™ Tegaderm™ Foam Adhesive Dressing is indicated for pressure, arterial, neuropathic (diabetic) and venous leg ulcers, including use under compression wraps, difficult body contours; toes, heel, and elbow, as well as skin tears, abrasions, skin grafts, and donor sites.

CONTRAINDICATIONS

- None known.

APPLICATION

- Cleanse wound and surrounding skin according to facility policy. If periwound skin is fragile or exposure to wound exudate is likely, apply a barrier film. Allow the barrier film to dry before dressing application.
- Hold the dressing by the side tab and remove the printed liner, exposing the adhesive border.
- Grasp the paper tab on the top of the dressing and position the dressing over the wound.
- Gently press the adhesive border tabs to the skin, overlapping the tabs to conform to contours. Avoid stretching the adhesive tabs or skin during application.
- Remove the paper tab.
- Firmly press and conform the adhesive border to the skin.
- Dressing change frequency will depend on the type of wound, volume of exudate, and clinical situation. Change at least every 7 days, or as indicated per treatment protocol.

REMOVAL

- Gently lift the adhesive film border while pressing down on the skin.
- If there is difficulty lifting the film border, apply tape to the edge of the dressing and use the tape to lift.

REFERENCE

1. https://www.3m.com/3M/en_US/company-us/all-3m-products/~/3M-Tegaderm-Foam-Adhesive-Dressing-90615-Mini-Wrap?N=5002385±3294775113&rt=rud.

FOAMS

3M™ Tegaderm™ High Performance Foam Adhesive Dressing

3M™ Health Care

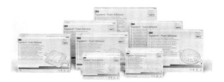

HOW SUPPLIED

Square	3 1/2″ × 3 1/2″ (2″ × 2″ pad)	A6212
Square	5 5/8″ × 5 5/8″ (4″ × 4″ pad)	A6212
Oval	4″ × 4 1/2″ (2 1/2″ × 3″ pad)	A6213
Oval	5 5/8″ × 6 1/8″ (4″ × 4 1/2″ pad)	A6212
Oval	7 1/2″ × 8 3/4″ (5 1/2″ × 6 3/4″ pad)	A6213
Heel/Elbow	5 1/2″ × 5 1/2″ (3″ × 3″ pad)	A6212

ACTION

3M™ Tegaderm™ High Performance Foam Adhesive Dressing provides total fluid management by a combination of fast wicking, high absorbency, and breathability. The innovative spoke delivery system allows fast, easy application for wounds over body contours. Oval and square dressings are constructed from a conformable polyurethane foam pad, an additional absorbent nonwoven layer, and a top layer of transparent adhesive film. This film is moisture-vapor permeable, which prevents wound exudate strike-through and acts as a barrier to outside contamination. The dressing maintains a moist environment, which has been shown to enhance wound healing. The dressing is supplied sterile.

INDICATIONS

For use as a primary dressing for low to highly exuding partial- and full-thickness dermal wounds, including pressure injuries, venous leg ulcers, abrasions, arterial ulcers, skin tears, and diabetic (neuropathic) ulcers.
- Can be used as a secondary (cover) dressing in conjunction with wound fillers (such as gauze or alginate dressings). Can be used under compression wrap systems for venous leg ulcer treatment.

CONTRAINDICATIONS

- Not designed, sold, or intended for use except as indicated.

APPLICATION

- Cleanse wound and surrounding skin according to facility policy. If periwound skin is fragile or exposure to wound exudate is likely, apply a barrier film. Allow the barrier film to dry before dressing application.
- Hold the dressing by the side tabs, and remove the printed liner, exposing the adhesive border.
- Position the dressing over the wound while holding the tabs.
- Gently press the adhesive border to the skin. Avoid stretching the dressing or skin.
- Remove the paper frame from the dressing while smoothing down the edges of the dressing.

FOAMS

REMOVAL

- Carefully lift the dressing edges from the skin. If there is difficulty lifting the dressing, apply tape to the edge of the dressing and use the tape to lift. Continue lifting edges until all are free from the skin surface.
- The change frequency will depend on the type of wound, volume of exudate, and clinical situation. Change at least every 7 days, or as indicated per treatment protocol.
- Observe the dressing frequently. As the dressing absorbs, exudate will wick to the top of the dressing, and discoloration may be noticeable. When the exudate spreads to the edges of the dressing or the dressing begins to leak, a dressing change is indicated.

REFERENCE

1. https://www.3m.com/3M/en_US/company-us/all-3m-products/~/3M-Tegaderm-High-Performance-Foam-Adhesive-Dressing?N=5002385±3293321924&rt=rud.

FOAMS

3M™ Tegaderm™ High Performance Foam Non-Adhesive Dressing

3M™ Health Care

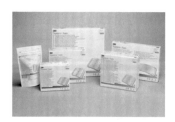

HOW SUPPLIED

Square	2" × 2"	A6209
Square	4" × 4"	A6209
Square	8" × 8"	A6211
Rectangle	4" × 8"	A6210
Fenestrated	3 1/2" × 3 1/2"	A6209
Roll	4" × 24"	A6211

ACTION

3M™ Tegaderm™ High Performance Foam Non-Adhesive Dressing is a highly absorbent, breathable, nonadherent wound dressing. It is constructed from conformable polyurethane foam covered with a highly breathable film backing. The film backing prevents exudate strike-through and acts as a barrier to outside contamination. The dressing maintains a moist wound environment, which has been shown to enhance wound healing. The dressing is sterile and may be cut to fit the needs of the user.

INDICATIONS

For use as a primary or secondary dressing for moderately to highly exuding partial- and full-thickness dermal wounds, including pressure injuries, venous leg ulcers, abrasions, arterial ulcers, skin tears, and neuropathic ulcers.

CONTRAINDICATIONS

- None known.

APPLICATION

- Cleanse wound and surrounding skin according to facility policy. If periwound skin is fragile or exposure to wound exudate is likely, apply a barrier film. Allow the barrier film to dry before dressing application.
- Remove the dressing from the package, and center it over wound, with the edges overlapping onto intact skin.
- Secure the dressing with adhesive tape, elastic or cohesive wrap, or other appropriate material.
- Note: Covering the entire foam dressing with an occlusive tape may reduce the breathability of the film backing. To maintain moisture vapor exchange, tape only edges of the dressing in picture frame manner.

REMOVAL

- Observe dressing frequently. As the dressing absorbs, exudates will wick to the top of the dressing, and discoloration may be noticeable. When exudates spread to the edges of dressing or dressing leaks, a dressing change is indicated. May remain in place for 7 days.

REFERENCE

1. https://www.3m.com/3M/en_US/company-us/all-3m-products/~/3M-Tegaderm-High-Performance-Foam-Non-Adhesive-Dressing?N=5002385±3293321962&rt=rud.

FOAMS

New Product: 3M™ Tegaderm™ Silicone Foam Adhesive Non-Bordered Dressing

3M™ Health Care

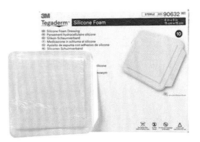

HOW SUPPLIED

Nonbordered Dressing	4″ × 4 1/4″	A6210
Nonbordered Dressing	6″ × 6″	A6210

ACTION

3M™ Tegaderm™ Silicone Foam Adhesive Non-Bordered Dressing is an absorbent, breathable, wound dressing. It is constructed from a conformable, polyurethane foam pad, absorbent nonwoven layers, a waterproof, breathable film backing, and gentle-to-skin silicone adhesive wound contact layer. The waterproof film backing is moisture vapor permeable, prevents wound exudate strike-through and acts as a barrier to outside contamination, including bacteria and viruses. In vitro testing shows that the transparent film provides a viral barrier from viruses 27 nm in diameter or larger while the dressing remains intact without leakage.

INDICATIONS

It is indicated for management of low to highly exuding partial- and full-thickness wounds such as pressure injuries, venous leg ulcers, neuropathic ulcers, arterial ulcers, skin tears, and surgical wounds. The dressing is suitable for use on fragile skin and with compression therapy.

CONTRAINDICATIONS

* The product is not designed, sold, or intended for use except as indicated.

APPLICATION

* Note: Follow facility guidelines for infection control.

Applying the dressing

* Cleanse wound and surrounding skin according to facility policy. If periwound skin is fragile or exposure to wound exudate is likely, apply a barrier film. Allow the barrier film to dry before dressing application.
* Select appropriate size dressing to ensure that the foam pad is larger than the wound area.
* Remove dressing from package. The dressing may be cut as necessary to accommodate wound contours.
* Remove white liner, exposing silicone adhesive.
* Position the dressing, silicone adhesive side down, over the wound with edges overlapping onto intact skin.
* Gently press the dressing to the skin. Secure with elastic or cohesive wrap, tape, or other methods as needed.
* When using the dressing for absorption and cushioning of tube sites (such as tracheostomy or gastric tubes), the dressing may be held in place by the silicone adhesive and tube itself, or additionally secured by taping the edges of the dressing in a picture frame manner.

FOAMS

Note: Covering the entire foam dressing with an occlusive tape may reduce the breathability of the film backing. To maintain moisture vapor exchange, tape only edges of the dressing in picture frame manner.

REMOVAL

- The dressing may remain in place up to 7 days. Dressing change frequency will depend on the type of wound, volume of exudate, and clinical situation. When the exudate spreads to the edges of the dressing or the dressing begins to leak, a dressing change is indicated.
- To remove dressing, first remove tape or other securement. Starting at the corners, carefully lift dressing from the skin. If the dressing is adhered to the wound surface, saturate with normal saline and gently loosen. Continue lifting until dressing is free from the skin surface and remove.

REFERENCE

1. https://www.3m.com/3M/en_US/company-us/all-3m-products/~/All-3M-Products/Health-Care/Medical/Skin-Wound-Care/Wound-Care-Dressings/Foam-Dressing/?N=5002385±8707795±8707798±8711017±8711098±8711132±8717785±3294857497&rt=r3&WT.mc_id=3m.com/siliconefoam.

New Product: 3M™ Tegaderm™ Silicone Foam Border Dressing

3M™ Health Care

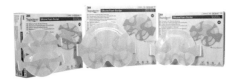

HOW SUPPLIED

Bordered Dressing	2″ × 2″	A6212
Bordered Dressing	3″ × 3″	A6212
Bordered Dressing	4″ × 4″	A6212
Bordered Dressing	6″ × 6″	A6213
Heel and Contour	6″ × 6″	A6212
Small Sacral	6″ × 6.75″	A6212
Large Sacral	7.25″ × 8.75″	A6213

ACTION

3M™ Tegaderm™ Silicone Foam Border Dressing is an absorbent, breathable, wound dressing. It is constructed from a conformable, polyurethane foam pad, absorbent nonwoven layers, a waterproof, breathable film backing, and gentle-to-skin silicone adhesive wound contact layer. The waterproof film backing is moisture vapor permeable, prevents wound exudate strike-through, and acts as a barrier to outside contamination, including bacteria and viruses.[1]

The use of 3M™ Tegaderm™ Silicone Foam Border Dressing may help prevent skin damage as part of a comprehensive pressure ulcer prevention program. The dressing may be lifted and repositioned to allow for skin assessment. In vitro testing shows that the transparent film provides a viral barrier from viruses 27 nm in diameter or larger while the dressing remains intact without leakage.

INDICATIONS

3M™ Tegaderm™ Silicone Foam Border Dressing is designed for management of low to highly exuding partial and full thickness wounds such as pressure injuries, venous leg ulcers, neuropathic ulcers, arterial ulcers, skin tears, and surgical wounds. The dressing is suitable for use on fragile skin and with compression therapy.

CONTRAINDICATIONS

- None known.

APPLICATION

- Note: Follow facility guidelines for infection control.

Before using the dressing

- Cleanse wound and surrounding skin according to facility policy. Dry surrounding skin.
- Assess wound. Select appropriate size dressing to ensure that the foam pad is larger than the wound area.

FOAMS

Applying the dressing

- Remove dressing from package. Hold the dressing by one of the side tabs, remove the white liner and position the dressing over the wound.
- Gently press the dressing to the skin. Avoid stretching the dressing or the skin.
- Beginning at the center of the dressing, grasp the blue paper delivery system one section at a time and remove by pulling toward the outer edge of the dressing. Press dressing to conform to the skin.

Sacral application

- Remove dressing from package. Fold dressing in half. Hold the tabs together. Remove the white liner. Spread the buttocks to get better placement. While holding the side tabs, position the dressing over the wound.
- Beginning at the gluteal cleft, gently press the dressing to the skin from the center outward. Avoid stretching the dressing or the skin.
- Beginning at the center of the dressing, grasp the blue paper delivery system one section at a time and remove by pulling toward the outer edge of the dressing. Press dressing to conform to the skin.

Heel application

- Remove dressing from package. Hold the dressing by one of the side tabs, remove the white liner and position the dressing over the wound.
- Beginning on the plantar aspect of the heel, gently press the bottom half of the dressing to the skin. Remove blue paper delivery system over this half of the dressing by pulling the tabs from the center toward the outer edge of the dressing.
- Mold the remaining the dressing over the posterior aspect of the heel, overlap the edges of the dressing if necessary. Avoid stretching the dressing or the skin.
- Remove blue paper delivery system over this half of the dressing by pulling the tabs from the center toward the outer edge of the dressing. Press to conform to the skin.

REMOVAL

- 3M™ Tegaderm™ Silicone Foam Border Dressing may remain in place up to 7 days.
- Dressing change frequency will depend on the type of wound, volume of exudate, and clinical situation. When the exudate spreads to the edges of the dressing or the dressing begins to leak, a dressing change is indicated.
- To remove dressing, carefully lift the edge of the dressing from the skin. If the dressing is adhered to the wound surface, saturate with normal saline and gently loosen. Continue lifting until dressing if free from the skin surface and removed.

REFERENCE

1. https://www.3m.com/3M/en_US/company-us/all-3m-products/~/All-3M-Products/Health-Care/Medical/Skin-Wound-Care/Wound-Care-Dressings/Foam-Dressing/?N=5002385±8707795±8707798±8711017±8711098±8711132±8717785±3294857497&rt=r3&WT.mc_id=3m.com/siliconefoam.

Hydrocolloids

ACTION

Hydrocolloids are occlusive or semiocclusive dressings composed of such materials as gelatin, pectin, and carboxymethyl cellulose. The composition of the wound contact layer may differ considerably among dressings. These dressings provide a moist healing environment that allows clean wounds to granulate and necrotic wounds to debride autolytically. Some hydrocolloids may leave a residue in the wound, and others may adhere to the skin around the wound. Hydrocolloids are manufactured in various shapes, sizes, adhesive properties, and forms, including wafers, pastes, and powders.

INDICATIONS

Hydrocolloid dressings may be used as primary or secondary dressings to manage select pressure ulcers, partial- and full-thickness wounds, wounds with necrosis or slough, and wounds with light to moderate exudate.

ADVANTAGES

- Are impermeable to bacteria and other contaminants.
- Facilitate autolytic debridement.
- Are self-adherent and mold well.
- Provide light to moderate absorption.
- Minimize skin trauma and disruption of healing.
- Allow observation of the healing process, if transparent.
- May be used under compression products (compression stockings, wraps, pumps, and Unna's boot).

DISADVANTAGES

- Are not recommended for wounds with heavy exudate, sinus tracts, or infections; wounds surrounded by fragile skin; or wounds with exposed tendon or bone.
- Can make wound assessment difficult, if opaque.
- May be dislodged if the wound produces heavy exudate.
- Provide an occlusive property that limits gas exchange between the wound and the environment.
- May curl at edges.
- May injure fragile skin upon removal.

HCPCS CODE OVERVIEW

The HCPCS codes normally assigned to hydrocolloid wound covers without an adhesive border are:
A6234—pad size <16 in^2.
A6235—pad size >16 in^2 but <48 in^2.
A6236—pad size >48 in^2.
The HCPCS codes normally assigned to hydrocolloid wound covers with an adhesive border are:
A6237—pad size <16 in^2.
A6238—pad size >16 in^2 but <48 in^2.
A6239—pad size >48 in^2.
The HCPCS codes normally assigned to hydrocolloid wound fillers are:
A6240—paste, per ounce.
A6241—dry form, per gram.

AMERX® Bordered Hydrocolloid Dressing

AMERX Health Care Corp.

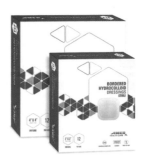

HOW SUPPLIED

Dressing	*2″ × 2″*	A6234
Dressing	*4″ × 4″*	A6234

ACTION

AMERX Bordered Hydrocolloid semi-transparent dressings easily conform to the skin surface, manage wound exudate, and create a moist wound environment for partial- and full-thickness wounds. Ideal for dry and light exudating, chronic and acute wounds and for areas subject to friction.

INDICATIONS

For use as a primary dressing over dry and light exudating, chronic and acute wounds.

CONTRAINDICATIONS

- Third-degree burns or if known sensitivities to dressing components.

APPLICATION

- Dressing size should extend a minimum of 1/2″ beyond the wound border.
- Cleanse the wound with sterile saline solution.
- Remove the dressing from the package and remove the paper liner.
- Place the dressing directly over the wound and surrounding skin without tension.
- Remove the remaining film in the direction of the blue arrows.
- Carefully smooth the edge of the dressing to ensure proper contact with the surrounding skin.

AMERX® Hydrocolloid Dressings—Thin

AMERX Health Care Corp.

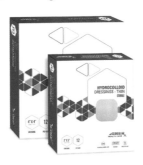

HOW SUPPLIED

Dressing	2″ × 2″	A6234
Dressing	4″ × 4″	A6234

ACTION

AMERX Thin Hydrocolloid semi-transparent dressings easily conform to the skin surface, manage wound exudate and create a moist wound environment for partial and full-thickness wounds. Ideal for dry and light exudating chronic and acute wounds and for areas subject to friction.

INDICATIONS

For use as a primary dressing over dry and light exudating, chronic and acute wounds.

CONTRAINDICATIONS

- Third-degree burns or if known sensitivities to dressing components.

APPLICATION

- Dressing size should extend a minimum of 1/2″ beyond the wound border.
- Cleanse the wound with sterile saline solution.
- Remove dressing from the package and remove the paper liner.
- Place dressing directly over the wound and surrounding skin without tension.
- Remove remaining film in the direction of the blue arrows.
- Carefully smooth the edge of the dressing to ensure proper contact with surrounding skin.

HYDROCOLLOIDS

Comfeel® Plus Contour Dressing; Comfeel® Plus Sacral Dressing

Coloplast

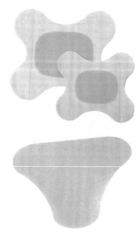

HOW SUPPLIED

Comfeel® Plus Ulcer Dressing

Butterfly-shaped	24 sq. in.	A6237
Butterfly-shaped	42 sq. in.	A6237
Sacral	7″ × 8″	A6235

ACTION

Comfeel® Plus hydrocolloid dressings provide an optimal, moist healing environment.

INDICATIONS

Comfeel Plus dressings are primarily indicated for the treatment of low to moderately exuding leg ulcers and pressure ulcers. Comfeel Plus Contour Dressing is primarily indicated for use in the treatment of pressure ulcers in difficult-to-dress sites. Comfeel Plus Sacral Dressing may be used on sacral wounds.

CAUTION

- May be used on patients with local and systemic infections under the discretion of a health care professional.
- Wounds which are solely or mainly caused by an arterial insufficiency or diabetic wounds (primarily lower leg and foot) should be inspected by a health care professional on a daily basis.

APPLICATION

- Rinse the wound with physiological saline or tap water. Gently pat dry the skin around the wound.
- Choose a dressing that 1 to 2 cm larger than the wound.

Comfeel Plus Contour Dressing

- Remove the protective paper from the center of the dressing, and place the dressing on the wound.
- Remove the protective paper from the wings, and gently press the wings one at a time to ensure that the dressing adheres to the skin.

Comfeel Plus Sacral Dressing

- Remove the protective paper from the center of the dressing.
- Spread the gluteal fold, place the dressing's narrow end into the deepest depression of the gluteal fold, and secure it in place. Ensure that the wound has 1″ (2.5 cm) of intact periwound skin and that the dressing adheres to the skin.
- Remove the second protective paper from the dressing, and secure the dressing in place.

HYDROCOLLOIDS

REMOVAL

- As Comfeel Plus dressings absorb wound exudate, a whitish gel is formed. When the gel reaches the upper film surface of the dressing, the appearance will become "marbled" or transparent. Comfeel Plus dressings should be changed when they are completely transparent.
- In case of leakage or nonadherence, change the dressing immediately.
- Comfeel Plus dressings are odor proof. A characteristic odor may develop under the dressing. This is normal and the odor will disappear once the wound is rinsed.

REFERENCES

Comfeel Plus Contour Dressing

1. https://www.coloplast.us/comfeel-plus-ulcer-en-us.aspx#section=product-description_3

Comfeel Plus Sacral Dressing

2. https://www.coloplast.us/comfeel-plus-ulcer-en-us.aspx#section=product-description_3

HYDROCOLLOIDS

Comfeel® Plus Ulcer Dressing; Comfeel® Plus Transparent Dressing

Coloplast

HOW SUPPLIED

Comfeel® Plus Ulcer Dressing

Wafer	1 1/2" × 2 1/2"	A6234
Wafer	4" × 4"	A6234
Wafer	6" × 6"	A6235
Wafer	8" × 8"	A6235

Comfeel® Plus Transparent Dressing

Wafer	2" × 2 3/4"	A6234
Wafer	4" × 4"	A6234
Wafer	3 1/2" × 5 1/2"	A6235
Wafer	6" × 6"	A6235

ACTION

Comfeel® Plus hydrocolloid dressings provide an optimal, moist healing environment.

INDICATIONS

Primarily indicated for the treatment of low to moderately exuding leg ulcers and pressure ulcers; may be used for superficial burns, partial-thickness burns, donor sites, postoperative wounds, and skin abrasions.

CAUTION

- May be used on patients with local and systemic infections under the discretion of a health care professional.
- Wounds which are solely or mainly caused by an arterial insufficiency or diabetic wounds (primarily lower leg and foot) should be inspected by a health care professional on a daily basis.

APPLICATION

- Rinse the wound with physiological saline or tap water. Gently pat dry the skin around the wound.
- Choose a dressing that 1 to 2 cm larger than the wound.
- Use the handles on the dressing to ensure aseptic application. Remove the protective paper.
- Place the adhesive side to the wound. Remove the handle.

REMOVAL

- As Comfeel Plus dressings absorb wound exudate, a whitish gel is formed. When the gel reaches the upper film surface of the dressing, the appearance will become "marbled" or transparent. Comfeel Plus dressings should be changed when they are completely transparent.

HYDROCOLLOIDS

- In case of leakage or nonadherence, change the dressing immediately.
- Comfeel Plus dressings are odor proof. A characteristic odor may develop under the dressing. This is normal and the odor will disappear once the wound is rinsed.

REFERENCES

Comfeel Plus Ulcer Dressing

1. https://www.coloplast.us/Wound/wound-/solutions/#section=Comfeel%c2%ae-Plus_82168

Comfeel Plus Transparent Dressing

2. https://www.coloplast.us/Wound/wound-/solutions/#section=Comfeel%c2%ae-Plus_82168

HYDROCOLLOIDS

DermaFilm HD

DermaRite Industries, LLC

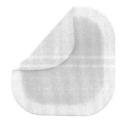

HOW SUPPLIED

Hydrocolloid Wound Dressing	4″ × 4″	A6234
Hydrocolloid Wound Dressing	6″ × 6″	

ACTION

DermaFilm® HD is a hydrocolloid wound dressing with a foam backing for use on shallow non-infected wounds and shallow pressure ulcers. DermaFilm HD provides protection and maintains body temperature at the wound, supports a moist wound environment, and aids in autolytic debridement.

INDICATIONS

May be used as a primary or secondary dressing. For the management of low-exuding noninfected shallow wounds including partial-thickness and shallow full-thickness ulcers.

CONTRAINDICATIONS

- DermaFilm HD should not be used on people who are sensitive or allergic to the dressing and its components.

APPLICATION

- Cleanse wound with advised liquid to remove residue according to local infection control protocol. Deep wounds should be well irrigated.
- Skin around wound should be clean and dry, use skin barrier prep as needed.
- Warm packaged dressing in hands prior to application.
- Remove dressing from package.
- Dressing may be cut to size prior to application.
- Remove backing paper from dressing.
- Apply sticky side of dressing to moist wound bed overlapping 1 to 2 inches of dry skin; gently smooth into place. Hold in place for several seconds to improve adhesion.
- Secure edges with tape if desired.

REMOVAL

- Dressing may be moistened to ease removal.
- Carefully remove adhesive dressings by holding the edge of the dressing and slowly pulling it parallel to the skin.
- Dispose of in accordance with local guidance.

REFERENCE

1. http://dermarite.com/product/dermafilm/

DermaFilm Thin

DermaRite Industries, LLC

HOW SUPPLIED

Thin Bordered Hydrocolloid Wound Dressing	2" × 2"	A6237
Thin Bordered Hydrocolloid Wound Dressing	4" × 4"	
Thin Bordered Hydrocolloid Wound Dressing	6" × 6"	
Thin Bordered Hydrocolloid Wound Dressing, Triangle	6" × 7"	
Thin Bordered Hydrocolloid Wound Dressing, Sacral	6" × 7"	A6238
Thin Bordered Hydrocolloid Wound Dressing, Heel	3.5" × 5"	

ACTION

DermaFilm® Thin is a thin bordered hydrocolloid wound dressing for shallow noninfected wounds and shallow pressure ulcers. DermaFilm provides thermal insulation and protection, maintains a moist wound environment and aids in autolytic debridement.

INDICATIONS

May be used as a primary or secondary dressing. For the management of low-exuding noninfected shallow wounds including partial-thickness and shallow full-thickness ulcers.

CONTRAINDICATIONS

- DermaFilm should not be used on people who are sensitive or allergic to the dressing and its components.

APPLICATION

- Cleanse wound with advised liquid to remove residue according to local infection control protocol. Deep wounds should be well irrigated.
- Skin around wound should be clean and dry, use skin barrier prep as needed.
- Warm packaged dressing in hands prior to application.
- Remove dressing from package.
- Remove backing paper from dressing.
- Apply sticky side of dressing to moist wound bed overlapping 1 to 2 inches of dry skin; gently smooth into place. Hold in place for several seconds to improve adhesion.

REMOVAL

- Dressing may be moistened to ease removal.
- Carefully remove adhesive dressings by holding the edge of the dressing and slowly pulling it parallel to the skin.
- Dispose of in accordance with local guidance.

REFERENCE

1. http://dermarite.com/

HYDROCOLLOIDS

New Product: DermaFilm X-Thin Clear

DermaRite Industries, LLC

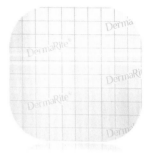

HOW SUPPLIED

Clear Hydrocolloid Wound Dressing with Grid	2" × 4"	
Clear Hydrocolloid Wound Dressing with Grid	4" × 4"	A6234
Clear Hydrocolloid Wound Dressing with Grid	6" × 6"	
Clear Hydrocolloid Wound Dressing with Grid, Oval Spots	1.75" × 1.5"	
Clear Hydrocolloid Wound Dressing with Grid, Oval	4" × 6"	

ACTION

DermaFilm® X-Thin Clear is a transparent hydrocolloid wound dressing for shallow noninfected wounds and shallow pressure ulcers. DermaFilm X-Thin Clear allows visualization of the wound, provides protection and normothermia, maintains a moist wound environment, and supports autolytic debridement.

INDICATIONS

May be used as a primary or secondary dressing. For the management of low-exuding noninfected shallow wounds including partial-thickness and shallow full-thickness ulcers.

CONTRAINDICATIONS

- DermaFilm should not be used on infected wounds or on people who are sensitive or allergic to the dressing and its components.

APPLICATION

- Cleanse wound with advised liquid to remove residue according to local infection control protocol. Deep wounds should be well irrigated.
- Skin around wound should be clean and dry, use skin barrier prep as needed.
- Warm packaged dressing in hands prior to application.
- Remove dressing from package.
- Dressing may be cut to size prior to application.
- Remove backing paper from dressing.
- Apply sticky side of dressing to moist wound bed overlapping 1 to 2 inches of dry skin; gently smooth into place. Hold in place for several seconds to improve adhesion.

REMOVAL

- Dressing may be moistened to ease removal.
- Carefully remove adhesive dressings by holding the edge of the dressing and slowly pulling it parallel to the skin.
- Dispose of in accordance with local guidance.

REFERENCE

1. http://dermarite.com/

HYDROCOLLOIDS

Dermatell

Gentell

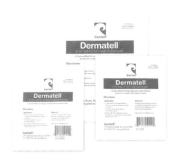

HOW SUPPLIED

Wafer	4″ × 4″ (2.5″ pad)	A6237
Wafer	6″ × 6″ (4.5″ pad)	A6238
Wafer	4″ × 4″ Nonbordered	A6235
Wafer	6″ × 7″ Sacral	A6238

ACTION

Gentell Dermatell™ Hydrocolloid Dressings consist of a soft, pliable hydrocolloid wafer that enhances patient comfort and protection. Dermatell™ is most effective when kept in place for a minimum of three days. Dermatell™ is available with our water-resistant adhesive border that is flexible and conforms easily to the body, and in a non-bordered hydrocolloid that naturally adheres to wounds with exudate.

INDICATIONS

- Gentell Dermatell should remain on the patient for at least three days and may be used on Stage 2 or Stage 3 wounds.

CONTRAINDICATIONS

- Dermatell™ is not indicated for use on heavily exuding wounds, Stage 4 pressure ulcers, infected wounds, or third-degree burns.

APPLICATION

- Irrigate the wound with Gentell Wound Cleanser and gently dry the skin surrounding the wound site.
- As a primary dressing, apply directly to the wound surface.
- As a secondary dressing, apply directly over primary treatment.

REMOVAL

- Change every 3 days or as ordered by a physician.

HYDROCOLLOIDS

DuoDERM® CGF Border Dressing*

ConvaTec

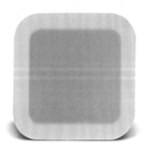

HOW SUPPLIED

Sterile Dressing	Square: 2.5" × 2.5" dressing plus 3/4" adhesive border	A6237
Sterile Dressing	4" × 4" dressing plus 3/4" adhesive border	A6237
Sterile Dressing	4" × 5" dressing plus 1" adhesive border	A6237
Sterile Dressing	Triangle: 6" × 6" plus 1" adhesive border	A6238
Sterile Dressing	6" × 7" plus 1" adhesive border	A6238

ACTION

DuoDERM® CGF Border Dressing creates a moist wound environment that supports the healing process and autolytic debridement and allows for nontraumatic removal. It helps isolate the wound against bacterial and other external contamination while remaining intact and without leakage.

INDICATIONS

To manage dermal ulcers, diabetic foot ulcers, and leg ulcers; may also be used on pressure ulcers (stages 1 to 4), full-thickness wounds, minor abrasions, second-degree burns, and donor sites.

CONTRAINDICATIONS

- Contraindicated for patients with sensitivity to the dressing or its components.

APPLICATION

- Dressing is sterile; handle appropriately.
- Clean the wound according to facility guidelines, and dry the surrounding skin to ensure that it is grease-free.
- Before applying the dressing, remove eschar that is particularly thick or fused to the wound margins.
- Choose a dressing size that is at least 1 1/4" (3 cm) larger than the wound margins.
- Remove only the top backing paper.
- Apply the dressing over the wound. Smooth into place, especially at the edges of the center adhesive. *Note:* The triangle-shaped dressing can be applied in several directions, depending on the location of the ulcer. For sacral ulcers, fold the dressing in half length-wise to make it easy to apply in the sacral fold.
- Fold back the border, and remove the release papers; press the borders into place. Additional taping is not required.
- Obtain a bacterial culture of the site if infection develops, and start appropriate medical treatment as ordered. Continue using the dressing as directed by the primary care provider.

REMOVAL

- Leave the dressing in place for up to 7 days unless it is uncomfortable or leaking, or infection develops.
- Press down on the skin, and carefully lift an edge of the dressing. Continue lifting around the dressing until all edges are free.
- The wound should be cleaned at each dressing change. (It is unnecessary to remove all residual dressing material from the surrounding skin.)

*See package insert for complete instructions for use.

DuoDERM® CGF Dressing*

ConvaTec

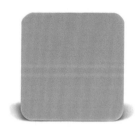

HOW SUPPLIED

Dressing	4″ × 4″	A6234
Dressing	6″ × 6″	A6235
Dressing	6″ × 8″	A6235
Dressing	8″ × 8″	A6236
Dressing	8″ × 12″	A6236

ACTION

DuoDERM® CGF (Control Gel Formula) Dressing is an adhesive (hydrocolloid) wound contact dressing. The self-adherent dressing absorbs wound fluid and provides a moist environment, which supports the body's healing process and aids in the removal of unnecessary material from the wound (autolytic debridement) without damaging new tissue. The dressing acts as a barrier to the wound against bacterial, viral, and other external contamination while intact and without leakage.

INDICATIONS

To manage minor abrasions, lacerations, minor cuts, minor scalds and burns, leg ulcers (venous stasis ulcers, arterial ulcers, and leg ulcers of mixed etiology); diabetic ulcers and pressure ulcers (partial- and full-thickness), surgical wounds (postoperative left to heal by secondary intention, donor sites, dermatologic excisions), second-degree burns, and traumatic wounds.

CONTRAINDICATIONS

- Not for use on individuals who are sensitive to or who have had an allergic reaction to the dressing or its components.

APPLICATION

- Choose a dressing size to ensure that the dressing is 1 1/2″ (3 cm) larger than the wound area.
- Remove the release paper from the back, being careful to minimize finger contact with the adhesive surface.
- Hold the dressing over the wound, and line up the center of the dressing with the center of the wound. Place the dressing directly over the wound.
- For difficult-to-dress areas, such as heels or the sacrum, a supplementary securing device, such as tape, may be required.
- Discard any unused portion of the product after dressing the wound.

REMOVAL

- Dressing may remain in place up to 7 days. The dressing should be changed when clinically indicated or when strikethrough occurs. The wound should be cleaned at each dressing change.
- Press down gently on the skin, and carefully lift one corner of the dressing until it no longer adheres. Continue until all edges are free.

*See package insert for complete instructions for use.

HYDROCOLLOIDS

DuoDERM® Extra Thin Dressing*

ConvaTec

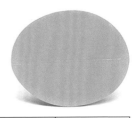

HOW SUPPLIED

DuoDERM Extra Thin Spots	1 1/4 × 1 1/2″	A6234
DuoDERM ExtraThin Dressing	2″ × 4″	A6234
DuoDERM ExtraThin Dressing	2″ × 8″	A6234
DuoDERM ExtraThin Dressing	3″ × 3″	A6234
DuoDERM ExtraThin Dressing	4″ × 4″	A6234
DuoDERM ExtraThin Dressing	4″ × 6″	A6235
DuoDERM ExtraThin Dressing	6″ × 6″	A6235
DuoDERM ExtraThin Dressing (Triangle)	6″ × 7″	A6235

ACTION

DuoDERM® Extra Thin dressing creates a moist environment that supports the healing process and autolytic debridement, and allows for nontraumatic removal. It acts as a barrier to help isolate the wound against bacterial and other contamination while intact and without leakage. This dressing is particularly suitable for use in areas subject to friction or those requiring contouring, such as elbows or heels.

INDICATIONS

To act as a protective dressing and manage superficial, dry to lightly exuding dermal ulcers and postoperative wounds.

CONTRAINDICATIONS

- Not for use on individuals who are sensitive to or who have had an allergic reaction to the dressings or their components.

APPLICATION

- Dressing is sterile; handle appropriately.
- Clean the wound and dry the surrounding skin to ensure that it is grease-free.
- Choose a dressing size that extends beyond the wound margin at least 1 1/4″ (3 cm).
- Minimize finger contact with the adhesive surface.
- Apply in a rolling motion; avoid stretching.
- Smooth into place, especially around the edges.
- Use tape to secure the edges, if necessary.
- For a heel or elbow, cut a slit about one third across each side of the dressing to make application easier.
- For a sacral ulcer, press the dressing into the anal fold. Depending on the location and depth of the ulcer, the triangle-shaped dressing can be applied in different directions.
- Obtain a bacterial culture of the wound site if infection develops, and start appropriate medical treatment, as ordered. Continue using the dressing as directed by the physician. Using an occlusive dressing in the presence of necrotic material may initially increase wound size and depth when the necrotic debris is cleaned away.

HYDROCOLLOIDS

REMOVAL

- Leave the dressing in place for up to 7 days unless it is uncomfortable or leaking or infection develops.
- Press down on the skin, and carefully lift an edge of the dressing. Continue lifting around the dressing until all edges are free.
- The wound should be cleaned at each dressing change. (It is unnecessary to remove all residual dressing material from the surrounding skin.)

*See package insert for complete instructions for use.

HYDROCOLLOIDS

DuoDERM® Signal Dressing*

ConvaTec

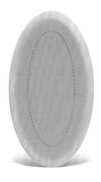

HOW SUPPLIED

DuoDERM® Signal Dressing (Oval)	4.5″ × 7.5″	A6235
DuoDERM® Signal Dressing (Sacral)	8″ × 9″	A6236
DuoDERM® Signal Dressing (Heel)	7.5″ × 7.8″	A6235
DuoDERM® Signal Dressing (Triangle)	6″ × 7″	A6238
DuoDERM® Signal Dressing (Triangle)	8″ × 9″	A6238
DuoDERM® Signal Dressing (Squares)	4″ × 4″	A6237
DuoDERM® Signal Dressing (Squares)	5.5″ × 5.5″	A6238
DuoDERM® Signal Dressing (Squares)	8″ × 8″	A6238

ACTION

DuoDERM® Signal creates a moist environment that supports healing and autolytic debridement, and allows for nontraumatic dressing removal. An indicator line on the dressing helps to determine when to change the dressing. The dressing acts as a barrier to the wound against bacterial, viral, and other external contamination provided the dressing remains intact and there is no leakage.

INDICATIONS

Over-the-counter type used for minor abrasions, lacerations, minor cuts, minor scalds, burns; under a physician's supervision, for leg ulcers (venous stasis ulcers, arterial ulcers, and leg ulcers of mixed etiology), diabetic ulcers and pressure ulcers, sores (partial- and full-thickness), surgical wounds (postoperative left to heal by secondary intention, donor sites, dermatologic excisions), second-degree burns, and traumatic wounds.

CONTRAINDICATIONS

- Not for use on patients who are sensitive to or who have had an allergic reaction to the dressing or its components.

APPLICATION

- Clean the wound surface and surrounding skin with SAF-Clens® AF Dermal Wound Cleanser or normal saline solution, and dry the surrounding skin.
- Debride if necessary.
- Choose a dressing size and shape to ensure that the dressing is 1 1/2″ (3 cm) larger than the wound area.
- Hold the dressing by its corner, and pull back the release paper about halfway.
- Apply the dressing from the outside edge toward the wound, completely removing the paper backing.
- Mold the entire dressing gently but firmly into place.

REMOVAL

- To remove the dressing, gently press down on the skin with one hand.
- Carefully peel up one edge of the dressing with the other hand.
- Continue until all edges are free.

*See package insert for complete instructions for use.

Exuderm Odorshield

Exuderm LP

Exuderm RCD

Exuderm Satin

Medline Industries, Inc.

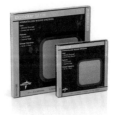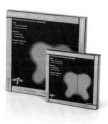

HOW SUPPLIED

Exuderm Satin

Wafer	2″ × 2″	A6234
Wafer	4″ × 4″	A6234
Wafer	6″ × 6″	A6235
Wafer	8″ × 8″	A6236
Sacral	3.6″ × 4″	A6234
Sacral	6″ × 5″	A6235

Exuderm Odorshield

Wafer	2″ × 2″	A6234
Wafer	4″ × 4″	A6234
Wafer	6″ × 6″	A6235
Wafer	8″ × 8″	A6236
Sacral	3.6″ × 4″	A6234
Sacral	6″ × 5″	A6235

Exuderm LP

Wafer	4″ × 4″	A6234
Wafer	6″ × 6″	A6235

Exuderm RCD

Wafer	4″ × 4″	A6234
Wafer	6″ × 6″	A6235
Wafer	8″ × 8″	A6236

ACTION

Exuderm reacts with wound exudate to create a moist healing environment while absorbing wound exudate. Exuderm OdorShield has a tapered-edge, no-residue formula plus added odor management via cyclodextrins. Exuderm Satin has a tapered-edge, low-profile, translucent appearance. The smooth satin backing resists rollup. Exuderm LP's low-profile design is used to protect against skin breakdown or to dress superficial wounds. Exuderm Regulated Colloidal Dispersion (RCD) is used to manage and absorb exudate with minimal meltdown.

HYDROCOLLOIDS

All Exuderm dressings provide a protective, occlusive barrier, facilitating granulation or autolytic debridement, if necessary.

INDICATIONS

To manage dermal ulcers, leg ulcers, pressure ulcers (stages 2 to 4), partial-thickness wounds, minor abrasions, first- and second-degree burns, donor sites, or wounds with slough or necrosis.

CONTRAINDICATIONS

- Contraindicated for third-degree burns.

APPLICATION

- Clean the application site with normal saline solution or another appropriate cleanser, such as Skintegrity Wound Cleanser. Dry the surrounding area to ensure that it is free from any greasy substance.
- Select the appropriate-sized dressing to allow 1 1/4″ to 1 1/2″ (3 to 4 cm) for attachment to healthy periwound skin.

Exuderm Satin, Exuderm Odorshield, Exuderm LP, Exuderm RCD

- Remove the paper carrier from the dressing.
- Center Exuderm over the site, and apply to skin using a rolling motion.
- Smooth the dressing into place, especially around the edges, and hold for 5 seconds to maximize adhesive qualities.
- For traditional hydrocolloids, such as Exuderm RCD, "picture framing" (taping down all sides with a skin-friendly tape, such as Medfix) can help prevent rollup.

REMOVAL

- Dressing may remain in place for 2 to 7 days, depending on the amount of wound drainage. If the dressing begins to lift or leak, change it immediately.
- An adhesive remover may be used to loosen the dressing.
- Carefully press down on the skin, and lift an edge of the dressing. Continue around the dressing until all edges are free.
- Remember that the wound should be cleaned at each dressing change.

REFERENCES

1. Exuderm Satin: https://www.medline.com/product/Exuderm-Satin-Hydrocolloid/Hydrocolloids/Z05-PF53360?question=exuderm&index=P4&indexCount=4
2. Exuderm Odorshield: https://www.medline.com/product/Exuderm-Odorshield-Hydrocolloid/Hydrocolloids/Z05-PF00173?question=exuderm&index=P1&indexCount=1
3. Exuderm LP: https://www.medline.com/product/Exuderm-Thin-Hydrocolloid/Hydrocolloids/Z05-PF00175?question=exuderm&index=P2&indexCount=2
4. Exuderm RCD: https://www.medline.com/product/Exuderm-RCD-Hydrocolloid/Hydrocolloids/Z05-PF00174?question=exuderm&index=P3&indexCount=3

HYDROCOLLOIDS

Procol Hydrocolloid Dressing

DeRoyal

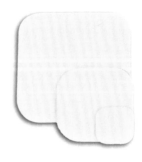

HOW SUPPLIED

Wafer	2″ × 2″	A6237
Wafer	4″ × 4″	A6237
Wafer	6″ × 6″	A6238
Procol X-Thin	2″ × 2″	A6237
Procol X-Thin	4″ × 4″	A6237
Procol X-Thin	6″ × 6″	A6238

ACTION

Procol is a self-adherent, hydrocolloid wound dressing that creates a moist environment conducive to local wound healing. It protects against wound dehydration, acts as a bacterial barrier, and helps to control wound drainage. Procol's matrix formulation helps reduce the residue left in the wound and also helps avoid damaging newly formed tissue during dressing changes.

INDICATIONS

For use as a primary or secondary dressing to manage dermal ulcers, superficial wounds, lacerations, abrasions, first- and second-degree burns, donor sites, and postoperative wounds.

CONTRAINDICATIONS

- Contraindicated for third-degree burns.

APPLICATION

- Clean the wound site with normal saline solution.
- If necessary, cut Procol Hydrocolloid Dressing to the desired size.
- Remove the dressing's release liner, and apply the exposed side to the wound.
- Because the dressing adheres to the skin around the wound, extra tape is not necessary.

REMOVAL

- Gently lift edges, and peel the dressing off.

HYDROCOLLOIDS

REPLICARE Hydrocolloid Dressing
REPLICARE Thin Hydrocolloid Dressing
REPLICARE Ultra Advanced Hydrocolloid Alginate Dressing

Smith & Nephew, Inc.
Wound Management

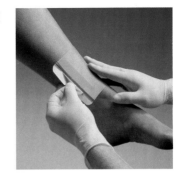

HOW SUPPLIED

REPLICARE

Wafer	1 1/2″ × 2 1/2″	A6234
Wafer	4″ × 4″	A6234
Wafer	6″ × 6″	A6235
Wafer	8″ × 8″	A6236

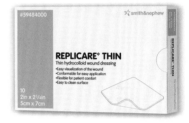

REPLICARE Thin

Wafer	2″ × 2 3/4″	A6234
Wafer	3 1/2″ × 5 1/2″	A6235
Wafer	6″ × 8″	A6235

REPLICARE Ultra

Wafer	4″ × 4″	A6234
Wafer	6″ × 6″	A6235
Wafer	8″ × 8″	A6236
Sacral Dressing	7″ × 8″	A6235

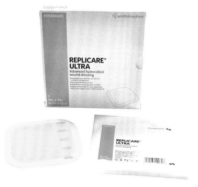

ACTION

These products support the creation and maintenance of a moist wound environment, which has been established as the optimal environment for management of the wound. They provide physical separation between the wound and external environments to help prevent bacterial contamination of the wound.

REPLICARE

REPLICARE is a hydrocolloid dressing that contains a dense concentration of absorbent material in a thin dressing for superior absorption in the management of exuding wounds. REPLICARE's cohesive properties keep the wound free from dressing residue. With the one-handed application system, the product will not stick to gloves. REPLICARE has a waterproof film exterior that helps prevent bacterial contamination. The top film can be wiped clean easily.

REPLICARE Thin

REPLICARE Thin is a hydrocolloid dressing made from a polyurethane film with a thin layer of absorbent colloid. REPLICARE Thin maintains a moist wound environment that assists in promoting autolytic debridement while managing low levels of exudate.

REPLICARE Ultra

REPLICARE Ultra is an advanced hydrocolloid dressing with alginate, which offers superior exudate management and increased absorption capability. REPLICARE Ultra's improved design provides better evaporation through an adaptable polyurethane top film that regulates moisture vapor transmission rate. This allows excess moisture to evaporate while maintaining the proper moist wound environment. The top film is waterproof, easy to clean, and aids in the prevention of bacterial contamination. Unique microthin edges and enhanced adhesive offer better adherence, reduced leakage potential, and reduced chance of edge roll. REPLICARE Ultra can remain in place for up to 7 days for convenience, fewer dressing changes, and a reduction in nursing costs. In addition, it's offered in a sacral design to conform to the difficult to dress sacral region.

INDICATIONS

REPLICARE

For exudate absorption and management of partial- to full-thickness wounds such as ulcers (venous, arterial, diabetic); pressure sores; donor sites; surgical incisions and excisions; and first- and second-degree burns.

REPLICARE Thin

For exudate absorption and management of partial- to full-thickness wounds such as ulcers (venous, arterial, diabetic); pressure sores; donor sites; surgical incisions and excisions; and first- and second-degree burns.

REPLICARE Ultra

Under a physician's supervision, for stage 1 through stage 4 wounds with light to moderate exudate, such as pressure ulcers, leg ulcers, superficial and partial-thickness burns, superficial wounds, donor sites, and skin abrasions.

CONTRAINDICATIONS

REPLICARE

- Contraindicated for use on third-degree or full-thickness burns.

REPLICARE Thin

- Contraindicated for use on third-degree burns.

REPLICARE Ultra

- Not to be continued if any signs of irritation (reddening, inflammation), maceration (overhydration of the skin), hypergranulation (excess tissue), or sensitivity (allergic reactions) appear; consult a health care professional.
- Not to be used if packaging is open or damaged.
- Not to be reused.
- Not for use on ulcers resulting from infection, such as tuberculosis, syphilis, and deep fungal infections; lesions in patients with acute vasculitis, such as periarteritis nodosa, systemic lupus erythematosus, and cryoglobulinemia; or third-degree burns.
- Must be removed before radiation therapy.

APPLICATION

REPLICARE

- Cleanse the wound with saline solution or an appropriate wound cleanser. Cleanse and dry the periwound skin. If the periwound skin is particularly friable, it may be protected from trauma by applying Skin-Prep.

- Choose a dressing large enough to cover the wound with 1″ (2.5 cm) of overlap on all sides of the wound. Remove the printed backing paper, exposing the adhesive surface.
- Center the dressing over the wound, and press the edges firmly to the surrounding skin. Remove the small plastic application tab from the underside of the dressing, and press all the sides firmly to the skin.

REPLICARE Thin

- Cleanse the wound with saline solution or an appropriate wound cleanser. Cleanse and dry the periwound skin. If the periwound skin is particularly friable, it may be protected from trauma by applying Skin-Prep.
- Choose a dressing large enough to cover the wound with 1″ of overlap on all sides of the wound. Remove the printed backing paper, exposing the adhesive surface.
- Center the dressing over the wound, and press the edges firmly to the surrounding skin. Remove the small plastic application tab from the underside of the dressing, and press all the sides firmly to the skin.

REPLICARE Ultra

- The following are designed to act as general guidelines and should only be used under the supervision of a health care professional.
  - Cleanse the wound using sterile saline or a recommended commercial brand of wound cleanser such as Dermal Wound Cleanser. Gently pat dry the skin around the wound. Skin-Prep is recommended to protect the periwound skin.
  - Choose a dressing that allows for 1/2″ to 1″ (1.25 to 2.5 cm) overlap of the wound.
  - Remove the protective paper, exposing the adhesive surface. Use the clear, plastic handle to ensure aseptic application.
  - Place the adhesive side to the wound, and remove the handle.
  - During the body's normal healing process, unnecessary material is removed from the wound, which will make the wound appear larger after the first few dressing changes. If the wound continues to get larger after the first few dressing changes, discontinue use and consult a health care professional.

REMOVAL
REPLICARE, REPLICARE Thin

- Change the dressing every 4 days or when transparent or leaking.
- Support the dressing with one hand while using the other hand to pull the edges laterally (parallel to the skin surface) away from the center.

REPLICARE Ultra

- As REPLICARE Ultra absorbs wound exudate, a gel is formed. When the gel reaches the upper film surface of the dressing, the dressing becomes white or opaque. Maximum absorbency is reached when the dressing becomes opaque and the exudate extends 1/2″ (1.25 cm) from the edges of the dressing.
- To remove the REPLICARE Ultra dressing, lift one corner of the dressing and gently pull the dressing away from the wound. To aid in removal of the dressing, Remove Adhesive Remover may be used.
- Gently cleanse the wound with tap water, sterile saline, or recommended commercial brand wound cleanser such as Dermal Wound Cleanser.
- Follow package instructions for applying a fresh dressing.

HYDROCOLLOIDS

Restore™ Extra Thin Hydrocolloid Dressing*

Hollister Wound Care

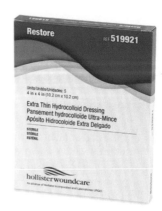

HOW SUPPLIED

Sheet	4″ × 4″	A6234
Sheet	6″ × 8″	A6235
Sheet	8″ × 8″	A6236

ACTION

Restore™ extra thin hydrocolloid dressing is a sterile, occlusive dressing. The flexible outer layer helps isolate the wound against bacterial and viral human immunodeficiency virus (HIV-1) and hepatitis B virus (HBV) contaminants and other external contamination such as urine and feces while the dressing remains intact without leakage. The self-adhesive dressing helps maintain a moist environment for wound healing. Disposable wound measuring guide included.

INDICATIONS

To protect skin from friction injury and to manage superficial wounds with minimal or no exudate.

CONTRAINDICATIONS

- Not for use on patients with active vasculitis or ulcers involving muscle, tendon, or bone.
- Contraindicated on patients with deep systemic infections.
- Contraindicated on patients with signs of active local infection at the wound site (erythema, cellulitis, or purulent discharge).

APPLICATION

- To ensure attachment to healthy skin, the dressing should extend at least 1″ (2.5 cm) beyond the wound edge. Dressings may be overlapped or cut to accommodate the wound site.
- Remove the printed release paper from the patient side of the dressing. Center the dressing over the wound site. Press the dressing to the skin and smooth it to remove all wrinkles.

REMOVAL

- Carefully lift an edge of the dressing, and peel away from the skin. The dressing should be left in place until one or more of the following occurs: leakage of exudate, loosening of the edges of the dressing, tenderness or signs of infection, 7 days have elapsed, or there is no longer a clinical need for the dressing.

*See package insert for complete instructions for use.

HYDROCOLLOIDS

Restore™ Hydrocolloid Dressing*

Hollister Wound Care

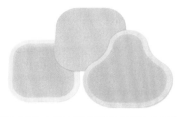

HOW SUPPLIED

Dressing	4" × 4" without tapered edges	A6234
Dressing	6" × 8" without tapered edges	A6235
Dressing	8" × 8" without tapered edges	A6236
Dressing	4" × 4" with tapered edges	A6234
Dressing	6" × 6" with tapered edges	A6235
Dressing	6" × 8" with tapered edges	A6235
Dressing	8" × 8" with tapered edges	A6236
Dressing	With tapered edges, triangle-shaped 17 in^2	A6235
Dressing	With tapered edges, triangle-shaped 26.5 in^2	A6235

ACTION

Restore™ hydrocolloid dressings are sterile, occlusive dressings. The flexible outer layer helps isolate the wound against bacterial and human immunodeficiency virus (HIV-1) and hepatitis B virus (HBV) contaminants and other external contamination such as urine and feces while the dressing remains intact without leakage. The self-adhesive inner layer maintains a moist wound environment while absorbing excess wound exudate to prevent fluid pooling. Disposable wound measuring guide included.

INDICATIONS

For use on dermal ulcers including partial- and full-thickness wounds with light to moderate amounts of exudate. Also for diabetic ulcers, pressure ulcers (stages I–IV), leg ulcer management, superficial wounds, second-degree burns, and donor sites; partial- and full-thickness wounds; moist to moderately exudative wounds.

CONTRAINDICATIONS

- Not for use on third-degree burns.

APPLICATION

- Rinse or irrigate the wound area. The skin should be clean and dry for secure application. To ensure attachment to healthy skin, the dressing should extend at least 1" (2.5 cm) beyond the wound edge. Dressings may be overlapped or cut to accommodate the size of the wound.
- Partially remove the release paper from the dressing, exposing the center of the dressing. Do not remove the paper completely at this point.
- Center the adhesive side of the dressing over the wound site. Be careful not to touch the adhesive side of the dressing (side applied to the wound).
- Remove the remaining pieces of the release paper from the dressing, and press the dressing margins to the skin.
- If clinical signs of infection are present, appropriate medical treatment should be initiated. Management of the wound with Restore hydrocolloid dressings may be continued at the discretion of the clinician.

REMOVAL

- Carefully lift an edge of the dressing while pressing gently down on the skin.
- Continue this procedure around the wound bed until all edges of the dressing are free. Wash the wound area to remove any residual materials. Remove excess moisture, and apply a new dressing. The dressing should be left in place (not more than 7 days) unless it is uncomfortable, leaking, or there are clinical signs of infection.

*See package insert for complete instructions for use.

Restore™ Hydrocolloid Dressing with Foam Backing*

Hollister Wound Care

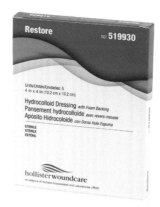

HOW SUPPLIED

Sheet	4" × 4"	A6234
Sheet	6" × 8"	A6235
Sheet	8" × 8"	A6236

ACTION

Restore™ hydrocolloid dressings are sterile, occlusive dressings. The heat-activated, self-adhesive inner layer maintains a moist environment while absorbing excess wound exudate. Product includes a disposable wound measuring guide.

INDICATIONS

The dressings are designed for use on dermal ulcers and partial-thickness wounds with light to moderate amounts of exudate. Also for venous stasis ulcers, superficial wounds, pressure ulcers (stages 1 and 2), arterial ulcers, diabetic ulcers, surgical incisions, and traumatic wounds.

CONTRAINDICATIONS

- Not for use on patients with active vasculitis, infection, or stage 3 or 4 pressure ulcers.

APPLICATION

- To ensure proper adhesion, the dressing should extend at least 1" (2.5 cm) beyond the wound edge. Dressings may be overlapped or cut to accommodate the wound site.
- Remove the release paper from the dressing. Center the dressing over the wound, being careful to minimize touching the adhesive side. Press the dressing in place. Initial tack may be improved by warming the dressing with your hands prior to application or after dressing is in place.

REMOVAL

- Carefully lift an edge of the dressing while pressing down on the skin adjacent to the edge. Continue this procedure around the wound until all of the edges are free of the skin. Gently lift the dressing off the wound.
- Gently rinse or irrigate the wound as needed, remove excess moisture, and apply a new dressing.

*See package insert for complete instructions for use.

HYDROCOLLOIDS

Triad™ Hydrophilic Wound Dressing

Coloplast

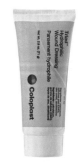

HOW SUPPLIED

Tube	2.5-oz	A6240
Tube	6-oz	A6240

ACTION

Triad™ Hydrophilic Wound Dressing is a zinc oxide-based hydrophilic paste that absorbs moderate levels of exudate, promotes a moist wound healing environment and facilitates autolytic debridement; and it is an ideal alternative for difficult-to-dress wounds.

INDICATIONS

For the local management of pressure and venous stasis ulcers, dermal lesions/injuries, superficial wounds, scrapes, first- and second-degree burns, partial- and full-thickness wounds.

CONTRAINDICATIONS

- Contraindicated for third-degree burns.
- Contraindicated for infected wounds.

APPLICATION

- **For shallow wounds.**
  - Apply Triad (thickness of a dime) directly on wound.
  - Cover Triad with a secondary dressing, such as Biatain® Foam Dressing, as needed.
  - Amount of wound exudate dictates frequency of dressing changes; change Triad every 5 to 7 days.
- **For deep wounds.**
  - Impregnate gauze (4 × 4″ or ribbon) with Triad.
  - Loosely pack impregnated gauze into wound.
  - Cover with a secondary dressing, such as Biatain Foam Dressing.
  - Impregnated gauze dressings are usually changed every 24 hours or per existing wound protocols.
- **Facilitating autolytic debridement.**
  - Apply Triad (thickness of a dime) over necrotic tissue and periwound area.
  - To help absorb liquefied necrotic tissue, cover Triad with an absorbent secondary dressing, such as Biatain Foam Dressing, as needed.
  - Amount of wound exudate dictates frequency of dressing changes; change Triad every 5 to 7 days.

REMOVAL

- Carefully unsecure the secondary dressing. Remove any impregnated gauze dressings, if applicable.
- Spray wound and periwound area with a pH-balanced wound cleanser.
- Gently wipe Triad off with a clean piece of gauze.
- If necessary, repeat the process.

REFERENCE

1. https://www.coloplast.ca/wound/wound/solutions/#section=Triad%e2%84%a2Hydrophilic-Wound-Dressing_168395

HYDROCOLLOIDS

3M™ Tegaderm™ Hydrocolloid Dressing

3M™ Tegaderm™ Hydrocolloid Thin Dressing

3M™ Tegaderm™ Hydrocolloid Dressing Sacral Design

3M™ Health Care

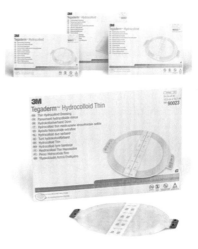

HOW SUPPLIED

3M™ Tegaderm™ Hydrocolloid Dressing

Oval	2 3/4" × 3 1/2" (gel pad)	A6237
Oval	4" × 4 3/4" (gel pad)	A6238
Oval	5 1/2" × 6 3/4" (gel pad)	A6238
Square	4" × 4" (gel pad)	A6234
Square	6" × 6" (gel pad)	A6235
Sacral	6 3/4" × 6 3/8" (gel pad)	A6238

3M™ Tegaderm™ Hydrocolloid Thin Dressing

Oval	2 3/4" × 3 1/2" (gel pad)	A6237
Oval	4" × 4 3/4" (gel pad)	A6238
Oval	5 1/2" × 6 3/4" (gel pad)	A6238
Square	4" × 4" (gel pad)	A6234

ACTION

3M™ Tegaderm™ Hydrocolloid Dressing and 3M™ Tegaderm™ Hydrocolloid Thin Dressing are sterile wound dressings which consist of a hypoallergenic, hydrocolloid adhesive with an outer clear adhesive cover film. The film is moisture vapor permeable, waterproof, and impermeable to liquids, bacteria, and viruses.[1] 3M™ Tegaderm™ Hydrocolloid Dressing supports wound management in two ways. First, the inner layer of hydrocolloid adhesive absorbs exudate—providing significantly higher absorbency during the first 48 hours than the leading competitive hydrocolloid. In addition to excellent absorbency, the breathable outer film layer provides a consistently high rate of moisture vapor transmission, reducing the potential for skin maceration. Together, these features ensure an optimal moist wound environment, minimize the chance for damage to healthy periwound skin, and provide cost-effective wear time for up to 7 days. The dressings also offer protection from the contaminants: The outer film barrier protects the wound and surrounding skin from contaminants and body fluids. Over the wound site, 3M™ Tegaderm™ Hydrocolloid Dressing interact with wound fluid to create a soft, semi-transparent, absorbent mass. The dressings maintain a moist wound environment, which has been shown to enhance wound healing.

HYDROCOLLOIDS

INDICATIONS

3M™ Tegaderm™ Hydrocolloid Dressings are indicated to manage partial- and full-thickness dermal ulcers, superficial wounds, abrasions, first- and second-degree burns, and donor sites. 3M™ Tegaderm™ Hydrocolloid Thin Dressing is indicated for partial- and full-thickness dermal ulcers, leg ulcers, superficial wounds, abrasions, first- and second-degree burns, donor sites, and to protect at-risk, undamaged skin or skin beginning to show signs of damage from friction or shear. 3M™ Tegaderm™ Hydrocolloid Dressing Sacral Design are very useful in body areas that are problems for dressing shape and conformance. Examples of such areas are breasts, and the sacral area of the buttocks.

CONTRAINDICATIONS

- Treatment of any skin ulcer should be part of a well-defined plan for ulcer management and under the supervision of a health care professional.

APPLICATION

- Clip excess hair at the wound site, thoroughly clean the wound and surrounding skin, and allow the skin to dry.
- If the patient's skin is easily damaged or drainage is expected to go beyond the wound edge, a skin protectant or a skin barrier film may be applied.
- Select a dressing that extends 1″ (2.5 cm) beyond the wound edge.

Oval dressing

- Remove the paper liner from the dressing by lifting and pulling one of the square end tabs marked "1," exposing the adhesive surface. Minimize contact with the border or the adhesive side of the dressing.
- Center the dressing over the wound. Then, gently press the adhesive side against the wound. Press from the center outward, and avoid stretching the dressing or the skin.
- Smooth the film edges to ensure good adherence.
- Remove the top delivery film by lifting one of the center tabs marked "2," and pulling it toward the edge of the dressing. Smooth down the dressing edges as you remove the film. Remove the other side of the top film in the same way.
- Gently tear off the square end tabs marked "1" at the perforations in a downward direction and discard. Avoid lifting the film edge while removing the tabs. Secure the entire film edge by pressing firmly.

Applying the dressing to heels or elbows

- Cut each corner of the dressing from the edge toward the center.
- Remove the adhesive (bottom) liner, grasping both slit sides of one corner.
- Place the dressing on the heel or elbow. Press from the center toward the two cut sides.
- Overlap the remaining piece, and press the edges to prevent leakage.
- Place tape around the edges of the dressing, pressing the tape firmly.

Square dressing

- Remove the top liner from the back of the dressing. 3M™ Tegaderm™ Hydrocolloid Thin Dressing may be cut to size before removing its top liner.
- Peel the dressing from its paper liner, minimizing contact with the dressing adhesive surface.
- Center the dressing over the wound, and gently press the adhesive side against the wound. Press from the center outward, and avoid stretching the dressing or the skin.
- Apply tape firmly around the edges of the dressing.

Sacral dressing

- Before removing the printed liner, fold the dressing in half.
- Hold the tabs together, and remove the printed liner on one-half of the dressing until the adhesive is exposed.
- Continue to remove the printed liner from the other half until the adhesive surface is completely exposed.
- While still holding both tabs, position the dressing over the wound, tilting the dressing toward the anal area. Spread the buttocks to get better placement. Secure the dressing notch in the anal region first to minimize risk of incontinence contamination or wrinkling.
- Gently press the adhesive side of the dressing down from the center outward. Avoid stretching the dressing or the skin.
- Remove the dressing frame, starting at the top and pulling down. Do not lift the film edge. Reinforce and smooth the dressing from the center outward.
- Repeat until all sections of the frame are removed.

REMOVAL

- The dressing should be changed if it is leaking, falling off, or has been on the wound for 7 days.
- Carefully lift the dressing edges from the skin. For easy removal, apply tape to the edge of the dressing, and use the tape to lift.
- Continue lifting the edges until all are free from the skin surface.
- Remove the dressing slowly, folding it over itself. Pull carefully in the direction of hair growth.
- Note that it is not unusual for wounds to have an odor. This may be noticed when the dressing is removed or when leakage occurs. The odor should disappear after the wound is cleaned.

REFERENCES

1. https://www.3m.com/3M/en_US/company-us/search/?Ntt=hydrocolloids&LC=en_US&co=cc&gsaAction=scBR&type=cc
2. https://www.3m.com/3M/en_US/company-us/all-3m-products/~/All-3M-Products/Health-Care/Medical/Pressure-Ulcer/Pressure-Injury/?N=5002385±8707795±8707798±8711017±8745208±3294857497&rt=r3

HYDROCOLLOIDS

Hydrogels

ACTION

Hydrogels are water- or glycerin-based amorphous gels, impregnated gauzes, or sheet dressings. Because of their high water content, some cannot absorb large amounts of exudate. Hydrogels help maintain a moist healing environment, promote granulation and epithelialization, and facilitate autolytic debridement.

INDICATIONS

Hydrogel dressings may be used as primary dressings (amorphous and impregnated gauzes) or as primary or secondary dressings (sheets). They may also be used to manage partial- and full-thickness wounds, deep wounds (amorphous, impregnated gauzes), wounds with necrosis or slough, minor burns, and tissue damaged by radiation.

ADVANTAGES

- Are soothing and reduce pain.
- Rehydrate the wound bed.
- Facilitate autolytic debridement.
- Fill in dead space (amorphous, impregnated gauzes).
- Provide minimal to moderate absorption.
- Are applied and removed easily from the wound.
- Can be used when infection is present.

DISADVANTAGES

- Are not usually recommended for wounds with heavy exudate.
- Dehydrate easily if not covered.
- Some require secondary dressing.
- Some may be difficult to secure.
- Some may cause maceration.

HCPCS CODE OVERVIEW

The HCPCS codes normally assigned to hydrogel wound covers without an adhesive border are:
A6242—pad size <16 in^2.
A6243—pad size >16 in^2 but ≤48 in^2.
A6244—pad size >48 in^2.
    The HCPCS codes normally assigned to hydrogel wound covers with an adhesive border are:
A6245—pad size <16 in^2.
A6246—pad size >16 in^2 but ≤48 in^2.
A6247—pad size >48 in^2.
    The HCPCS code normally assigned to hydrogel wound fillers is:
A6248—gel, per fluid ounce.
    The HCPCS codes normally assigned to gauze, impregnated, hydrogel, for direct wound contact are:
A6231—pad size <16 in^2.
A6232—pad size >16 in^2 but ≤48 in^2.
A6233—pad size >48 in^2.

AMERIGEL® Hydrogel Wound Dressing

AMERX Health Care Corp.

HOW SUPPLIED

Tube	1 oz	A6248
Tube	3 oz	A6248

ACTION

The #1 physician-rated wound/ulcer topical since 2006, AMERIGEL Hydrogel Wound Dressing provides a moist wound environment. This dressing sustains moisture longer than standard hydrogels, is noncytotoxic to healthy tissues, and contains Oakin® (an oak extract), meadowsweet extract, zinc acetate, polyethylene glycol 400 and 3350, and water.

INDICATIONS

For use as a wound dressing to manage pressure ulcers stages I to IV, stasis ulcers, skin irritation, cuts, abrasions, and skin irritations associated with peristomal care.

CONTRAINDICATIONS

- Contraindicated in patients who are sensitive or allergic to any ingredient.

APPLICATION

- Irrigate the wound with a sterile saline solution, and blot dry.
- Apply a thin layer of AMERIGEL Hydrogel Wound Dressing to the wound bed and overlap onto the periwound skin.
- Cover with appropriate secondary dressing.

REMOVAL

- Remove secondary dressing and irrigate with a sterile saline solution daily.

REFERENCES

1. http://www.japmaonline.org/doi/10.7547/8750-7315-104.6.617?url_ver=Z39.88-2003&rfr_dat=cr_pub%3Dpubmed&rfr_id=ori:rid:crossref.org&code=pmas-site
2. http://www.magonlinelibrary.com/doi/abs/10.12968/jowc.2014.23.Sup2a.S4

HYDROGELS

Anasept® Antimicrobial Skin and Wound Gel

Anacapa Technologies, Inc.

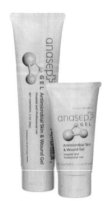

HOW SUPPLIED

Tube	3-oz	A6248
Tube	1.5-oz	A6248

PRODUCT DESCRIPTION

Anasept Antimicrobial Skin and Wound Gel is a clear, amorphous iso-tonic hydrogel that helps maintain moist wound environment that is conducive to healing, by either absorbing wound exudates or donating moisture while delivering 0.057% broad spectrum antimicrobial sodium hypochlorite. Anasept Gel inhibits the growth of microorganisms, such as *Staphylococcus aureus, Pseudomonas aeruginosa, Proteus mirabilis, Serratia marcescens, Acinetobacter baumannii, Clostridium difficile,* including antibiotic-resistant strains methicillin-resistant *S. aureus* (MRSA), vancomycin-resistant *Enterococcus faecalis* (VRE), and carbapenem-resistant *Escherichia coli* (CRE), that are commonly found in the wound bed, as well as fungi such as *Candida albicans* and *Aspergillus niger.*

INDICATIONS FOR USE

OTC

Anasept Antimicrobial Skin and Wound Gel is intended for OTC use for management of skin abrasions, lacerations, minor irritations, cuts, exit sites, and intact skin.

Professional use

Anasept Antimicrobial Skin and Wound Gel is intended for use under the supervision of a health care professional for the management of wounds such as stage I to IV pressure ulcers, partial- and full-thickness wounds, diabetic foot ulcers, postsurgical wounds, first- and second-degree burns, grafted and donor sites.

CONTRAINDICATIONS

- Not compatible with wound care products containing silver.

APPLICATION

Skin

- Cleanse the site with an appropriate skin cleanser.
- Apply a thin layer of Anasept® Gel to the intended site. Repeat as necessary.

Wounds

- Cleanse and/or debride the wound as necessary.
- Apply a generous amount of Anasept Gel directly onto the wound bed (1/8″ to 3/16″ thick).
- Cover the wound with a sterile gauze or other appropriate wound dressing and secure in place (avoid wound dressings containing silver and other metals). Maintain a moist wound environment between dressing changes.

HYDROGELS

REMOVAL

- Remove the secondary dressing.
- Cleanse with an appropriate skin and wound cleanser as necessary.

CLINICAL INFORMATION

- **Bactericidal:** Including the antibiotic-resistant strains such as MRSA, VRE, and CRE.
- **Sporicidal:** Effective against *C. difficile* spores which is known to be resistant to a wide range of biocides and antibiotics, a health hazard that reached epidemic proportions in long-term care facilities.
- **Fungicidal:** Effective against the well-known pathogenic fungi *C. albicans* and *A. niger.*
- **Virucidal:** Effective against HIV-Type 1 (human immunodeficiency virus).
- **Rapid antimicrobial action:** Kills most organisms in 2 minutes.
- **Biofilm:** Effective against the polymicrobial biofilm, a primary cause of chronic nonhealing wounds.
- **Debridement:** Exceptional and powerful debriding action in effectively solubilizing necrotic wound slough for easy removal. Anasept Gel has been shown to be equal or better than enzymatic wound debriding agents at a fraction of the cost.
  Clinical case study: Case study series – **Sodium Hypochlorite Debrides Necrotic Wound Tissue**, Martin Winkler, MD, FACS Creighton University Department of Surgery, Omaha, NE University of Nebraska Department of Surgery (Contributed Service), Omaha, NE.
  Laura Wesnieski, RN, CWS Bergan. Mercy Wound Care Clinic, Omaha, Nebraska.
  Sara M. Winkler. Dept. of Biomedical Engineering, Stanford University, Palo Alto, CA.
- **Wound odor control:** Anasept is unmatched in wound odor control.
- **No known microbial resistance** to Anasept Antimicrobial Skin and Wound Gel.

Safety

Anasept has been subjected to rigorous safety testing at an independent laboratory and shown to meet the criteria for safe use:

- Modified primary skin irritation (FSHA method—7-day exposure with repeated insult to intact and abraded skin).
- Cytotoxicity (ISO agarose overlay method).
- Systemic toxicity (ISO acute systemic toxicity).
- ISO sensitization study.
- ISO vaginal irritation study.

Shelf-life

- Two years when stored at normal room temperature 25°C (77°F).

Other features and benefits

- Proudly manufactured in the United States in an FDA-registered and ISO-certified facility.
- Nonflammable and can be used in hyperbaric chambers.
- Significant reduction in the treatment of chronic and recalcitrant wounds.
- No untoward or adverse reactions reported in over 10 years of use.

HYDROGELS

New Product: AquaDerm

DermaRite Industries, LLC

HOW SUPPLIED

Hydrogel Sheet Wound Dressing	2″ × 2″	A6242
Hydrogel Sheet Wound Dressing	4″ × 4″	A6242

ACTION

AquaDerm® is a translucent, flexible, absorbent hydrogel sheet dressing for partial- or full-thickness wounds. AquaDerm absorbs exudate and maintains its shape while supporting a moist wound-healing environment. AquaDerm leaves no residue and minimizes dressing-change–related pain.

INDICATIONS

For the management of partial- or full-thickness wounds including pressure ulcers, minor burns, surgical wounds, skin abrasions, and radiation tissue damage.

CONTRAINDICATIONS

- AquaDerm should not be used on full-thickness burns or on people who are sensitive or allergic to the dressing and its components.

APPLICATION

- Cleanse the wound with the advised liquid to remove residue according to the local infection control protocol. Deep wounds should be well irrigated.
- The skin around the wound should be clean and dry. Use skin barrier prep as needed.
- Remove the dressing from the package.
- The dressing may be cut to size prior to application.
- Remove the backing paper from the dressing.
- Apply the gel surface directly to the wound, overlapping 1 to 2 inches of dry skin.
- Cover with the appropriate secondary dressing that maintains a moist wound bed.

REMOVAL

- The dressing may be moistened to ease removal.
- Carefully remove adhesive dressings by holding the edge of the dressing and slowly pulling it parallel to the skin.
- Dispose of in accordance with local guidance.

REFERENCE

1. http://dermarite.com/product/aquaderm/

HYDROGELS

CarraDres Clear Hydrogel Sheet

Medline Industries, Inc.

HOW SUPPLIED

Sheet	4″ × 4″	A6242

ACTION

CarraDres Clear Hydrogel Sheet consists of 89.5% water combined with a cross-linked polyethylene matrix in sterile hydrogel polymer sheets especially formulated for managing partial- and full-thickness wounds. The hydrophilic dressings absorb at least three times their weight in fluid. The products have a high specific heat to provide a cooling effect; the sheets may be refrigerated for maximum cooling.

INDICATIONS

To dress and manage pressure ulcers (stages 1 to 4), venous stasis ulcers, first- and second-degree burns, cuts, abrasions, skin irritations, radiation dermatitis, diabetic ulcers, foot ulcers, postsurgical incisions, and skin conditions associated with peristomal care. May also be used on partial- and full-thickness wounds, tunneling wounds, infected and noninfected wounds, wounds with moderate exudate, wounds with serosanguineous drainage, and red, yellow, or black wounds.

CONTRAINDICATIONS

- Heavily draining wounds.

APPLICATION

- Flush the wound with a suitable cleanser, such as Skintegrity Wound Cleanser.
- Remove the dressing's blue backing and apply moist side of the dressing to the wound bed.
- Cover with a secondary dressing, such as OptiFoam Gentle or Stratasorb.

REMOVAL

- Change the dressing according to the wound condition and amount of exudate, or as directed by the physician.
- The dressing may remain in place up to 3 days.
- Gently lift to remove.

REFERENCE

1. http://www.medline.com/product/CarraDres-Clear-Hydrogel-Sheets/Sheet-Dressings/Z05-PF00184

HYDROGELS

Carrasyn Gel Wound Dressing

Carrasyn Spray Gel Wound Dressing

Carrasyn V

Medline Industries, Inc.

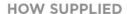

HOW SUPPLIED

Carrasyn gel wound dressing

Tube	3 oz	A6248

Carrasyn spray gel wound dressing

Bottle	8 oz	A6248

Carrasyn V

Tube	3 oz	A6248

ACTION

Carrasyn hydrogel products provide a moist environment to support healing. All three are nonoily hydrogels with a high water content and aloe. Carrasyn V is a thicker, more viscous formulation to better remain in place in the wound bed.

INDICATIONS

All three products manage pressure ulcers (stages 1 to 4), venous stasis ulcers, first- and second-degree burns, cuts, abrasions, skin irritations, radiation dermatitis, diabetic ulcers, foot ulcers, postsurgical incisions, and skin conditions associated with peristomal care. They may also be used on partial- and full-thickness wounds, tunneling wounds, infected and non-infected wounds, wounds with serosanguineous drainage, and red, yellow, or black wounds.

CONTRAINDICATIONS

- Contraindicated in patients with known sensitivity to aloe vera extract.
- Heavily draining wounds.

APPLICATION

- Flush the wound with a suitable wound cleanser, such as CarraKlenz, UltraKlenz, or MicroKlenz.

Carrasyn gel wound dressing and Carrasyn V (when a thicker formulation of gel is desired)

- Apply a generous amount of gel to the wound area in a layer about 1/4″ (0.5 cm) thick.
- Apply a secondary dressing. If using gauze as a secondary dressing, moisten it first.

Carrasyn spray gel wound dressing

- Adjust the nozzle setting on the bottle to either spray or stream.
- Apply a generous amount of gel, about 1/4″ (0.5 cm) thick, to the wound and wound margins.

- Apply spray gel as often as needed, usually daily.
- Apply a secondary dressing. If using gauze as a cover dressing, moisten it first.

REMOVAL

- Change all hydrogel dressings as often as needed, usually daily.
- Flush the wound with normal saline solution or an appropriate wound cleanser, such as Skintegrity Wound Cleanser.

REFERENCE

1. https://www.medline.com/product/Carrasyn-Hydrogel/Hydrogel-Dressings/Z05-PF00176

DermaGauze

DermaRite Industries, LLC

HOW SUPPLIED

Hydrogel-Impregnated Gauze Wound Dressing	2″ × 2″	A6231
Hydrogel-Impregnated Gauze Wound Dressing	4″ × 4″	A6231

ACTION

DermaGauze™ is a gauze dressing impregnated with a vitamin-E–enriched hydrogel. DermaGauze helps maintain a moist healing environment in partial- and full-thickness wounds.

INDICATIONS

DermaGauze is a primary dressing that may be used for the management of acute or chronic partial- and full-thickness wounds that are dry or have minimal exudate.

CONTRAINDICATIONS

- DermaGauze should not be used on people who are sensitive or allergic to the dressing and its components. Bleeding should be controlled before applying the dressing.

APPLICATION

- Cleanse the wound with the advised liquid to remove the residue according to the local infection control protocol. Deep wounds should be well irrigated.
- The skin around the wound should be clean and dry. Use skin barrier prep as needed.
- Remove the dressing from the package.
- Apply the dressing to the wound bed; loosely fill empty space in deep wounds.
- Secure with the appropriate cover dressing that manages drainage and maintains a moist wound environment.

REMOVAL

- The dressing may be moistened to ease removal.
- Carefully remove adhesive dressings by holding the edge of the dressing and slowly pulling it parallel to the skin.
- Dispose of in accordance with local guidance.

REFERENCE

1. http://dermarite.com/product/dermagauze/

HYDROGELS

DermaGel Hydrogel Sheet

Medline Industries, Inc.

HOW SUPPLIED

Sheet	4" × 4"	A6242

ACTION

DermaGel Hydrogel Sheet is a soft, flexible, semiocclusive hydrogel dressing that creates a moist healing environment. It is 65% glycerin so that it does not liquefy into the wound, and it absorbs about five times its own weight in exudate.

INDICATIONS

To manage leg ulcers, pressure ulcers (stages 1 to 4), superficial wounds, lacerations, cuts, abrasions, donor sites, partial- and full-thickness wounds, infected and noninfected wounds, and wounds with light to moderate drainage.

CONTRAINDICATIONS

- Heavily draining wounds.
- Contraindicated for patients with known hypersensitivity to glycerin.

APPLICATION

- Clean the application site with normal saline solution or an appropriate wound cleanser, such as Skintegrity Wound Cleanser. Dry the surrounding area to ensure that it is free from greasy substances.
- Remove the clear plastic cover from the dressing, and apply the pad to the wound. Leave the cloth backing in place.
- Tape the edges of the dressing to keep it in place or use an elastic net to secure it without adhesive.
- If waterproofing is desired, cover with a transparent film.

REMOVAL

- Change the dressing every 2 to 5 days, depending on the amount of drainage.
- Carefully press down on the skin, and lift an edge of the dressing. Continue around the dressing until all edges are free.
- Remember to clean the wound with each dressing change.

REFERENCE

1. https://www.medline.com/product/DermaGel-Hydrogel-Sheets/Sheet-Dressings/Z05-PF00185

HYDROGELS

DermaSyn

DermaRite Industries, LLC

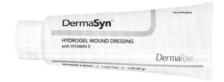

HOW SUPPLIED

Hydrogel Wound Dressing with Vitamin E	3 oz	A6248
Hydrogel Wound Dressing with Vitamin E	8 oz	A6248

ACTION

DermaSyn® is a nonoily amorphous hydrogel wound dressing enriched with vitamin E that assists with autolytic debridement while providing and/or maintaining a moist wound environment.

INDICATIONS

Wound treatments should be under the supervision of a healthcare professional. Use for the management of partial- and full-thickness dry to minimally draining wounds including:
- Diabetic ulcers.
- Vascular ulcers.
- Pressure ulcers.
- Abrasions and lacerations.
- Minor burns.
- Minor cuts.
- Sunburn.

CONTRAINDICATIONS

- DermaSyn hydrogel should not be used on people who are sensitive or allergic to the dressing and its components.

APPLICATION

- Flush the wound with a cleanser and per the infection control protocol.
- Leave the wound bed moist. Pat the periwound area dry.
- Apply hydrogel directly to the wound at 1/4th inch thickness, avoid overlapping onto the skin.
- Apply the cover dressing that manages the wound drainage and maintains a moist wound bed.

REMOVAL

- Reapply every 24 to 72 hours.
- Change if drainage shows through the back of the dressing or if the edge of the dressing becomes loose; or if the condition of the wound or the surrounding skin causes concern; or as directed by a qualified healthcare professional.
- Initially the wound may appear larger and deeper as autolysis occurs.
- The dressing may be moistened to ease removal.
- Carefully remove the adhesive dressing by holding the edge of the dressing and slowly pulling it parallel to the skin.
- Dispose of in accordance with local guidance.

REFERENCE

1. http://dermarite.com/product/dermasyn/

Elasto-Gel™
Elasto-Gel™ Plus

Southwest Technologies, Inc.

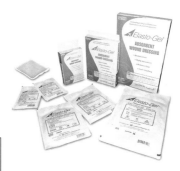

HOW SUPPLIED
Elasto-Gel™

Sheet Without Tape	2″ × 3″ (5 cm × 7.5 cm); (5 ea/box, 40 boxes/ case)	A6242
Sheet Without Tape	4″ × 4″ (10 cm × 10 cm); (5 ea/box, 20 boxes/ case)	A6242
Sheet Without Tape	5″ × 5″ (12.7 cm × 12.7 cm); (5 ea/box, 20 boxes/ case)	A6243
Sheet Without Tape	6″ × 8″ (15 cm × 20 cm); (5 ea/box, 5″boxes/case)	A6243
Sheet Without Tape	8″ × 16″ (20 cm × 40 cm); (5 ea/box, 5 boxes/case)	A6244
Sheet Without Tape	12″ × 12″ (30 cm × 30 cm); (5 ea/box, 5 boxes/case)	A6244

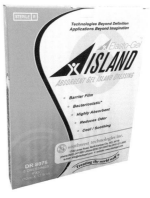

Elasto-Gel Plus

Sheet with Tape	4″ × 4″ (10 cm × 10 cm) (5 ea/box, 20 boxes/ case), bill tape separately	A6242
Sheet with Tape	2″ × 3″ (5 cm × 7.5 cm) (5 ea/box, 20 boxes/ case) tape not affixed, bill tape separately	A6242
Sheet with Tape	8″ × 8″ (20 cm × 20 cm) horseshoe-shaped tape affixed; (5 ea/box, 5 boxes/case)	A6247

ACTION

Elasto-Gel™ absorbs exudate and seals, protects, and cushions the wound. It permits water vapor transmission and is bacteriostatic*. It also reduces odor, acts as a thermal barrier, and reduces pressure.

INDICATIONS

To manage first- and second-degree burns, cuts, abrasions, surgical incisions, foot and leg ulcers, pressure ulcers (stages 1 to 4), partial- and full-thickness wounds, wounds with moderate drainage, wounds with serosanguineous drainage, and red, yellow, or black wounds.

---

*Elasto-Gel™ has not been proven to prevent infection at the wound site.

HYDROGELS

CONTRAINDICATIONS

- Contraindicated for highly exuding wounds that may require packing.

APPLICATION

- Clean the wound with normal saline solution or suitable wound cleanser. Select the appropriate size dressing or cut one to the desired size or shape. It should extend 1″ to 2″ (2.5 to 5 cm) beyond the wound opening. Leave the clear plastic film on the gel while cutting.
- Remove the clear plastic film, and apply the exposed gel directly on the wound. Don't remove the white fabric backing.
- Secure the dressing with tape, elastic or gauze wrap, or stretch netting.
- If the dressing is exposed to moisture, protect it from contamination with a waterproof covering, such as the tape supplied with the dressing.

REMOVAL

- Change the dressing when it is saturated with exudate.

Elasto-Gel™ Island

Southwest Technologies, Inc.

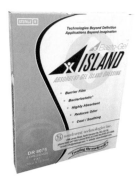

HOW SUPPLIED

Sheet with Adhesive Border, Gel	4″ × 5″ (10 cm × 12.7 cm) (5 ea/box, 20 boxes/case)	A6246

ACTION

Elasto-Gel™ Island is designed to provide effective management of a wide variety of wounds and to protect the skin and newly formed tissue. The gel's high glycerin content facilitates the natural wound-healing process. Glycerin is a main component in every fat molecule and is a natural moisturizing agent. Elasto-Gel™ Island provides cool, soothing relief when applied to an open wound. It will not dry out and is bacteriostatic*. Latex free with gel and adhesive.

INDICATIONS

To manage first- and second-degree burns, cuts, abrasions, surgical incisions, foot and leg ulcers, pressure ulcers (stages 1 to 4), partial-thickness wounds, wounds with moderate drainage, wounds with serosanguineous drainage, and red, yellow, or black wounds.

CONTRAINDICATIONS

- Contraindicated for highly exuding wounds that may require packing with additional dressing or other highly absorbent material.

APPLICATION

- Clean the wound with normal saline solution or an appropriate wound cleanser.
- Remove the sterile gel dressing from the package.
- Remove the protective cover to expose the gel and adhesive.
- Apply the dressing to the wound, being sure that the gel fully covers the wound area.
- Gently press the adhesive border to assure a watertight seal.
- Change the dressing as needed (if leaking occurs and/or the dressing becomes highly saturated with exudate).
- Consult a physician if signs of infection occur (such as redness, swelling, or fever).

REMOVAL

- Change the dressing when it is saturated with exudate.

*Elasto-Gel™ Island has not been proven to prevent infection at the wound site.

HYDROGELS

Elasto-Gel™ Island Mini

Southwest Technologies, Inc.

HOW SUPPLIED

Tape	1.25″ square affixed to a T-shaped tape	A6245

ACTION

Because of its high glycerin content, Elasto-Gel™ Island Mini assists in the natural wound-healing process. The soft gel pad provides a protective cushion to the injury, is highly absorbent, won't dry out, and is bacteriostatic*. Elasto-Gel™ Island Mini absorbent dressing is a uniquely formulated glycerin gel pad attached to a hypoallergenic, water-resistant, adhesive T-shaped tape.

INDICATIONS

To manage small wounds on the digits, face, elbows, heels, and feet. Use on wounds with moderate drainage, wounds with serosanguineous drainage, and red or yellow wounds.

CONTRAINDICATIONS

- Contraindicated for highly exuding wounds that may require packing with additional dressing or other highly absorbent material.

APPLICATION

- Prepare the wound site by cleaning the wound, as needed.

Securing the digit area

- Fold the dressing under the digit first and then overlap the tape to make a waterproof seal.
- Wrap one side of the dressing down around the digit and then repeat with the other side of the dressing.
- Don't get the gel wet. Make a waterproof seal to protect the gel from getting wet. The product may be worn in the shower if the tape is properly secured.
- When using on small wounds other than the digit, the gel square may be ripped from the "T" portion of the tape and then that tape can be used as extra securing over the square.

REMOVAL

- Change the dressing if leaking occurs or if the dressing becomes highly saturated with exudate. When applied to intact skin or directly to the toenail, the dressing may be left in place for up to 7 days.

HYDROGELS

---

*Elasto-Gel™ Island Mini has not been proven to prevent infection at the wound site.

Gold Dust®

Southwest Technologies, Inc.

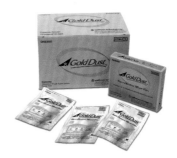

HOW SUPPLIED

Hydrogel Wound Filler with Super Aabsorbent Properties	3 g per packet; (10 packets/box, 10 boxes/case)	A6248

ACTION

Gold Dust is a highly absorbent hydrophilic polymer capable of absorbing 100 times its own weight (over 300 mL) and retaining the exudate in the matrix, even under high pressures. Therefore, when used as a wound dressing, Gold Dust protects the wound and the surrounding periwound area from maceration and degradation. Once the granules interact with the wound exudate, the powder turns into a gel filling the dead space.

INDICATIONS

To manage heavy drainage.

CONTRAINDICATIONS

• Not for use on wounds without drainage.

APPLICATION

• Premoisten Gold Dust® granules to form a gel to avoid overdrying the tissue. Mix the packet with 30 cc of water, mix rapidly to form a gel.
• Fill the cavity with the gel from step one.
• It is recommended that Gold Dust® be covered with a nonadherent dressing.

REMOVAL

• The product doesn't have to be changed daily.
• Gold Dust may be flushed using a saline solution or an irrigation system.

HYDROGELS

Hydrogel

Gentell

HOW SUPPLIED

Filler	4-oz tube	A6248
Filler	8-oz bottle	A6248

ACTION

Gentell Hydrogel is an Aloe Vera-based hydrating wound gel that protects the wound bed. Because it contains less water than other hydrogels, Gentell Hydrogel is more viscous and less "runny." Aloe is also a source of ace mannin, in addition to other mono- and polysaccharides, amino acids, glycoproteins, vitamins, and enzymes.

INDICATIONS

Use Gentell Hydrogel on Stage 2–4 wounds with little or no drainage, diabetic skin ulcers, venous stasis ulcers, first and second-degree burns, post-surgical incisions, cuts, and abrasions.

CONTRAINDICATIONS

- Gentell Hydrogel is not indicated for infected wounds or those with heavy exudate.

APPLICATION

- Irrigate the wound with Gentell Wound Cleanser and gently dry the skin surrounding the wound site.
- Apply a 1/8 inch layer of Gentell Hydrogel to the entire surface of the wound using an appropriate clean applicator or gauze to sufficiently cover the wound bed.
- Cover the wound with a secondary dressing like Gentell Bordered Gauze or Gentell Comfortell™.

REMOVAL

- Change daily or as ordered by a physician.

Hydrogel Gauze

Gentell

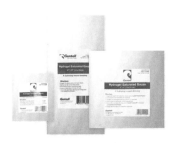

HOW SUPPLIED

Gauze	2″ × 2″	A6231
Gauze	4″ × 4″	A6231
Gauze	4″ × 8″	A6243

ACTION

Gentell Hydrogel Saturated Gauze is 12-ply gauze fully saturated in crystal-clear, viscous Aloe Vera-based hydrating wound gel. Hydrogel Gauze protects the wound bed and enhances the environment essential to the healing process. Aloe Vera is also a source of ace mannin, in addition to other mono- and polysaccharides, amino acids, glycoproteins, vitamins, and enzymes.

INDICATIONS

Use Gentell Hydrogel on Stage 2–4 wounds with little or no drainage, diabetic skin ulcers, venous stasis ulcers, first- and second-degree burns, post-surgical incisions, cuts, and abrasions.

CONTRAINDICATIONS

- Gentell Hydrogel is not indicated for infected wounds or those with heavy exudate.

APPLICATION

- Irrigate the wound with Gentell Wound Cleanser and gently dry the skin surrounding the wound site.
- To apply, peel open the pouch and remove the Hydrogel Gauze pad.
- Following your standard protocol, cover or pack the wound loosely with Gentell Hydrogel Gauze.
- Cover the wound with a secondary dressing such as Gentell Bordered Gauze or Gentell Comfortell™.

REMOVAL

- Change daily or as ordered by a physician.

HYDROGELS

INTRASITE Gel Hydrogel Wound Dressing

Smith & Nephew, Inc.
Wound Management

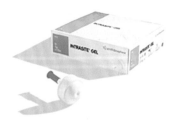

HOW SUPPLIED

Applipaks	8 g	A6248
Applipaks	15 g	A6248
Applipaks	25 g	A6248

ACTION

INTRASITE Gel is an amorphous hydrogel that gently rehydrates necrotic tissue, facilitating autolytic debridement, while being able to loosen and absorb slough and exudate. It can also be used to provide the optimum moist wound management environment during the later stages of wound closure. It is nonadherent and doesn't harm viable tissue or the skin surrounding the wound. This makes INTRASITE Gel ideal for every stage in the wound management process.

INDICATIONS

INTRASITE Gel is used to create a moist wound environment for the treatment of conditions such as minor burns, superficial lacerations, cuts and abrasions (partial-thickness wounds), and skin tears. Under the direction of a health care professional, INTRASITE Gel is used to create a moist wound environment for the management of venous ulcers (leg ulcers), surgical incisions, diabetic foot ulcers, and pressure ulcers (including stage 4). INTRASITE creates a moist wound environment, which assists in autolytic debridement of wounds covered with necrotic tissues.

CONTRAINDICATIONS

- Contraindicated in patients who are sensitive to INTRASITE Gel or any of its ingredients.
- Should be used with care in the vicinity of the eyes and in deep wounds with narrow openings (e.g., fistulas) where removal of the gel may be difficult.
- For external use only; not to be taken internally.

APPLICATION

- Prepare the wound site. Remove the secondary dressing. Irrigate the wound with sterile saline solution to clean the site.
- Prepare the pack. Remove the blue protective cap from the nozzle. Swab the snap-off tip and nozzle of the pack with a suitable antiseptic swab. Snap the patterned tip off the nozzle.
- Introduce INTRASITE Gel into the wound. Keeping the nozzle tip clear of the wound surface, gently press the bowl of the pack to dispense gel into the wound. Smooth INTRASITE Gel over the surface of the wound to a depth of about 5 mm (0.2″). Discard any unused gel.
- Dress the wound. Cover with a secondary dressing of choice, for example:
  - Necrotic stage: Site Flexigrid Moisture Vapour Permeable Adhesive Film Dressing.
  - Sloughy stage: Allevyn Hydrocellular Hydrophilic Wound Dressing/Melolin Low-Adherent Absorbent Dressing.
  - Granulating stage: Allevyn/Melolin/OpSite Flexigrid.

HYDROGELS

REMOVAL

- INTRASITE Gel can be removed from the wound by rinsing with sterile saline solution.
- On necrotic and sloughy wounds, it is recommended that the dressing be changed at least every 3 days.
- On clean granulating wounds, the frequency of dressing changes depends on the clinical condition of the wound and the amount of exudate produced.

Prontosan® Wound Gel

B. Braun Medical Inc.

HOW SUPPLIED

| Gel | 30 mL | A6248 |

ACTION

Prontosan® Wound Gel:

When the PHMB (polyhexanide) comes in contact with bacteria, the outer cell wall of the bacteria is disrupted, resulting in leakage of cytoplasm and cell death. As a consequence, cell replication ceases and mutation cannot occur. A clear, colorless, and virtually odorless aqueous wound cleanser with surfactants. The preservative contained within the Gel disrupts the bacteria on and within the Gel to help provide a bacteria-free wound dressing.

INDICATIONS

Prontosan® Wound Gel is intended to cleanse and moisten wound beds and for the management of ulcers, first- and second-degree burns, cuts, partial- and full-thickness wounds, and surgical incisions. It can be used during wound dressing changes to soften encrusted wound dressings.
- Prontosan® Wound Gel may be used:
  - For cleansing wounds or wound coatings even when surfaces are difficult to access such as deep wound cavities, fissures, and wound pockets.
  - For cleansing and moistening chronic skin wounds.
  - For moistening of bandages and wound dressings, such as compresses, gauze, pads, sponges, etc.
  - During dressing changes to loosen encrusted bandaging or other encrusted wound dressings.

CONTRAINDICATIONS

- Prontosan® Wound Gel should not be used if there is a history of allergy to any of the ingredients.
- Do not use in the presence of a hyaline cartilage.
- Do not use in combination with anionic tensides as these may impair preservation.
- Mixing Prontosan Wound Gel with other wound-cleansing soaps, lotions, ointments, oils, or enzymes may lower efficacy. When such substances need to be removed from a wound, ensure the entire wound area is thoroughly rinsed with a cleansing solution such as Prontosan Wound Irrigation Solution.

APPLICATION

For general use

- Rinsing and cleansing the wound and surrounding area are recommended prior to application of Prontosan Wound Gel. Prontosan Wound Irrigation Solution can be used for this purpose. Refer to cleansing solution instructions for use.
- Apply a 3- to 5-mm coating of Prontosan Wound Gel directly to shallow flat wound surfaces or deep wound fissures. Bandages or dressings soaked in Prontosan Wound Gel can be used for cleaning as required.

HYDROGELS

- Prontosan Wound Gel can be used to sustain wound moisture for the duration of time between dressing changes per institutional protocol.

Directions

- Use aseptic technique.
  - To open, screw the cap down fully to pierce the container.
  - Remove the cap and proceed with use as required in accordance with the institutional protocol.
  - Replace the cap after use in accordance with the institutional protocol.

REMOVAL

- Prontosan Wound Gel is water soluble. To remove, irrigate with Saline or Prontosan Irrigation Solution when changing dressing according to institutional protocol.

REFERENCES

Preservative Testing[1]
No microbial growth was observed at 7, 14, and 28 days for the following organisms:
Acinetobacter baumannii.
Enterobacter cloacae.
Enterococcus faecalis.
Vancomycin-resistant *Enterococcus faecalis* (VRE).
Escherichia coli.
Proteus mirabilis.
Pseudomonas aeruginosa.
Serratia marcescens.
Staphylococcus aureus.
Methicillin-resistant *S. aureus* (MRSA).
Staphylococcus epidermidis.
Candida albicans.
[1]Preservative effectiveness demonstrated using USP 51, with an expanded list of organisms, to support the role of PHMB as a preservative to inhibit microbial growth within the product during shelf storage.
   Antimicrobial Effectiveness Testing Successfully Meets USP 51 Category 2 Criteria.

Organisms	Result Day 14	Result Day 28
Escherichia coli (ATCC 8739)	Greater than 2.0 log reduction from the initial count	No increase from the 14 days count
Pseudomonas aeruginosa (ATCC 9027)	Greater than 2.0 log reduction from the initial count	No increase from the 14 days count
Staphylococcus aureus (ATCC 6538)	Greater than 2.0 log reduction from the initial count	No increase from the 14 days count
Candida albicans (ATCC 10231)	No increase from the initial calculated count	No increase from the initial calculated count
Aspergillus niger (ATCC 16404)	No increase from the initial calculated count	No increase from the initial calculated count

HYDROGELS

New Product: Prontosan® Wound Gel X

B. Braun Medical Inc.

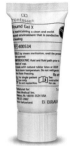

HOW SUPPLIED

Prontosan® Wound Gel X is a clear, colorless, and virtually odorless aqueous amorphous hydrogel wound dressing	250 g	A6248

Prontosan Wound Gel X contains 0.1% polyaminopropyl biguanide (polyhexanide [PHMB]), alkylamidopropyl betaine, purified water, hydroxyethyl cellulose, and glycerol. PHMB is added to the product as a preservative to inhibit the growth of microorganisms within the product.

ACTION

Prontosan Wound Gel X:
- Is an effective microbial barrier.
- Resists microbial colonization within the dressing.
- Reduces microbial penetration through the dressing.
- Softens necrotic tissue facilitating autolytic debridement.

INDICATIONS

Prontosan Wound Gel X is indicated for the management of ulcers (including diabetic foot and leg ulcers and pressure ulcers), first- and second-degree burns, partial- and full-thickness wounds, large surface area wounds, and surgical incisions.

CONTRAINDICATIONS

- Prontosan Wound Gel X should not be used if there is a history of allergy to any of the ingredients.
- Do not use in the presence of a hyaline cartilage.
- Do not use in combination with anionic surfactants as these may impair preservation.
- Mixing Prontosan Wound Gel X with other wound-cleansing soaps, lotions, ointments, oils, or enzymes may lower efficacy.
- Do not use in the middle or inner ear.
- Do not use in the eyes.

APPLICATION

Instructions for use

- For general use:
  - Rinsing and cleansing the wound and surrounding area is recommended prior to the application of Prontosan Wound Gel X. Prontosan Wound Irrigation Solution can be used for this purpose. Refer to cleansing solution instructions for use.
  - Apply a generous amount of Prontosan Wound Gel X directly to the wound.
  - Prontosan Wound Gel X can be used to sustain wound moisture for the duration of time between dressing changes per institutional protocol.
- Use an aseptic technique.
  - Remove the cap from the tube.
  - Invert the screw cap and press the keyed indent on the cap top onto the keyed sealed tube. Ensure the cap is firmly seated. Rotate the cap to open the seal on the tube.
  - Proceed with use as required in accordance with the institutional protocol.
  - Replace the cap after use in accordance with the institutional protocol.

HYDROGELS

REMOVAL

- Gel X is water soluble. To remove, irrigate with saline or Prontosan Irrigation Solution when changing dressing according to institutional protocol.

REFERENCES

1. American Burn Association. Burn incidence and treatment in the United States: 2015. Available at http://www.ameriburn.org/resources_factsheet.php. Accessed February 15, 2016.
2. American Burn Association. *National Burn Repository 2015 Report*. Chicago, IL: American Burn Association; 2015.
3. Selig HF, Lumenta DB, Giretzlehner M, et al. The properties of an "ideal" burn wound dressing—what do we need in daily clinical practice? Results of a worldwide online survey among burn care specialists. *Burns*. 2012;38(7):960–966.
4. Sussman G. Management of the wound environment with dressings and topical agents. In: Sussman C, Bates-Jensen BM, eds. *Wound Care: A Collaborative Practice Manual*. 4th ed. Baltimore, MD: Lippincott Williams & Wilkins; 2012:502–520.
5. *Wound Gel X DOF*. Bethlehem, PA: B. Braun; 2014.
6. Bradbury S, Fletcher J. Prontosan made easy. *Wounds Int*. 2011;2(2):1–6.
7. Vowden K, Vowden P. Debridement made easy. *Wounds Int*. 2011;7(4):1–4.
8. Valenzuela AR, Perucho NS. [The effectiveness of a 0.1% polyhexanide gel]. *Rev Enferm*. 2008;31(4):7–12.
9. *Prontosan Wound Gel X IFU*. Bethlehem, PA: B. Braun. 2014.
10. Dabiri G, Damstetter E, Phillips T. Choosing a wound dressing based on common wound characteristics. *Adv Wound Care (New Rochelle)*. 2016;5(1):32–41.

HYDROGELS

Purilon® Gel

Coloplast

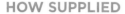

HOW SUPPLIED

Tube	0.28 oz (8 g)	A6248
Tube	0.5 oz (15 g)	A6248
Tube	0.88 oz (25 g)	A6248

ACTION

Purilon® Gel is a sterile, clear, cohesive, amorphous hydrogel with hydrating and absorbing properties that provides effective autolytic debridement of necrotic tissue, while maintaining a moist wound environment.

INDICATIONS

To treat necrotic and sloughy wounds, such as leg ulcers, pressure ulcers, and noninfected diabetic foot ulcers, which can only heal with secondary intent. May also be used on first- and second-degree burns. The gel may be used throughout the healing process to provide a moist healing environment in all types of wounds, except those mentioned under cautions.

CAUTION

- May be used on patients with local or systemic infections under the discretion of a healthcare professional.
- Wounds which are solely or mainly caused by an arterial insufficiency or diabetic wounds (primarily lower leg and foot) should be inspected by a healthcare professional, depending on the clinical condition.

APPLICATION

- Clean the wound with physiological saline or tap water. Gently dry the skin around the wound.
- Remove the label from the accordion pack by pulling the corner, as indicated on the package. Swab the nozzle below the snap-off tip with a suitable antiseptic; remove the tip.
- Gently press the base of the accordion pack to apply Purilon Gel to the wound, in a layer no higher than the periwound skin.
- Cover with a secondary dressing. For slightly to moderately exuding wounds, choose a hydrocolloid as a secondary dressing, for example, Comfeel® Plus. For moderately to severely exuding wounds, choose a highly absorbent or highly permeable dressing to cover the wound, for example, Biatain® Dressings.

REMOVAL

- For necrotic and sloughy wounds, change Purilon Gel at least every 3 days. For clean wounds, change Purilon Gel according to the amount of exudate.
- To remove the gel from the wound, rinse with physiological saline or tap water.

REFERENCE

1. https://www.coloplast.us/wound/wound-/solutions/#section=Purilon%c2%ae_82170

RadiaDres Gel Sheet

Medline Industries, Inc.

HOW SUPPLIED

Sheet	4″ × 4″	A6242

ACTION

RadiaDres Gel Sheet is a sterile, clear, oxygen-permeable gel sheet for radiation-related skin reactions. The sheet is composed of a high water content, cross-linked polymer matrix that facilitates the formation of a moist wound-healing environment, while preventing bacteria and foreign matter from entering the wound. The RadiaDres Gel Sheet may be refrigerated for maximum cooling effect.

INDICATIONS

For management of pressure ulcers (stages 1 to 4), partial-thickness draining and nondraining wounds, first- and second-degree burns, radiation reactions, and noninfected wounds.

CONTRAINDICATIONS

- Heavily draining wounds.
- Contraindicated for infected wounds.

APPLICATION

- Before application, thoroughly cleanse the wound with an appropriate wound cleanser, such as Skintegrity Wound Cleanser. Gently dry the skin surrounding the wound.
- Peel open the package and remove RadiaDres Gel Sheet using a clean technique.
- Grab the tabbed edges of the pink polyethylene film backing to remove. Discard the backing.
- Apply the uncovered hydrogel side to the wound. RadiaDres Gel Sheet may overlap intact skin if desired.
- The dressing may be trimmed or overlapped, if preferred, to more closely approximate the wound size and shape.
- Apply a secondary dressing, such as Medline Bordered Gauze or Stratasorb.

REMOVAL

- To remove, carefully lift an edge of the dressing while gently pressing against the skin.
- Change as often as necessary until the wound is healed. May be left on up to 3 days.
- Before applying a new dressing, cleanse the wound with a suitable cleanser, such as Skintegrity Wound Cleanser.

REFERENCE

1. https://www.medline.com/product/RadiaDres-Clear-Hydrogel-Sheets/Hydrogel-Dressings/Z05-PF00186

HYDROGELS

Restore™ Hydrogel Dressing*

Hollister Wound Care

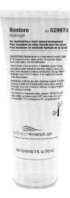

HOW SUPPLIED

Amorphous/tube	3 oz	A6248

ACTION

Restore™ hydrogel maintains a moist wound environment.

INDICATIONS

For maintenance of a moist environment in partial- and full-thickness wounds.

CONTRAINDICATIONS

- For external use only.
- Not for contact with eyes.

APPLICATION

- Cleanse the wound if indicated.
- Apply to cover the wound to a minimum depth of 1/5″ (5 mm). Cover with a secondary dressing as required and secure.

REMOVAL

- Change the dressing every 24 to 72 hours or as required to maintain a moist environment.
- If the condition worsens or doesn't improve within 7 days, consult a physician. Keep out of reach of children. In case of ingestion, seek professional help.

*See package insert for complete instructions for use.

Skintegrity Amorphous Hydrogel

Skintegrity Hydrogel Impregnated Gauze

Medline Industries, Inc.

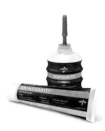

HOW SUPPLIED

Bellows bottle	1 oz	A6248
Tube	4 oz	A6248
Impregnated gauze	2" × 2"	A6231
Impregnated gauze	4" × 4"	A6231
Impregnated gauze	4" × 4", 2 per pack	A6231

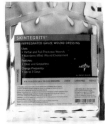

ACTION

Skintegrity Hydrogel dressings are greaseless and maintain a moist healing environment. Skintegrity Hydrogel Impregnated Gauze is a compression-saturated gauze sponge, which ensures thorough hydration. A special formulation balances viscosity and hydration, added aloe vera aids healing, and the greaseless formulation irrigates easily from the wound bed.

INDICATIONS

To manage pressure ulcers (stages 2 to 4), partial- or full-thickness wounds, venous stasis ulcers, first- and second-degree burns, cuts, abrasions, skin irritations, postoperative incisions, infected and noninfected wounds, and wounds with no drainage or light drainage.

CONTRAINDICATIONS

- Heavily draining wounds.
- Contraindicated in patients who are hypersensitive to components of the gel.

APPLICATION

- Clean the wound with normal saline solution or appropriate wound cleanser, such as Skintegrity Wound Cleanser.
- Dry the periwound skin.

Skintegrity amorphous hydrogel

- Apply a generous layer of hydrogel to all wound surfaces.
- Cover with an appropriate secondary dressing, such as Stratasorb or Medline Bordered Gauze.
- Repeat every 72 hours or as necessary to maintain a moist wound bed.

Skintegrity hydrogel–impregnated gauze

- Unfold the hydrogel gauze pad and loosely pack it in the wound bed, filling any undermining and tunneling areas.
- Cover with an appropriate secondary dressing, such as Stratasorb or Medline Bordered Gauze.
- Change the dressing every 72 hours or as necessary to maintain a moist wound bed.

HYDROGELS

REMOVAL

- Carefully remove the secondary dressing and irrigate the wound bed with a normal saline solution or appropriate wound cleanser, such as Skintegrity Wound Cleanser. Dry the periwound skin.
- If the dressing has dried to the wound edge or the base of the wound, moisten with Skintegrity Wound Cleanser or normal saline solution until it loosens, then remove it.

REFERENCES

1. Skintegrity Amorphous Hydrogel. https://www.medline.com/product/Skintegrity-Hydrogel/Gel/Z05-PF00182
2. Skintegrity Impregnated Gauze. https://www.medline.com/product/Skintegrity-Hydrogel-Impregnated-Gauze/Hydrogel-Dressings/Z05-PF00235

HYDROGELS

SOLOSITE Wound Gel
SOLOSITE Gel Conformable Wound Dressing

Smith & Nephew, Inc.
Wound Management

HOW SUPPLIED
SOLOSITE Wound Gel

Tube	3 oz	A6248
Push-Button Applicators	2 oz	A6248
Push-Button Applicators	7 oz	A6248

SOLOSITE gel conformable wound dressing

Gel Pad	2″ × 2″	A6231
Gel Pad	4″ × 4″	A6231

ACTION
SOLOSITE wound gel

SOLOSITE is a hydrogel wound dressing with preservatives. It can donate moisture to rehydrate nonviable tissue. It absorbs exudate while retaining its structure in the wound. It rehydrates and helps deslough dry eschar, absorbs exudate, and assists autolytic debridement. It is nonirritating, nonsensitizing, gentle to fragile granulation tissue.

SOLOSITE gel conformable wound dressing

SOLOSITE Gel Conformable is designed to keep the gel in intimate contact with the wound bed. It is ideal for packing into and around the sides of the wound. While wound gels alone tend to pool at the base of deeper wounds leaving portions of the wound bed uncovered, SOLOSITE Gel Conformable maintains close contact between the wound surface and the gel. It keeps the gel in intimate contact with the wound surface, absorbs excess exudate, creates a moist wound-healing environment, which may promote desloughing, meets USP requirements for cytotoxicity, and is nonsensitizing.

INDICATIONS

Used to create a moist wound environment for the treatment of minor conditions such as minor burns, superficial lacerations, cuts and abrasions (partial-thickness wounds), and skin tears; under the direction of a health care professional, used to create a moist wound environment for the management of venous ulcers (leg ulcers), surgical incisions, diabetic foot ulcers, and pressure ulcers (including stage 4); creates a moist wound environment, which assists in autolytic debridement of wounds covered with necrotic tissues.

CONTRAINDICATIONS
SOLOSITE wound gel

- For external use only.
- If condition worsens or doesn't improve within 7 days, consult a physician.

SOLOSITE gel conformable wound dressing

- Contraindicated for the management of full-thickness burns.

HYDROGELS

APPLICATION

SOLOSITE wound gel

- Cleanse the wound with saline or an appropriate wound cleanser.
- Apply SOLOSITE Gel to cover the wound bed 1/4 9 (5-mm) thick and cover with a gauze, foam, or transparent film dressing.

SOLOSITE gel conformable wound dressing

- Gently and thoroughly cleanse the wound area of necrotic (damaged) tissue or dressing residue with sterile saline or other appropriate wound cleanser.
- Remove the pouch from the outer packaging.
- Tear open the pouch using the notched opening.
- Remove the dressing from the pouch and carefully unfold the dressing.
- Carefully place the dressing in the wound so that the entire wound bed is covered.
- Don't overlay the dressing on the healthy skin surrounding the wound because this could lead to maceration (overhydration) of the healthy skin.
- Secure the dressing in place by placing a secondary dressing of the following type over the total wound area:
  - A transparent film such as OPSITE or OPSITE FLEXIGRID, especially where the wound is necrotic (full of damaged tissue) or sloughy (full of wound fluid).
  - A nonwoven, nonsensitizing (nonallergic) dressing such as COVRSITE or retention tape such as Hypafix where there is little wound drainage.
  - Gauze held in place with a conforming bandage, a net bandage, or a cohesive bandage such as Coban, where there are skin tears and an adhesive secondary dressing is inappropriate.
- If you are unsure of which secondary dressing to use, consult a health care professional.

REMOVAL

- Change the dressing each day or as directed by the physician.

3M™ Tegaderm™ Hydrogel Wound Filler

3M™ Health Care

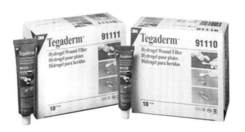

HOW SUPPLIED

Tube	15 g	A6248
Tube	25 g	A6248

ACTION

3M™ Tegaderm™ Hydrogel Wound Filler is a sterile, nonpreserved, amorphous hydrogel wound dressing. The product helps provide a moist healing environment, prevent wound desiccation, assists with autolytic debridement by hydrating devitalized tissue, and fills the dead space in full-thickness wounds.

INDICATIONS

3M™ Tegaderm™ Hydrogel Wound Filler is indicated for the management of nondraining to minimally draining dermal wounds, including pressure injuries, venous ulcers, arterial ulcers, diabetic (neuropathic) ulcers, dehisced surgical wounds, skin tears, abrasions, radiation, dermatitis, wounds exhibiting dry eschar and fibrinous slough, and malignant lesions; may be used with gauze to lightly pack tunneling or undermined chronic wounds. Can be used on infected wounds only under the care of a health professional.

CONTRAINDICATIONS

- Not designed, sold, or intended for use except as indicated.

APPLICATION

- Clean skin and wound thoroughly according to facility policy.
- If periwound skin is fragile or exposed to wound exudate is likely, apply a barrier film.
- Apply enough wound filler to cover the wound base and necrotic tissue, to a depth of approximately 5 mm thick, with no overlap to the surrounding skin. Or saturate a sterile gauze pad with wound filler and place in the wound.
- Apply appropriate cover dressing to help manage the wound drainage and maintain a moist wound environment.

REMOVAL

- Gently lift off cover dressing and discard. The frequency of changing the dressing will depend on factors such as the type of wound and the volume of drainage.
- Remove saturated gauze or rinse away the remaining gel with wound cleanser or sterile normal saline if necessary. Monitor periwound skin for maceration.
- At the time of dressing change, if the dressing is adhered to the wound surface, saturate with wound cleanser or sterile normal, allow the dressing to soften, and gently remove.
- Avoid forceful removal of the dressing to minimize disruption of the wound.

REFERENCE

1. https://www.3m.com/3M/en_US/company-us/all-3m-products/~/3M-Tegaderm-Hydrogel-Wound-Filler?N=5002385±3293321940&rt=rud

HYDROGELS

Negative-Pressure Wound Therapy

ACTIONS

Negative-pressure wound therapy (NPWT) systems include a vacuum pump, drainage tubing, and a dressing set. The pump may be stationary or portable, relies on AC or battery power, allows for regulation of the suction strength, has alarms to indicate loss of suction, and has a replaceable collection canister. The dressing sets may contain either foam or gauze dressing to be placed in the wound and an adhesive film drape for sealing the wound. The drainage tubes come in a variety of configurations depending on the dressings used or wound being treated. NPWT may also include automated instillation and provides wounds with the benefits of both NPWT and wound irrigation.

INDICATIONS

NPWT is primarily intended for chronic wounds that have been resistant to other forms of wound care, and for minimizing scarring on acute wounds by promoting healing through granulation tissue formation and re-epithelialization ("secondary intention"). Therefore, it may be used as either a primary or secondary line of treatment, depending on the type of wound.

CONTRAINDICATIONS

- Contraindications to NPWT for chronic wounds include, but may not be limited to:
  - Exposed vital organs (treatment may proceed after the organ has been covered by vicryl absorbable mesh).
  - Inadequately debrided wounds; granulation tissue that will not form over necrotic tissue.
  - Untreated osteomyelitis or sepsis within the vicinity of the wound.
  - Presence of untreated coagulopathy.
  - Necrotic tissue with eschar.
  - Malignancy in the wound (negative-pressure therapy may lead to cellular proliferation).
  - Allergy to any component required for the procedure.
- NPWT should be used cautiously when there is active bleeding, when the patient is on anticoagulants, when there is difficult wound hemostasis, or when placing the dressing in proximity to blood vessels.
- *Note:* It is the clinician's responsibility to understand the actions, indications, advantages, disadvantages, and reimbursement information for each NPWT product prior to its use. Each product under this category description may be assigned a different code based on its physical size and characteristics; or the manufacturer has not yet received or applied for a code. Please refer to individual product listings for further information about each product and verify coding of each product with the product's manufacturer.

ANASEPT® Antimicrobial Wound Irrigation Solution

Anacapa Technologies, Inc.

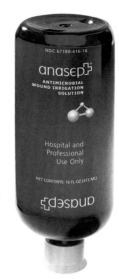

PRODUCT DESCRIPTION

Anasept Antimicrobial Wound Irrigation Solution is a clear, isotonic liquid that helps in the mechanical removal of the debris from the application site while delivering 0.057% broad-spectrum antimicrobial sodium hypochlorite to the application site via negative-pressure wound therapy (NPWT) device. Anasept Antimicrobial Wound Irrigation Solution inhibits the growth of bacteria such as *Acinetobacter baumannii, Clostridium difficile, Escherichia coli, Pseudomonas aeruginosa, Proteus mirabilis, Staphylococcus aureus, Serratia marcescens,* carbapenem-resistant *E. coli* (CRE), methicillin-resistant *S. aureus* (MRSA), vancomycin-resistant *Enterococcus faecalis* (VRE), as well as fungi such as *Candida albicans* and *Aspergillus niger* that are commonly found in the wound bed.

INDICATIONS FOR USE

Anasept Antimicrobial Wound Irrigation Solution is intended for use under the supervision of a health care professional for cleansing of foreign materials including micro-organisms from wounds such as stage I to IV pressure ulcers, diabetic foot ulcers, postsurgical wounds, first- and second-degree burns, grafted and donor sites.

CONTRAINDICATIONS

* None.

DIRECTIONS FOR USE

Must be used with a vented spike adapter set:
* Remove the dust cover from the cap.
* Insert the vented spike.
* Pull up the sling and hang on a pole or NPWT device.
* Use Anasept Antimicrobial Wound Irrigation Solution via NPWT device (follow the device manufacturers' installation instructions).
* Do not rinse.
* Repeat as necessary.

REMOVAL

* No removal necessary. See directions for use above.

OTHER CLINICAL INFORMATION

* **Bactericidal:** Including the antibiotic-resistant strains such as MRSA, VRE, and CRE.
* **Sporicidal:** Effective against *C. difficile* spores which is known to be resistant to a wide range of biocides and antibiotics. A health hazard that reached epidemic proportions in long-term care facilities.
* **Fungicidal:** Effective against the well-known pathogenic fungi *C. albicans* and *A. niger*.
* **Virucidal:** Effective against *HIV-Type 1* (human immuno deficiency virus).

- **Rapid Antimicrobial Action:** Kills most organisms in 2 minutes.
- **Biofilm:** Effective against polymicrobial biofilm, a primary cause of chronic nonhealing wounds.
- **Debridement:** Effective in solubilizing necrotic wound slough for easy removal.
- **Wound Odor Control:** Anasept is unmatched in wound odor control.
- **No known microbial resistance:** To Anasept Antimicrobial Wound Irrigation Solution.

SAFETY

Anasept has been subjected to rigorous safety testing at an independent laboratory and shown to meet the criteria for safe use:
- Modified primary skin irritation (FSHA method—7-day exposure with repeated insult to intact and abraded skin).
- Cytotoxicity (ISO agarose overlay method).
- Systemic toxicity (ISO acute systemic toxicity).
- ISO sensitization study.

CLINICALLY TESTED

Anasept has been clinically proven to reduce wound bioburden levels and improve the rate of healing.

J. Lindfors: A Comparison of an Antimicrobial Wound Cleanser to Normal Saline in Reduction of Bioburden and its Effect on Wound Healing. Ostomy/Wound Management 2004;50 (8): 28–41.

SHELF-LIFE

Two years when stored at normal room temperature 25°C (77°F). Once opened Anasept is stable for 14 weeks.

PREVENA™ Incision Management System

KCI, An ACELITY™ Company

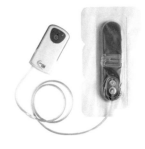

HOW SUPPLIED

PREVENA™	45ml Canister	97607, 97608
PREVENA PEEL & PLACE™ Dressing Kit	20cm, 5 pack	97607, 97608
PREVENA PEEL & PLACE™ System Kit	20cm	97607, 97608
PREVENA PEEL & PLACE™ Dressing Kit	13cm, 5 pack	97607, 97608
PREVENA PEEL & PLACE™ System Kit	13cm	97607, 97608
PREVENA PLUS™	150ml Canister	97607, 97608
PREVENA PLUS CUSTOMIZABLE™ System Kit		97607, 97608
PREVENA PLUS CUSTOMIZABLE™ Dressing Kit	5 pack	97607, 97608
PREVENA PEEL & PLACE™ Dressing Kit	35cm, 5 pack	97607, 97608
PREVENA PLUS™ System with PEEL & PLACE™ Dressing	35cm	97607, 97608
PREVENA DUO™ System with PEEL & PLACE™ Dressings	13cm/13cm	97607, 97608
PREVENA PLUS DUO™ System with PEEL & PLACE™ Dressings	13cm/20cm	97607, 97608
PREVENA PLUS DUO™ System with PEEL & PLACE™ Dressings	20cm/20cm	97607, 97608
PREVENA™ Therapy V.A.C.® Connector		97607, 97608

ACTION

The PREVENA™ Incision Management System[1] consists of a single-use therapy unit, canister, and dressing that is applied over clean, closed sutured, or stapled incisions in a simple peel-and-place process. The dressing has a built-in pressure indicator and a skin interface layer with 0.019% ionic silver, which wicks fluid from the skin surface. PREVENA™ Incision Dressing is an integrated one-piece dressing comprised of a polyurethane film with acrylic adhesive that provides adhesion of the dressing to the skin surrounding the incision and a polyurethane shell that encapsulates the foam bolster and interface layer, providing a closed system. The dressing is uniquely designed to be skin-friendly over clean, closed surgical incisions. The PREVENA™ 125 Therapy Unit delivers negative pressure that is preset to deliver -125 mm Hg to the incision site. The system also contains a sterile PREVENA™ 45ml Canister for collection of incision exudate and PREVENA™ Patch Strips, which may be used to help seal leaks around the dressing.

---

[1]See PREVENA™ Incision Management System Clinician Guide (Instructions for Use) for complete information regarding safety and application instructions.

INDICATIONS

The PREVENA™ Incision Management System is marketed in the United States as a device that is intended to manage the environment of surgical incisions (sutured or stapled) that continue to drain following sutured or stapled closure by maintaining a closed environment and removing the exudate via the application of negative-pressure wound therapy.

CONTRAINDICATIONS

- Should not be used on patients with sensitivity to silver.
- Should not be placed over drains or wires. Improper placement/cuts made to the dressing to accommodate drains or wires can lead to leak alerts.
- Should not be used to treat open or dehisced surgical incisions or patients who have excessive amounts of exudate from the incision area that may exceed the 45-mL canister limit. V.A.C.® Therapy should be considered for treatment of these wounds or incisions.
- Is not appropriate for all incisions. It may not be effective in addressing complications associated with ischemia to the incision or incision area, untreated or inadequately treated infection, inadequate hemostasis of the incision, or cellulitis of the incision area.

APPLICATIONS

- Open the sterile dressing package and remove the dressing and patch strips using an aseptic technique. Do not use if package has been torn or if sterile seal has been compromised.
- Gently peel back the center strip on the back of the dressing, exposing the pull tabs and adhesive.
- Center and apply the dressing over the closed wound or incision, ensuring that the adhesive will not contact or cover the surgical closure. Orient the dressing on the patient to eliminate sharp bends/kinks in the tubing. Remove the remaining bottom adhesive covers by grasping the bottom tabs and gently pulling. Firmly press around the dressing to ensure a good seal where the adhesive contacts the skin. Remove top stabilization layers.
- Remove the PREVENA™ 45ml Canister from the sterile package. Do not use if package has been torn or if sterile seal has been compromised. Connect the dressing tubing to the canister tubing by twisting the connectors until they lock.
- Insert the canister into the PREVENA™ 125 Therapy Unit, and slide inward until the canister clicks. The canister is fully inserted when the side tabs are flushed with the body of the therapy unit. Therapy can now begin (see section Beginning Therapy).

Beginning therapy

- To begin therapy, press and hold the ON/OFF button for **2 seconds**; an audible beep will confirm that therapy is on. A green LED on the front of the unit indicates that therapy is on. *Note:* Pressing the ON/OFF button begins the 192-hour (8-day) life cycle of the therapy unit. Turning the therapy unit off stops the life-cycle counter. Turning the therapy unit on for purposes other than delivering therapy reduces the life cycle of the therapy unit. It is not recommended to press the ON/OFF button until therapy is ready to begin. To turn therapy unit off, press and hold ON/OFF button for **5 seconds**.
- With therapy on, assess the dressing to ensure integrity of the seal.
  - The dressing should have a wrinkled appearance and the foam bolster should be compressed.
  - The pressure indicator on the dressing should be in the collapsed position.
- Place the therapy unit into the PREVENA™ System carrying case. Make sure that the display is visible through the opening in the carrying case when the front flap is lifted. The PREVENA™ System carrying case has an integrated belt loop and a separate adjustable strap to allow for versatile positioning. *Caution: Do not wear the strap around the neck.*

Duration of therapy

- Therapy should be continuous for a minimum of 2 days and up to a maximum of 7 days.
- Therapy unit will automatically time out after 192 hours (8 days) of cumulative run time.
- Patients should be instructed not to turn therapy off unless:
  - advised by the treating physician.
  - bleeding develops suddenly or in large amounts during therapy.
  - there are serious signs of allergic reaction or infection.
  - the canister is full of fluid.
  - batteries need to be changed.
  - system alerts must be addressed.
- The patient should be instructed to contact the treating physician if:
  - bleeding develops.
  - signs of infection are present.
  - therapy unit turns off and cannot be restarted before therapy is scheduled to end.
  - canister becomes full of fluid.
- At the end of therapy, the patient should return to the treating physician for dressing removal.

Indicators and alerts

- **Visual Alerts:** Flashing LEDs cannot be turned off or paused by the user. Visual alerts will only stop when the alert condition has been corrected.
- **Audible Alerts:** Repeated beeps (which in some cases will increase in volume) can be temporarily muted (paused) by pressing the ON/OFF button once. The audible alert will recur after 60 minutes unless the alert condition has been corrected.

REMOVAL (DRESSING)

- *Note*: If the dressing is lifted to observe the wound, do not readhere the same dressing; a new dressing must be applied.
- *Warning:* Dressings should always be removed in-line with the sutures and ***never*** across the sutures.
- Turn the PREVENA™ Therapy Unit off by pressing and holding the ON/OFF button for 5 seconds.
- Gently stretch the drape/dressing horizontally to release the adhesive from the skin. Do not peel vertically. Remove the drape/dressing in-line with the sutures, ***never*** across the sutures.
- Clean any residual adhesive with an alcohol swab.
- If a new dressing is to be applied:
  - Ensure that the area is clean, using an alcohol swab or antiseptic wipe.
  - Allow the skin to completely dry before applying.
  - Follow Dressing Application instructions from above.

REFERENCES

1. Willy C, Agarwal A, Andersen CA, et al. Closed incision negative pressure therapy: international multidisciplinary consensus recommendations. *Int Wound J.* 2017;14(2):385–398.
2. Grauhan O, Navasardyan A, Tutkun B, et al. Effect of surgical incision management on wound infections in a poststernotomy patient population. *Int Wound J.* 2014;11 Suppl 1:6–9.
3. Matatov T, et al. Experience with a new negative pressure incision management system in prevention of groin wound infection in vascular surgery patients. *J Vasc Surg.* 2013;57(3):791–795.

Prontosan® Wound Irrigation Solution

B. Braun Medical Inc.

HOW SUPPLIED

Wound Irrigation Solution	1000 mL

ACTION

A clear, colorless, and virtually odorless aqueous wound cleanser with surfactants. Prontosan Wound Irrigation Solution cleanses the tissue surface, even when surfaces are difficult to access such as deep wound cavities, fissures, and wound pockets. Prontosan Wound Irrigation Solution contains: Purified water, 0.1% undecylenamidopropyl betaine, 0.1% polyaminopropyl biguanide (polyhexanide [PHMB]) and pH may be adjusted with sodium hydroxide.

INDICATIONS

Prontosan® Wound Irrigation Solution is intended for cleaning wounds and for moistening and lubricating absorbent wound dressings for the management of ulcers, burns, postsurgical wounds, and abrasions.
- Prontosan® Wound Irrigation Solution may be used:
  - For cleansing and moistening chronic skin wounds.
  - For moistening of bandages and wound dressings, such as compresses, gauze, pads, sponges, gels, hydrofibers, alginates, hydrocolloids, etc.
  - During dressing changes to loosen encrusted bandaging or other encrusted wound dressings.

CONTRAINDICATIONS

- Prontosan® Wound Irrigation Solution should not be used if there is a history of allergy to any of the ingredients.
- Do not use in the presence of a hyaline cartilage.
- Do not use in combination with anionic tensides as these may impair preservation.
- Mixing Prontosan Wound Irrigation Solution with other wound-cleansing soaps, lotions, ointments, oils, or enzymes may lower efficacy. When such substances need to be removed from a wound, ensure the entire wound area is thoroughly rinsed with Prontosan Wound Irrigation Solution.

APPLICATION

For general use

- Cleanse the wounds with Prontosan Wound Irrigation Solution before further treatment is carried out.
- Bandages or dressings soaked in Prontosan Wound Irrigation Solution can be used for cleaning as required.

Cleansing the wound site

- Cleansing of a large area around the whole wound site with Prontosan Wound Irrigation Solution is recommended.
- When required, wash and decontaminate the whole section of the body or the whole body of the person affected according to the institutional protocol.
- For wounds covering a large area and wounds difficult to access, bathe the whole section of the body with Prontosan Wound Irrigation Solution, for at least 15 minutes. The solution should be used in an undiluted form.

For use in the case of encrusted bandages or when changing dressings is problematic

- In cases where bandages are difficult to release, wetting the wound dressing with Prontosan Wound Irrigation Solution is advisable until the bandages can be gently released without traumatizing the surface of the wound. If stubborn, large encrustations are present, the whole section of the body with the dressing can be saturated or bathed in Prontosan Wound Irrigation Solution until the dressing ca be easily released.

Directions

- Use aseptic technique.
  - Remove cap.
  - Remove and discard white ring below cap.
  - Replace cap. Ensure cap is screwed down fully to pierce container.
  - Remove cap and proceed with use as required in accordance with the institutional protocol.
  - Replace cap after use in accordance with the institutional protocol.
  - Record the date opened on the bottle.
  - Solution may be used for up to 28 days.
  - Discard any unused solution and the bottle.

REFERENCES

Preservative Testing[1]
No microbial growth was observed at 7, 14, and 28 days for the following organisms:
Acinetobacter baumannii.
Enterobacter cloacae.
Enterococcus faecalis.
Vancomycin-resistant *E. faecalis* (VRE).
Escherichia coli.
Proteus mirabilis.
Pseudomonas aeruginosa.
Serratia marcescens.
Staphylococcus aureus.
Methicillin-resistant *S. aureus* (MRSA).
Staphylococcus epidermidis.
Candida albicans.
[1]Preservative effectiveness demonstrated using USP 51, with an expanded list of organisms, to support the role of PHMB as a preservative to inhibit microbial growth within the product during shelf storage.
   Antimicrobial Effectiveness Testing Successfully meets USP 51 Category 2 Criteria.

Organisms	Result Day 14	Result Day 28
Escherichia coli (ATCC 8739)	Greater than 2.0 log reduction from the initial count	No increase from the 14 days count
Pseudomonas aeruginosa (ATCC 9027)	Greater than 2.0 log reduction from the initial count	No increase from the 14 days count
Staphylococcus aureus (ATCC 6538)	Greater than 2.0 log reduction from the initial count	No increase from the 14 days count
Candida albicans (ATCC 10231)	No increase from the initial calculated count	No increase from the initial calculated count
Aspergillus niger (ATCC 16404)	No increase from the initial calculated count	No increase from the initial calculated count

V.A.C.® Therapy

KCI, An ACELITY™ Company

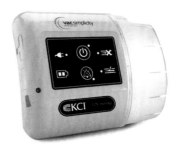

HOW SUPPLIED

V.A.C. SIMPLICITY™ Therapy Unit	E2402
V.A.C.ULTA™ Therapy Unit	E2402

ACTION

V.A.C.® Therapy is the controlled application of subatmospheric pressure to a wound using a therapy unit utilizing intermittent, continuous, or dynamic pressure control to convey negative pressure to a specialized wound dressing to help promote formulation of granulation tissue. The wound dressing is a resilient, reticulated open-cell foam surface dressing (such as GRANUFOAM™ Dressing), that assists in granulation tissue formation, or polyvinyl alcohol foam, that has a high tensile strength to allow for easy removal from tunnels and undermining and recommended when granulation tissue needs to be controlled for a more comfortable dressing change, and is sealed with an adhesive drape. Specially engineered Therapeutic Regulated Accurate Care (T.R.A.C.) technology enhances patient safety by regulating the pressure at the wound site. Specifically, the open cells of the foam enable equal distribution of the negative pressure across the surface of the wound, while tubing transfers accumulated fluids to a specially designed V.A.C.® Therapy canister.

INDICATIONS

The ACTIV.A.C.™, INFOV.A.C.™, V.A.C. ATS™, V.A.C. FREEDOM™, V.A.C. SIMPLICITY™, V.A.C.ULTA™, and V.A.C.VIA™ Therapy Systems are integrated wound management systems for use in acute, extended, and home care settings.

- They are intended to create an environment that promotes wound healing by secondary or tertiary (delayed primary) intention by preparing the wound bed for closure, reducing edema, promoting granulation tissue formation and perfusion, and by removing exudate and infectious material. They are indicated for patients with chronic, acute, traumatic, subacute, and dehisced wounds, partial-thickness burns, ulcers (such as diabetic, pressure, or venous insufficiency), flaps, and grafts.
- The V.A.C.® GRANUFOAM SILVER™ Dressing is an effective barrier to bacterial penetration and may help reduce infection in the above wound types.

CONTRAINDICATIONS

- Not for use on direct contact with exposed blood vessels, anastomotic sites, organs, or nerves.
- Not for use if there is a malignancy in the wound.
- Not for use with untreated osteomyelitis.
- Not for use with nonenteric and unexplored fistulas.
- Not for use with necrotic tissue with eschar (may be used after debridement of necrotic tissue and complete removal of eschar).
- Not for use on patients with a sensitivity to silver (V.A.C.® GRANUFOAM SILVER™ Dressing only).
- Please refer to V.A.C.® Therapy Clinical Guidelines for complete listing of contraindications, warnings, and precautions.

APPLICATION

- Never leave a V.A.C.® Dressing in place without active V.A.C.® Therapy for more than 2 hours. If negative pressure is off for more than 2 hours in a 24-hour period, remove old V.A.C.® Dressing and irrigate the wound. Either apply new V.A.C.® Dressing from an unopened sterile package and restart V.A.C.® Therapy or apply an alternative dressing, such as wet-to-moist gauze, as approved during times of extreme need by the treating clinician.
- Always use a V.A.C.® Dressing from an unopened sterile package. V.A.C.® Dressing components are disposable and are for single use only. They aren't to be reused.
- Remove and discard previous dressing per institution protocol. Thoroughly inspect the wound to ensure all pieces of dressing components have been removed.
- Debride all necrotic, nonviable tissue, including bone, eschar, or hardened slough, as prescribed by the physician.
- Perform thorough wound and periwound area cleaning per physician order or institution protocol prior to each dressing application.
- Ensure adequate hemostasis has been achieved.
- Protect vessels, organs, and nerves by covering them with natural tissues or several layers of fine-meshed, nonadherent dressing that form a complete barrier between the structures and the foam dressing.
- Consult a physician if bone fragments and/or sharp edges are present in the wound area, as these must be eliminated prior to dressing application.
- Clean and dry the periwound tissue. The use of a skin preparation product to protect the periwound tissue may also improve adhesion and assist with the integrity of the dressing seal.
- Assess wound dimensions and pathology, including the presence of undermining or tunnels.
- Use V.A.C. WHITEFOAM™ Dressing with explored tunnels and undermining. Do not place any foam dressing into blind/unexplored tunnels.
- Cut foam dressing to dimensions that will allow the foam to be placed gently into the wound, but not overlap onto intact skin.
- Do not cut the foam over the wound, as fragments may fall into the wound.
- Gently place the foam into the wound cavity, ensuring contact with all wound surfaces.
- Do not force the foam dressing into any area of the wound.
- Ensure foam-to-foam contact for even distribution of negative pressure.
- Always note the total number of pieces of foam used in the dressing and document on the drape and in the patient's chart.
- Superficial or retention sutures should be covered with a single layer of nonadherent dressing prior to drape placement.
- Trim and place the V.A.C.® Drape to cover the foam dressing and an additional 3- to 5-cm border of intact periwound tissue.
- V.A.C.® Drape may be cut into multiple pieces or strips for easier handling.
- Choose SENSAT.R.A.C.™ Dressing application site. Give particular consideration to fluid flow, tubing positioning to allow for optimal drainage, and avoiding placement over bony prominences or within creases in the tissue.
- Pinch the drape and cut a 2.5-cm hole (not a slit) through the drape. The hole should be large enough to allow for removal of fluid and/or exudate through the SENSAT.R.A.C.™ Dressing. It is not necessary to cut into the foam.
- Apply SENSAT.R.A.C.™ Dressing.
- Remove the canister from the sterile packaging and insert into the V.A.C.® Therapy Unit until it locks into place. If the canister is not fully engaged, V.A.C.® Therapy Unit will alarm.
- Connect the canister tubing, and ensure that the clamp on each tube is open. Position clamps away from the patient.
- Turn on the power to the V.A.C.® Therapy Unit and select the prescribed therapy setting. Refer to the V.A.C.® Therapy Clinical Guidelines for specific recommendations.
- Initiate V.A.C.® Therapy. Assess dressing to ensure seal integrity. The dressing should be collapsed.

- V.A.C.® GRANUFOAM™ and V.A.C. GRANUFOAM SILVER™ Dressings should have a wrinkled appearance. There should be no hissing sounds.
- If there is any evidence of nonintegrity, check SENSAT.R.A.C.™ Dressing and drape seals, tubing connections, and canister insertion, and ensure that clamps are open. Secure the excess tubing to prevent interference with patient mobility.
- If a leak source is identified, patch with additional drape to ensure seal integrity.
- Multiple layers of the V.A.C.® Drape may decrease the moisture vapor transmission rate, which may increase the risk of maceration, especially in small wounds, lower extremities, or load-bearing areas.
- For complete application instructions, please refer to the V.A.C.® Therapy Clinical Guidelines.

REMOVAL

- V.A.C.® Dressings should be changed routinely every 48 to 72 hours but no less than three times per week for noninfected wounds, with frequency adjusted by the clinician, as appropriate.
- Infected wounds must be monitored often and very closely; for these wounds, dressings may need to be changed more often than 48 to 72 hours; the dressing change intervals should be based on a continuing evaluation of the wound condition and the patient's clinical presentation, rather than a fixed schedule.
- To remove the dressing, raise the tubing connectors above the level of the therapy unit.
- Tighten the clamp on the dressing tubing.
- Separate the canister tubing and dressing tubing by disconnecting the connector.
- Allow the therapy unit to pull the exudate in the canister tubing into the canister. Then tighten the clamp on the canister tubing.
- Press the THERAPY ON/OFF button to deactivate the pump.
- Wait for 15 to 30 seconds to allow for the foam to decompress.
- Gently stretch the drape horizontally and slowly pull up from the skin. Don't peel.
- Gently remove the foam from the wound. *Note:* If the dressing adheres to the wound base, consider introducing sterile water or normal saline into the dressing, waiting 15 to 30 minutes, then gently removing the dressing from the wound. Consider placing a single layer, wide-meshed nonadherent material prior to placement of the V.A.C.® Dressing to potentially reduce further adherence, or consider more frequent dressing changes.
- Count the number of foam pieces removed; correlate the count with the number of foam pieces previously placed.
- Thoroughly inspect the wound to ensure that all pieces of dressing components have been removed.
- If the patient experiences pain during a dressing change, consider premedication, the use of a nonadherent interpost layer before foam placement, using V.A.C. WHITEFOAM™ Dressing to dress the wound, or manage the discomfort as prescribed by the treating physician.
- Discard disposables per facility protocol.
- For complete information on dressing removal, please refer to the V.A.C.® Therapy Clinical Guidelines.

REFERENCES

1. Armstrong DG, Lavery L. Negative pressure wound therapy after partial diabetic foot amputation: a multicentre, randomised controlled trial. *Lancet*. 2005;366(9498):1704–1710.
2. Vuerstaek JD, Vainas T, Wuite J, et al. State-of-the-art treatment of chronic leg ulcers: A randomized controlled trial comparing vacuum-assisted closure (V.A.C.) with modern wound dressings. *Journal of Vascular Surgery*. 2006;44(5):1029–1037.
3. Blume PA, Walters J, Payne W, et al. Comparison of negative pressure wound therapy using vacuum-assisted closure with advanced moist wound therapy in the treatment of diabetic foot ulcers—a multicenter randomized controlled trial. *Diabetes Care*. 2008;31(4):631–636.

V.A.C.® Therapy Dressings

KCI, An ACELITY™ Company

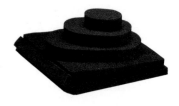

HOW SUPPLIED

V.A.C.® GRANUFOAM™ Dressing	*Small*	A6550
V.A.C.® GRANUFOAM™ Dressing	*Medium*	A6550
V.A.C.® GRANUFOAM™ Dressing	*Large*	A6550
V.A.C.® GRANUFOAM™ Dressing	*Extra Large*	A6550
V.A.C.® GRANUFOAM SILVER™ Dressing Kit	*Small*	A6550
V.A.C.® GRANUFOAM SILVER™ Dressing Kit	*Medium*	A6550
V.A.C.® GRANUFOAM SILVER™Dressing Kit	*Large*	A6550
V.A.C.® GRANUFOAM™ Dressing	*Bridge*	A6550
V.A.C.® GRANUFOAM™ Dressing	*Bridge XG*	A6550
V.A.C.® GRANUFOAM™ Dressing	*Thin*	A6550
V.A.C.® SIMPLACE™ Dressing	*Small*	A6550
V.A.C.® SIMPLACE™ Dressing	*Medium*	A6550
V.A.C. WHITEFOAM™	*Small (foam only)*	A6550
V.A.C. WHITEFOAM™	*Large (foam only)*	A6550
V.A.C. WHITEFOAM™ Dressing	*Small*	A6550
V.A.C. WHITEFOAM™ Dressing	*Large*	A6550

ACTION

The V.A.C.® GRANUFOAM™ Dressing is a black, polyurethane foam dressing with a reticulated open-cell design that provides uniform distribution of pressure at the wound site. The 400- to 600-micron pore size foam assists in promotion of granulation tissue formation and aids in wound contraction. It is a hydrophobic (moisture repelling) foam, which enhances exudate removal.

The V.A.C.® GRANUFOAM SILVER™ Dressing is also a reticulated, open-cell polyurethane foam that has been microbonded with metallic silver via a proprietary metallization process. During V.A.C.® Therapy, exposure of the dressing to wound fluid results in oxidation of metallic silver to ionic silver, allowing the continuous, sustained release of silver ions that acts as an effective barrier to bacterial penetration.

The V.A.C. WHITEFOAM™ Dressing is a polyvinyl alcohol foam with a dense, open-pore design, and a high tensile strength, ideal for use in tunnels and undermining. It is hydrophilic (or moisture retaining) and premoistened with sterile water. Its characteristics help to reduce the likelihood of adherence to the wound base. It can be used to assist in minimizing discomfort, over fresh split-thickness skin grafts, or in situations where hypergranulation responses are likely. The higher density of V.A.C. WHITEFOAM™ dressing requires a minimum pressure setting of -125 mm Hg.

V.A.C.® SIMPLACE™ Dressings are designed to simplify the V.A.C.® Therapy dressing placement process. The dressing uses the same black polyurethane foam as the V.A.C.® GRANUFOAM™ Dressing, and there are fewer steps for faster application. This spiral cut foam is simple to size, as it can be easily torn manually; scissors may not be necessary. The Simplace design allows for easy bridging and is proven to actively promote formation of granulation tissue.

The V.A.C.® GRANUFOAM™ Bridge Dressing allows for the application of negative-pressure wound therapy (NPWT) to those wounds, such as sacral wounds, wounds on the foot, or wounds requiring offloading or compression therapy which, because of their anatomical location, require that the SENSAT.R.A.C.™ Dressing be placed at a remote location. It also helps improve mobility, allowing patients to resume activities of daily living and facilitates patient transition to a nonacute care setting. It is also packaged as V.A.C.® GRANUFOAM™ Bridge XG dressing to simplify the bridging of large wounds.

INDICATIONS

These foams are indicated for use with the V.A.C.® family of NPWT systems to help promote formation of granulation tissue in chronic, acute, traumatic, subacute and dehisced wounds, partial-thickness burns, pressure and diabetic ulcers, flaps, and grafts. For optimal pressure distribution, it is recommended to use a V.A.C.® GRANUFOAM™ Dressing over V.A.C. WHITEFOAM™ Dressing. These foam dressings should only be used with appropriate V.A.C.® Therapy products.

CONTRAINDICATIONS

- Do not place directly on exposed blood vessels, anastomotic sites, exposed organs, or nerves.
- Contraindicated on patients with malignancy in the wound, untreated osteomyelitis, nonenteric and unexplored fistulas, necrotic tissue with eschar present, and those with sensitivity to silver (V.A.C.® GRANUFOAM SILVER™ Dressing only).
- For complete listing of all contraindications, warnings, and precautions, please refer to V.A.C.® Therapy Clinical Guidelines.

APPLICATIONS

- V.A.C.® Dressings, tubings, and drape are packaged sterile and are latex free.
- The decision to use clean versus sterile/aseptic technique is dependent on wound pathophysiology, physician/clinician preference, and institutional protocol.
- Do not place any foam dressing into blind or unexplored tunnels. The V.A.C. WHITEFOAM™ Dressing may be more appropriate for use with explored tunnels and undermining.
- Do not force foam dressings into any area of the wound, as this may damage tissue, alter delivery of negative pressure, or hinder exudate removal.
- Always count the total number of pieces of foam used in the dressing and document that number on the drape and in the patient's chart. Also, document the dressing change date on the drape.
- Consult a physician and review all V.A.C.® Therapy Instructions for Use and the V.A.C.® Therapy Clinical Guidelines before use.

REMOVAL

- V.A.C.® Dressings should be changed routinely every 48 to 72 hours but no less than three times per week for noninfected wounds, with frequency adjusted by the clinician, as appropriate.
- Infected wounds must be monitored often and very closely; for these wounds, dressings may need to be changed more often than 48 to 72 hours; the dressing change intervals should be based on a continuing evaluation of the wound condition and the patient's clinical presentation, rather than a fixed schedule.
- Always replace all disposable components with new sterile dressing components.
- For complete information regarding dressing removal, please refer to the V.A.C.® Therapy Clinical Guidelines.

New Product: V.A.C.® VERAFLO CLEANSE CHOICE

KCI, An ACELITY™ Company

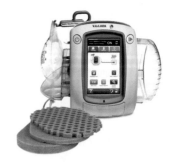

HOW SUPPLIED

V.A.C.ULTA™ Therapy Unit	E2402
V.A.C. VERAFLO CLEANSE CHOICE™ Dressing	E2402

ACTIONS

V.A.C. VERAFLO™ Therapy with V.A.C. VERAFLO CLEANSE CHOICE™ Dressing incorporates negative-pressure wound therapy (NPWT) with the instillation of topical wound solutions to promote wound healing. V.A.C. VERAFLO™ Therapy consists of NPWT coupled with automated, controlled delivery to and removal of topical wound solutions form the wound bed. This therapy uses dressings specifically designed for instillation therapy with NPWT. The dressings are less hydrophobic than the current V.A.C.® Therapy dressings and provide improved fluid distribution within and removal from the wound bed. V.A.C VERAFLO™ Therapy provides thorough wound coverage with topical solution during select dwell time and dilutes and helps solubilize infectious material and wound debris such as slough/devitalized tissue. V.A.C. VERAFLO CLEANSE CHOICE™ Dressing provides a wound cleansing option for clinicians when surgical debridement must be delayed or is not possible or appropriate.

INDICATIONS

V.A.C. VERAFLO™ Therapy is intended for use with V.A.C. VERAFLO™ Therapy disposables and topical wound treatment solutions and suspensions. Only use solutions or suspensions that are:

- Indicated for topical wound treatment according to solution manufacturer's instructions for use. Some topical agents may not be intended for extended tissue contact. If in doubt about the appropriateness of using a particular solution, contact the solution's manufacturer about its suitability for saturated topical wound exposure.
- Compatible with V.A.C.® Dressings and disposable components. Hypochlorous acid solutions applied frequently at high concentrations can lead to significant material degradation. Consider using concentrations as low as clinically relevant.

V.A.C VERAFLO™ Therapy is indicated for patients with chronic, acute, traumatic, subacute, and dehisced wounds, partial-thickness burns, ulcers (such as diabetic, pressure, and venous insufficiency), flaps, and grafts. V.A.C. VERAFLO™ Therapy is also indicated for use in patients who would benefit from vacuum-assisted drainage and controlled delivery of topical wound treatment solutions and suspensions over the wound bed.

CONTRAINDICATIONS

- Not for use on direct contact with exposed blood vessels, anastomotic sites, organs, or nerves.
- Not for use if there is a malignancy in the wound.
- Not for use with untreated osteomyelitis.
- Not for use with nonenteric and unexplored fistulas.

- Not for use with necrotic tissue with eschar (may be used after debridement of necrotic tissue and complete removal of eschar).
- Not for use with Octenisept (not available in the United States), hydrogen peroxide, or solutions that are alcohol-based or contain alcohol.
- Do not deliver fluids to the thoracic or abdominal cavity due to the potential risk to alter core body temperature and the potential for fluid retention within the cavity.
- Do not use V.A.C. VERAFLO™ Therapy unless the wound has been thoroughly explored due to the potential for inadvertent instillation of topical wound solutions to adjacent body cavities.
- Please refer to V.A.C.ULTA™ Negative Pressure Wound Therapy System Clinical Guidelines for complete listing of contraindications, warnings, and precautions.
- Do not use V.A.C. GRANUFOAM SILVER™ Dressings with V.A.C. VERAFLO™ Therapy as instillation of solutions may negatively impact the benefits of the dressing.

APPLICATIONS

- Refer to V.A.C.® Therapy Clinical Guidelines for detailed instructions for treating different wound types.
- Assess wound dimensions and pathology, including the presence of undermining or tunnels. The V.A.C. VERAFLO CLEANSE CHOICE™ Contact Layer with through holes is not recommended for use in tunnels or undermining. Do not place any foam dressing into blind/unexplored tunnels.
- Nonadherent materials can be used prior to foam dressing placement in order to facilitate future dressing removal. If adjunct materials are utilized under the V.A.C. VERAFLO™ Dressing, they must be compatible with solution in use and meshed, porous, or fenestrated to allow for effective fluid and exudate removal. Document on the drape, on the supplied foam-quantity label, and in the patient's chart to ensure the removal of nonadherent material with subsequent dressing changes.
- Select the layers (wound-contact and cover layer) of the dressing to be used in the wound. The choice of the cover layer (thick or thin) depends on the wound depth. Size the dressing layers as needed to allow gentle placement into the wound without firm packing of the foam, or overlapping onto intact skin.
  - Do not cut or tear the foam over the wound, as fragments may fall into the wound. Away from the wound sites, rub the foam edges to remove any fragments or loose particles that may fall into or be left in the wound upon dressing removal.
- Gently place the foam into the wound cavity, ensuring contact with all wound surfaces. Do not force the foam into any areas of the wound.
  - As required, use a cover layer to fill explored tunnels and undermined areas.
  - Place the wound contact layer with through holes directly into the wound bed.
  - Place the selected cover layer over the wound contact layer with holes.
  - Do not use the wound contact layer with holes into tunnels or undermined areas.
  - Do not force the dressing into any areas of the wound.
  - Do not overpack the wound cavity. Do not place multiple pieces of foam in tunnels to prevent the foam from being left behind at subsequent dressing changes.
  - If using multiple pieces of foam, ensure foam-to-foam contact between adjacent pieces of foam for even distribution of fluid and negative pressure.
- Record the total number of foam pieces used in the wound and document this in the patient's chart.
- Trim the V.A.C.® Advanced Drape to cover the foam and an additional 3- to 5-cm border of intact periwound tissue. V.A.C.® Drape may be cut into multiple pieces or strips for easier handling.
  - Proper sealing of the wound with the drape is essential for assuring therapy is delivered to the wound. The use of V.A.C. VERAFLO™ Therapy in wounds where large volumes

of instillation fluid are delivered to the wound or in wounds in anatomical locations that are difficult to seal required additional precautions to assure that the dressing is adequately sealed throughout therapy. Consider adjusting patient placement during instillation cycle, application of an additional layer of drape in tissue folds or areas more likely to be susceptible to leaks, and supporting the wound area with surface contact or pillow to prevent bulging of drape if the wound is in a dependent position.

- Choose V.A.C. VERAT.R.A.C.™ Pad application site. Give particular consideration to fluid flow, tubing positioning to allow for optimal drainage, and avoiding placement over bony prominences or within creases in the tissue.
  - To prevent periwound maceration with wounds that are smaller than the central disc pad, it is very important that the central disc not overhang the edge of the foam and that the periwound area is properly protected. Refer to the wound preparation section for periwound area protection instructions. Refer to the bridge application section in the application instructions and the V.A.C.® Therapy Clinical Guidelines for additional dressing application techniques.
- Pinch the drape, and cut a 2.5-cm hole (not a slit) through the drape. The hole should be large enough to allow for removal of fluid and/or exudate. It is not necessary to cut into the foam.
- Apply the V.A.C VERAT.R.A.C.™ Pad.
- Remove the V.A.C. VERALINK™ Cassette from packaging and insert into the V.A.C.ULTA™ Therapy Unit until it locks into place.
- Using the V.A.C. VERALINK™ Cassette spike, connect the instillation solution bottle/bag to the V.A.C. VERALINK™ Cassette.
- Hang instillation solution bottle/bag on the therapy unit's adjustable hanger arm. Refer to the V.A.C.ULTA™ Therapy System User Manual for detailed instructions.
- Connect the instillation line (smaller-diameter tube) of the V.A.C. VERAT.R.A.C.™ or instill the pad to the V.A.C. VERALINK™ Cassette tubing.
- Ensure both the tubing clamps are open and are positioned appropriately to prevent pressure points and/or skin irritation.
- Remove the canister from packaging and insert into the V.A.C.ULTA™ Therapy Unit until it locks into place.
- Connect the negative pressure line of the V.A.C VERAT.R.A.C.™ Pad or SensaT.R.A.C.™ Pad tubing to the canister tubing.
- Ensure the clamp on each tube is open and position clamps away from patients.
- Turn on the power to the V.A.C.ULTA™ Therapy Unit, select the prescribed therapy settings, and initiate therapy. Refer to the V.A.C.ULTA™ Therapy System User Manual for detailed instruction.
- The V.A.C. VERAFLO™ Dressing should have a wrinkled appearance shortly after therapy is initiated. There should be no hissing sounds. If there is any evidence of leaks, check the seals around the V.A.C VERAT.R.A.C.™ Pad or SensaT.R.A.C.™ Dressing, drape, tubing connections, canister connections, V.A.C. VERALINK™ Cassette connections, and ensure all tubing clamps are open.
- Secure excess tubing to prevent interference with patient mobility.

REMOVAL

- V.A.C. VERAFLO™ Dressings should be changed routinely every 48 to 72 hours but no less than three times per week for noninfected wounds, with frequency adjusted by clinician, as appropriate.
- Infected wounds must be monitored often and very closely; for these wounds, dressings may need to be changed more often than 48 to 72 hours; the dressing change intervals should be based on a continuing evaluation of the wound condition and the patient's clinical presentation, rather than a fixed schedule.

- Initiate the dressing soak tool on the V.A.C.ULTA™ Therapy Unit.
  - Ensure that both the canister tubing and instillation lines are properly connected and all four tubing clamps are open.
  - Ensure that the V.A.C VERALINK™ Cassette is properly installed and has adequate capacity remaining for the dressing change.
- Select Dressing Soak from the home screen and select the target dressing soak time.
- Confirm the settings and return to the home screen on the V.A.C.ULTA™ Therapy Unit. The therapy unit will complete the instill, soak, and fluid removal phases.
- Once the dressing soak/fluid removal phase is complete, the dressing can be removed.
- Raise the tubing connectors above the level of the therapy unit.
- Tighten the clamp on the dressing tubing.
- Separate canister tubing and dressing tubing by disconnecting the connector.
- Allow the therapy unit to pull the exudate in the canister tube into the canister, then tighten the clamp on the canister tubing.
- Press THERAPY ON/OFF to deactivate the pump.
- Wait 15 to 30 seconds to allow the foam dressing to decompress.
- Gently stretch the drape horizontally and slowly pull up from the skin. Do not peel.
- Gently remove the foam from the wound and count the number of foam dressings removed from the wound to ensure that no foam remains within the wound bed. Note: If the dressing adheres to the wound base, consider introducing sterile water or normal saline into the dressing, waiting 15 to 30 minutes, then gently removing the dressing from the wound. Consider placing a single-layer, wide-meshed, nonadherent material prior to placement of the V.A.C. foam dressing to potentially reduce further adherence, or consider more frequent dressing changes.
- Count the number of foam pieces removed; correlate the count with the number of foam pieces previously placed.
- Thoroughly inspect the wound to ensure that all pieces of dressing components have been removed.
- If the patient experiences pain during a dressing change, consider premedication, the use of a nonadherent contact layer before foam placement to dress the wound, or managing the discomfort as prescribed by the treating physician.
- Discard disposables per facility protocol.

REFERENCES

1. Kim PJ, Attinger CE, Steinberg JS, et al. Negative pressure wound therapy with instillation: Consensus guidelines. *Plastic and Reconstructive Surgery*. 2013;132(6):1569–1579.
2. Gupta S, Gabriel A, Lantis J, et al. Clinical recommendations and practical guide for negative pressure wound therapy with instillation. *Int Wound J*. 2016;13(2):159–174.
3. Teot L; Boissiere F; Fluieraru S. Novel foam dressing using negative pressure wound therapy with instillation to remove thick exudate. *Int Wound J*. 2017;14(5):842–848.
4. Fernandez L; Ellman C; Jackson P. Initial experience using a novel reticulated open cell foam dressing with through holes during negative pressure wound therapy with instillation for management of pressure ulcers. *J Trauma Treatment* 2017;6(5):410.

New Product: V.A.C. VERAFLO™ Therapy

KCI, An ACELITY™ Company

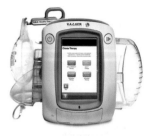

HOW SUPPLIED

V.A.C.ULTA™ Therapy Unit		E2402
V.A.C. VERAFLO™ Dressing	*5 Pack, Large*	A6550
V.A.C. VERAFLO™ Dressing	*Medium*	A6550
V.A.C. VERAFLO™ Dressing	*Small*	A6550
V.A.C. VERAFLO CLEANSE™ Dressing	*Medium*	E2402
V.A.C. VERALINK™ Cassette (canister for instillation fluid)		
V.A.C. VERAT.R.A.C. Duo™ Tube Set (two separate tubing lines and pads)		

ACTIONS

V.A.C. VERAFLO™ Therapy incorporates negative-pressure wound therapy (NPWT) with the instillation of topical wound solutions to promote wound healing. V.A.C. VERAFLO™ Therapy consists of NPWT coupled with automated, controlled delivery to and removal of topical wound solutions from the wound bed. This therapy uses dressings specifically designed for instillation therapy with NPWT. The dressings are less hydrophobic than the current V.A.C.® Therapy dressings and provide improved fluid distribution within and removal from the wound bed. V.A.C VERAFLO™ Therapy provides thorough wound coverage with topical solution during select dwell time and dilutes and helps solubilize infectious material and wound debris.

INDICATIONS

V.A.C. VERAFLO™ Therapy is intended for use with V.A.C. VERAFLO™ Therapy disposables and topical wound treatment solutions and suspensions. Only use solutions or suspensions that are:

- Indicated for topical wound treatment according to the solution's manufacturer's instructions for use. Some topical agents may not be intended for extended tissue contact. If in doubt about the appropriateness of using a particular solution, contact the solution's manufacturer about its suitability for saturated topical wound exposure.
- Compatible with V.A.C.® Dressings and disposable components. Hypochlorous acid solutions applied frequently at high concentrations can lead to significant material degradation. Consider using concentrations as low as clinically relevant.

V.A.C VERAFLO™ Therapy is indicated for patients with chronic, acute, traumatic, subacute, and dehisced wounds, partial-thickness burns, ulcers (such as diabetic, pressure, and venous insufficiency), flaps, and grafts. V.A.C. VERAFLO™ Therapy is also indicated for use in patients who would benefit from vacuum-assisted drainage and controlled delivery of topical wound treatment solutions and suspensions over the wound bed.

CONTRAINDICATIONS

- Not for use on direct contact with exposed blood vessels, anastomotic sites, organs, or nerves.
- Not for use if there is a malignancy in the wound.
- Not for use with untreated osteomyelitis.

- Not for use with nonenteric and unexplored fistulas.
- Not for use with necrotic tissue with eschar (may be used after debridement of necrotic tissue and complete removal of eschar).
- Not for use in with Octenisept (not available in the United States), hydrogen peroxide, or solutions that are alcohol-based or contain alcohol.
- Do not deliver fluids to the thoracic or abdominal cavity due to the potential risk to alter core body temperature and the potential for fluid retention within the cavity.
- Do not use V.A.C. VERAFLO™ Therapy unless the wound has been thoroughly explored due to the potential for inadvertent instillation of topical wound solutions to adjacent body cavities.
- Please refer to V.A.C.ULTA™ Therapy System Clinical Guidelines for complete listing of contraindications, warnings, and precautions.
- Do not use V.A.C. GRANUFOAM SILVER™ Dressings with V.A.C. VERAFLO™ Therapy as instillation of solutions may negatively impact the benefits of the dressing.

APPLICATIONS

- Refer to V.A.C.® Therapy Clinical Guidelines for detailed instructions for treating different wound types.
- Assess wound dimensions and pathology, including the presence of undermining or tunnels. Do not place any foam dressing into blind/unexplored tunnels.
- Ensure debridement of all necrotic, nonviable tissue including bone, eschar, or hardened slough, as prescribed by a physician.
- Perform a thorough wound and periwound area cleaning per physician order or institution protocol prior to dressing application.
- Protect fragile/friable periwound skin with additional V.A.C.® Advanced Drape, 3M™ Tegaderm™ Dressing, or other similar medical-grade transparent film, skin protectant, or hydrocolloid. Document on the drape, on the supplied foam-quantity label, and in the patient's chart to ensure the removal of nonadherent material with subsequent dressing changes.
- Size V.A.C. VERAFLO™ Dressing as needed:
  - V.A.C. VERAFLO™ Dressing—Small and Medium: Carefully tear the foam along the perforation to a size that will allow gentle placement into the wound without firm packing of the foam or overlapping onto intact skin.
  - V.A.C. VERAFLO™ Dressing—Large: Cut the foam to a size that will allow gentle placement into the wound without firm packing of the foam or overlapping onto the intact skin.
  - Do not cut or tear the foam over the wound, as fragments may fall into the wound. Away from the wound site, rub the foam edges to remove any fragments or loose particles that may fall into or be left in the wound upon dressing removal.
- Gently place the foam into the wound cavity, ensuring contact with all wound surfaces. Do not force the foam into any areas of the wound.
- Record the total number of foam pieces used in the wound and document this in the patient's chart.
- Trim the V.A.C.® Advanced Drape to cover the foam and an additional 3- to 5-cm border of intact periwound tissue. V.A.C.® Drape may be cut into multiple pieces or strips for easier handling.
  - Proper sealing of the wound with the drape is essential for assuring therapy is delivered to the wound. The use of V.A.C. VERAFLO™ Therapy in wounds where large volumes of instillation fluid are delivered to the wound or in wounds in anatomical locations that are difficult to seal require additional precautions to assure that the dressing is adequately sealed throughout the therapy. Consider adjusting patient placement during the instillation cycle, application of an additional layer of drape in tissue folds or areas more likely to be susceptible to leaks, and supporting the wound

area with surface contact or pillow to prevent bulging of the drape if the wound is in a dependent position.

- Choose V.A.C. VERAT.R.A.C.™ Pad application site. Give particular consideration to fluid flow, tubing positioning to allow for optimal drainage, and avoiding placement over bony prominences or within creases in the tissue.
  - To prevent periwound maceration with wounds that are smaller than the central disc pad, it is very important that the central disc not overhang the edge of the foam and that the periwound area is properly protected. Refer to the wound preparation section for periwound area protection instructions. Refer to the bridge application section in the application instructions and the V.A.C.® Therapy Clinical Guidelines for additional dressing application techniques.
- Pinch the drape, and cut a 2.5-cm hole (not a slit) through the drape. The hole should be large enough to allow for removal of fluid and/or exudate. It is not necessary to cut into the foam.
- Apply the V.A.C VERAT.R.A.C.™ Pad.
- Choose the pad application site for the SENSAT.R.A.C.™ Dressing.
  - Give particular consideration to fluid flow and tubing positioning to allow for optimal flow, and avoid placement over bony prominences or within creases in the tissue. Whenever possible, the SENSAT.R.A.C™ Dressing should be placed at a lower elevation than the instill pad.
  - To prevent periwound maceration with wounds that are smaller than the central disc pad, it is very important that the central disc not overhang the edge of the foam and that the periwound area is properly protected. Refer to the wound preparation section for periwound area protection instructions. Refer to the bridge application section in the application instructions and the V.A.C.® Therapy Clinical Guidelines for additional dressing application techniques.
- Pinch the drape, and cut a 2.5-cm hole (not a slit) through the drape. The hole should be large enough to allow for removal of fluid and/or exudate. It is not necessary to cut into the foam.
- Apply the SENSAT.R.A.C.™ Dressing.
- Remove the V.A.C. VERALINK™ Cassette from packaging and insert into the V.A.C.ULTA™ Therapy Unit until it locks into place.
- Using the V.A.C. VERALINK™ Cassette spike, connect the instillation solution bottle/bag to the V.A.C. VERALINK™ Cassette.
- Hang the instillation solution bottle/bag on the therapy unit's adjustable hanger arm. Refer to the V.A.C.ULTA™ Therapy System User Manual for detailed instructions.
- Connect the instillation line (smaller diameter tube) of the V.A.C. VERAT.R.A.C.™ or the instill pad to the V.A.C. VERALINK™ Cassette tubing.
- Ensure both the tubing clamps are open and are positioned appropriately to prevent pressure points and/or skin irritation.
- Remove the V.A.C.® Canister from packaging and insert into the V.A.C.ULTA™ Therapy Unit until it locks into place.
- Connect the V.A.C.® line of the V.A.C VERAT.R.A.C.™ Pad or SENSAT.R.A.C.™ Dressing tubing to the canister tubing.
- Ensure the clamp on each tube is open and position clamps away from patients.
- Turn on the power to the V.A.C.ULTA™ Therapy Unit, select the prescribed therapy settings, and initiate therapy. Refer to the V.A.C.ULTA™ Therapy System User Manual for detailed instructions.
- The V.A.C. VERAFLO™ Dressing should have a wrinkled appearance shortly after therapy is initiated. There should be no hissing sounds. If there is any evidence of leaks, check the seals around the V.A.C VERAT.R.A.C.™ Pad or SENSAT.R.A.C.™ Dressing, drape, tubing connections, canister connections, V.A.C. VERALINK™ Cassette connections, and ensure all tubing clamps are open.
- Secure excess tubing to prevent interference with patient mobility.

REMOVAL

- V.A.C. VERAFLO™ Dressings should be changed routinely every 48 to 72 hours but no less than three times per week for noninfected wounds, with frequency adjusted by the clinician, as appropriate.
- Infected wounds must be monitored often and very closely; for these wounds, dressings may need to be changed more often than 48 to 72 hours; the dressing change intervals should be based on a continuing evaluation of the wound condition and the patient's clinical presentation, rather than a fixed schedule.
- Initiate the dressing soak tool on the V.A.C.ULTA™ Therapy Unit.
  - Ensure that both the V.A.C.® Canister tubing and instillation lines are properly connected and all four tubing clamps are open.
  - Ensure that the V.A.C VERALINK™ Cassette is properly installed and has adequate capacity remaining for the dressing change.
  - Select Dressing Soak from the home screen and select the target dressing soak time.
  - Confirm the settings and return to the home screen on the V.A.C.ULTA™ Therapy Unit. The therapy unit will complete the instill, soak, and fluid removal phases.
  - Once the dressing soak–fluid removal phase is complete, the dressing can be removed.
  - Raise the tubing connectors above the level of the therapy unit.
  - Tighten the clamp on the dressing tubing.
  - Separate canister tubing and dressing tubing by disconnecting the connector.
  - Allow the therapy unit to pull the exudate in the canister tube into the canister, then tighten the clamp on the canister tubing.
  - Press THERAPY ON/OFF to deactivate the pump.
  - Wait 15 to 30 seconds to allow the foam dressing to decompress.
  - Gently stretch the drape horizontally and slowly pull up from the skin. Do not peel.
  - Gently remove the foam from the wound and count the number of foam dressings removed from the wound to ensure that no foam remains within the wound bed. *Note:* If the dressing adheres to the wound base, consider introducing sterile water or normal saline into the dressing, waiting 15 to 30 minutes, then gently removing the dressing from the wound. Consider placing a single layer, wide-meshed, nonadherent material prior to placement of the V.A.C.® Dressing to potentially reduce further adherence, or consider more frequent dressing changes.
  - Count the number of foam pieces removed; correlate the count with the number of foam pieces previously placed.
  - Thoroughly inspect the wound to ensure that all pieces of dressing components have been removed.
  - If the patient experiences pain during a dressing change, consider premedication, the use of a nonadherent contact layer before foam placement to dress the wound, or managing the discomfort as prescribed by the treating physician.
  - Discard disposables per facility protocol.

REFERENCES

1. Kim PJ, Attinger CE, Steinberg JS, et al. Negative pressure wound therapy with instillation: Consensus guidelines. *Plast Reconstr Surg.* 2013;132(6):1569–1579.
2. Gupta S, Gabriel A, Lantis J, et al. Clinical recommendations and practical guide for negative pressure wound therapy with instillation. *Int Wound J.* 2016;13(2):159–174.
3. Teot L, Boissiere F, Fluieraru S. Novel foam dressing using negative pressure wound therapy with instillation to remove thick exudate. *Int Wound J.* 2017;14(5):842–848.
4. Fernandez L, Ellman C, Jackson P. Initial experience using a novel reticulated open cell foam dressing with through holes during negative pressure wound therapy with instillation for management of pressure ulcers. *J Trauma Treatment.* 2017;6(5):410.

Specialty Absorptives

ACTION

Specialty absorptives are unitized, multilayered dressings that consist of highly absorptive layers of fibers, such as absorbent cellulose, cotton, or rayon. These dressings may or may not have an adhesive border.

INDICATIONS

Specialty absorptive dressings may be used as primary or secondary dressings to manage light to heavy drainage from partial- and full-thickness wounds, infected and noninfected wounds, and red, yellow, or black wounds.

ADVANTAGES

- Can be used as secondary dressing over most primary dressings.
- Are semiadherent or nonadherent.
- Are highly absorptive.
- Are easy to apply and remove.
- May have an adhesive border, making additional tape unnecessary.

DISADVANTAGES

- May not be appropriate as a primary dressing for undermining wounds.

HCPCS CODE OVERVIEW

The HCPCS codes normally assigned to specialty absorptive wound covers without an adhesive border are:

A6251—pad size <16 in^2.

A6252—pad size >16 in^2 but <48 in^2.

A6253—pad size >48 in^2.

The HCPCS codes normally assigned to specialty absorptive wound covers with an adhesive border are:

A6254—pad size <16 in^2.

A6255—pad size >16 in^2 but ≤48 in^2.

A6256—pad size >48 in^2.

Combine ABD Pads

DUKAL Corporation

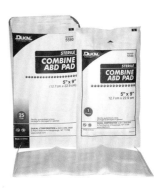

HOW SUPPLIED

Sterile Combine ABD Pads	5" × 9"	A6252
Sterile Combine ABD Pads	8" × 7.5"	A6252
Sterile Combine ABD Pads	8" × 10"	A6253

ACTION

- Highly absorbent multilayer dressing.
- Soft nonwoven outer facing wicks moisture into the cellulose core that quickly absorbs and disperses fluid.
- Moisture-resistant barrier prevents fluid strikethrough.
- All edges are sealed to prevent linting and leakage.
- Not made with natural rubber latex.

EXU-DRY

Smith & Nephew, Inc.
Wound Management

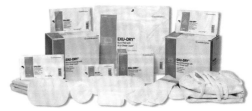

HOW SUPPLIED

Specialty Dressing	Arm 6″ × 9″	A6253
Specialty Dressing	Arm 9″ × 15″	A6253
Specialty Dressing	Arm/Shoulder	A6253
Specialty Dressing	Scalp/Face, Elbow/Knee/Heel, Boot/Foot L	A6252
Specialty Dressing	Hand, Boot/Foot M/S	A6251
Specialty Dressing	Neck, Buttocks, Leg, Burn Jacket/Vest	A6253
Slit Disk	3″	A6251
Slit Tube	2″ × 3″	A6251
Slit Tube	3″ × 4″	A6251
Slit Tube	4″ × 6″	A6252
Disk	2″	A6251
Disk	3″	A6251
Disk	3″ × 4″	A6251
Disk	4″ × 6″	A6252
Disk	6″ × 9″	A6253
Disk	9″ × 15″	A6253
Disk	15″ × 18″	A6253
Disk	15″ × 24″	A6253
Disk	20″ × 28″	A6253
Incision Dressing	3″ × 9″	A6252
Nonpermeable Pad	24″ × 36″	A6253
Nonpermeable Pad	36″ × 72″	A6253
Permeable Sheet	36″ × 72″	A6253
Pediatric Specialty Dressing	Scalp, Infant/Toddler Vest	A6252
Pediatric Specialty Dressing	Hand, Foot	A6251
Arm, Leg, Child Vest	6″ × 9″	A6253
Arm, Leg, Child Vest	9″ × 15″	A6253
Pad/Sheet	20″ × 28″ Crib Sheet (permeable)	A6253
Pad/Sheet	20″ × 28″ Receiving Blanket	A6253
Pad/Sheet	24″ × 36″ Pad (nonpermeable)	A6253

SPECIALTY ABSORPTIVES

ACTION

EXU-DRY's highly absorptive properties may reduce the need for frequent dressing changes. The dressings are designed to minimize adherence and improve patient comfort. The antishear layer helps to minimize friction and shear. It may be used wet or dry.

INDICATIONS

To manage exudate in partial- and full-thickness wounds, such as burns and donor or skin graft sites.

CONTRAINDICATIONS

- None provided by the manufacturer.

APPLICATION

- Select a dressing slightly larger than the wound.
- Place the dressing on the wound with the words "Use other side against wound" face up.
- Secure the dressing with gauze, tape, or netting.

REMOVAL

- Remove the gauze, tape, or netting.
- Lift off the dressing.

Multipad Non-Adherent Wound Dressing

DeRoyal

HOW SUPPLIED

Pad	2″ × 2″	A6251
Pad	4″ × 4″	A6251
Pad	4″ × 8″	A6252
Pad	7 1/2″ × 7 1/2″	

ACTION

Multipad Non-Adherent Wound Dressing is a thick, multilayered, absorbent wound dressing that won't stick to the wound site or damage fragile granulation tissue. It is composed of a highly absorptive nonwoven pad between two wound contact layers.

INDICATIONS

To manage pressure ulcers (stages 2 to 4), partial- and full-thickness wounds, donor sites, tunneling wounds, infected and noninfected wounds, and red, yellow, or black wounds.

CONTRAINDICATIONS

- None provided by the manufacturer.

APPLICATION

- Clean the wound and then position the dressing over it.
- Secure the dressing with tape, roll gauze, or tubular elastic bandages if using it as a primary dressing.
- If using Multipad as a secondary dressing, apply the primary dressing or filler before securing Multipad to the wound.

REMOVAL

- Remove any secondary dressing.
- Gently lift the dressing from the wound.

SPECIALTY ABSORPTIVES

Sofsorb Wound Dressing

DeRoyal

HOW SUPPLIED

Pad	3″ × 3″	A6251
Pad	4″ × 6″	A6252
Pad	4″ × 6″ with drain slit	A6252
Pad	4″ × 9″	A6253
Pad	6″ × 9″	A6253
Pad	9″ × 15″	A6253
Pad	15″ × 18″	A6253
Pad	15″ × 24″	A6253

SPECIALTY ABSORPTIVES

ACTION

Sofsorb Wound Dressing is a nonadherent, absorbent, multilayered, one-piece dressing used wet or dry to treat various wounds. The nonwoven layer permits passage of wound drainage into the absorbent pad and prevents it from returning. The center layer absorbs drainage. The cellulose layer wicks drainage horizontally along the pad to increase dressing capacity. The air-permeable backing provides strength and integrity.

INDICATIONS

For use as a postoperative dressing and as a primary or secondary dressing to manage burns, minor lacerations, abrasions, and heavily draining skin ulcers; may also be used on pressure ulcers (stages 2 to 4), partial- and full-thickness wounds, tunneling wounds, infected and noninfected wounds, wounds with heavy drainage, wounds with serosanguineous or purulent drainage, and red, yellow, or black wounds.

CONTRAINDICATIONS

- None provided by the manufacturer.

APPLICATION

- Apply the dry dressing with the wound contact layer toward the wound surface.
- Alternatively, soak the dressing with normal saline solution or another topical solution. Squeeze out excess fluid, and then apply the dressing with the wound contact layer toward the wound surface.
- Secure with a stretch net dressing, roll gauze, or tape.

REMOVAL

- Moisten with normal saline solution, if necessary.
- Carefully lift the dressing off the wound.

Super Absorbent Dressing

Gentell

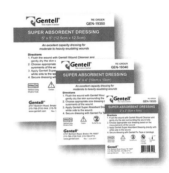

HOW SUPPLIED

Pad	2″ × 2″	A6196
Pad	4″ × 4″	A6196
Pad	5″ × 5″	A6197
Pad	8″ × 8″	A6198

ACTION

Gentell Super Absorbent Dressing offers excellent absorbent capacity for the treatment of moderate or heavy exudting wounds. The dressing consists of a breathable and waterproof non-woven backing, a super absorbent pad layer, and a hydro-penetrating non-woven contact layer.

INDICATIONS

Ideal for leg ulcers, pressure injuries, non-infected diabetic foot ulcers, dehisced surgical wounds, and donor sites.

CONTRAINDICATIONS

- Do not use this product on dry or light exuding wounds, eyes, mucous membranes, or in wound cavities because the dressing swells during absorption. Do not use on third-degree burns. Do not use on individuals with known allergy or hypersensitivity to the dressing or its components.

APPLICATION

- Irrigate the wound with Gentell Wound Cleanser and gently dry the skin surrounding the wound site.
- Choose the appropriate-size dressing based on the dimensions of the wound.
- Apply Gentell Super Absorbent Dressing with the white side to the wound and blue side up.
- Secure the dressing with Gentell FixTape™.

REMOVAL

- Change daily or as ordered by a physician.

Super Absorbent Dressing Adherent

Gentell

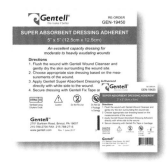

HOW SUPPLIED

Pad	2″ × 2″	A6196
Pad	5″ × 5″	A6197
Pad	8″ × 8″	A6198

ACTION

Gentell Super Absorbent Dressing Adherent offers excellent absorbent capacity for the treatment of moderate or heavy exuding wounds. It provides all the benefits of Gentell Super Absorbent Dressing with the addition of a comfortable silicone contact layer that provides gentle adherence and can speed up exudate absorption. The dressing consists of a breathable and waterproof, non-woven backing, a super absorbent pad layer, and a silicone contact layer.

INDICATIONS

Ideal for leg ulcers, pressure injuries, non-infected diabetic foot ulcers, dehisced surgical wounds, and donor sites.

CONTRAINDICATIONS

- Do not use this product on dry or light exuding wounds, eyes, mucous membranes, or in wound cavities because the dressing swells during absorption. Do not use on third-degree burns. Do not use on individuals with known allergy or hypersensitivty to the dressing or its components.

APPLICATION

- Irrigate the wound with Gentell Wound Cleanser and gently dry the skin surrounding the wound site.
- Choose the appropriate size dressing based on the dimensions of the wound.
- Apply Gentell Super Absorbent Dressing Adherent with the white side to the wound and blue side up.

REMOVAL

- Change daily or as ordered by a physician.

SPECIALTY ABSORPTIVES

New Product: 3M™ Tegaderm™ Superabsorber Dressing

3M™ Health Care

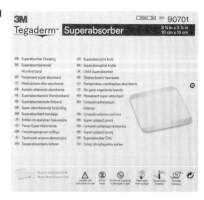

HOW SUPPLIED

Pad	4 1/2″ × 3 7/8″ (4 1/2″ × 2 7/8″ pad)	A6196
Pad	4 1/2″ × 7 7/8″ (4 1/2″ × 6 7/8″ pad)	A6197
Pad	7 7/8″ × 7 7/8″ (7 7/8″ × 6 7/8″ pad)	A6197
Pad	7 7/8″ × 11 3/4″ (7 7/8″ × 10 1/2″ pad)	A6198

ACTION

3M™ Tegaderm™ Superabsorber Dressing is a sterile, superabsorbent dressing for use on moderate to highly draining wounds. Absorbs drainage vertically into the dressing to minimize the risk of maceration of the wound edges.

INDICATIONS

Exuding wounds such as leg ulcers, pressure injuries, diabetic foot ulcers, and other wounds producing high levels of exudate. It should be used on moderate to heavily exuding wounds when there is a need for high absorption and fewer dressing changes. The dressing can be used both—as a primary dressing or as a secondary dressing. The backing on the dressing minimizes leakage.

CONTRAINDICATIONS

- None known.

APPLICATION

- Note: Follow facility guidelines for infection control.

Applying the dressing

- Cleanse the wound and surrounding skin according to facility policy. If the periwound skin is fragile or exposure to wound exudate is likely, apply a barrier film. Allow the barrier film to dry before dressing application.
- Choose a size of dressing depending on the wound size; the core edge of the dressing should overlap the wound by minimum 2 cm (0.8″).
- The dressing must be in close contact with the wound or the primary dressing.
- The dressing should be monitored regularly in accordance with best practice in the management of exuding wounds to avoid complete saturation.
- Do not reuse the dressing.

REMOVAL

- Dressing removal can be facilitated by moistening the dressing with saline solution. Dispose of dressing as of normal waste.
- May be used in combination with compression therapy.

REFERENCE

1. https://www.3m.com/3M/en_US/company-us/search/?Ntt=superabsorber&LC=en_US&co= cc&gsaAction=scBR&type=cc

Surgical Supplies, Miscellaneous

NOTE: The Pricing, Data Analysis and Coding (PDAC) contractor maintains the Durable Medical Equipment Coding System (DMECS). DMECS is an official source for Medicare Durable Medical Equipment Prosthetics, Orthotics and Supplies (DMEPOS) product code verification and assignment. Coding verification is the process that allows manufacturers/ distributors to request a coding decision on a DMEPOS item. It is the responsibility of the PDAC to review DMEPOS products to determine the appropriate Healthcare Common Procedure Coding System (HCPCS) code for Medicare billing.[1]

When the PDAC, or the former Statistical Analysis Durable Medical Equipment Regional Carrier (SADMERC) perform a Coding Verification Review and fail to reach a consensus coding decision based on the following definition, they sometimes assign the product or procedure to a general category[2]:

- Products where a single material comprises greater than 50% (by weight) of a product's composition are coded based upon the applicable specific HCPCS code for that material. If a specific HCPCS code does not exist for the predominant component, HCPCS code A4649 (Surgical Supply, miscellaneous) is used.
- Products where no single material comprises greater than 50% (by weight) of the composition are coded as A4649 (Surgical Supply, miscellaneous).

Therefore, various dissimilar products and procedures are usually assigned to this category. These products in this category do not have a universal definition, use, or payment guidelines. Yet, each product listed under this category has an individual action, indication, contraindication, and application and removal process. It remains the clinician's responsibility to understand each product before using it.

When submitting claims for products or procedures in this category, the provider and supplier must check with the payer for the supporting documentation that is required.

HCPCS CODE OVERVIEW

The HCPCS code normally assigned to miscellaneous surgical supplies is: A4649—Surgical supply; miscellaneous.

---

[1] Accessed June 4, 2018 https://www.dmepdac.com/review/index.html
[2] Accessed June 4, 2018 https://www.dmepdac.com/resources/articles/2015/08_19_15.html

New Product: Eclypse® Contour Super Absorbent Dressing

Advancis Medical/DUKAL Corporation

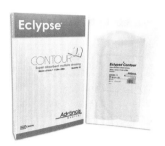

HOW SUPPLIED

Eclypse® Contour Super Absorbent Dressing	12″ × 20″	A4649

ACTION

- Super-absorbent dressing specifically designed to treat highly exuding wounds in difficult-to-dress areas, such as the underarm, abdomen, back, lower leg, and thigh.
- Molds to body contours, ensuring optimum contact with the wound and effective exudate management.
- Thin and conforming for comfort and reduces dressing changes.

INDICATIONS

- Moderate to heavily exuding wounds.
- Leg ulcers.
- Pressure ulcers.
- Sloughy or granulating wounds.
- Postoperative or dehisced wounds.
- Fungating wounds.
- Donor site management.

CONTRAINDICATIONS

- Do not use on arterial bleeds or heavily bleeding wounds.

APPLICATION

- Open out the dressing fully; the white side will be in contact with the wound surface, the beige backing will be uppermost.
- Secure the dressing with tape or appropriate bandage.
- Do not cut Eclypse® Contour.

REMOVAL

- Up to 7 days.

New Product: THERAHONEY®

Medline Industries, Inc.

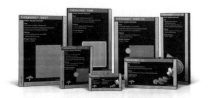

TheraHoney Gel	0.5-oz tube	A4649
TheraHoney Gel	1.5-oz tube	A4649
TheraHoney Sheet	4″ × 5″	A4649
TheraHoney HD Sheet	2″ × 2″	A4649
TheraHoney HD Sheet	4″ × 5″	A4649
TheraHoney Ribbon	1″ × 12″	A4649
TheraHoney Foam	4″ × 4″	A4649
TheraHoney Foam Flex	4″ × 4″	A6209

ACTION

Made of 100% manuka honey. Promotes autolytic debridement with high sugar level (87%). Helps rapidly reduce odor and creates a moist wound environment.

INDICATIONS

Partial- and full-thickness wounds, leg ulcers, pressure injuries, first- and second-degree burns, diabetic foot ulcers, surgical wounds and trauma wounds, minor abrasions, lacerations, minor cuts, minor scalds, and burns.

CONTRAINDICATIONS

- Contraindicated for third-degree burns.
- Individuals with a known sensitivity to honey.

APPLICATION

- Gel: Using a tongue-blade applicator, apply TheraHoney gel at 2- to 3-mm thickness. Then cover with an absorbent secondary dressing.
- Sheets or Rope: Cut or fold the dressing as needed to fit the wound bed. Then cover with an absorbent secondary dressing.
- Foam and Foam Flex: Place the dressing over the wound and secure with an adhesive tape or gauze.
- Apply skin protectant or barrier around wound edges to prevent maceration.

REMOVAL

- TheraHoney can be removed with saline or sterile water.
- Change in frequency will depend upon the amount of wound drainage. Check the secondary dressing for indications on time to change the dressing. TheraHoney sheet/rope should be changed/removed when it appears whitish. TheraHoney can be left in place for up to 7 days.

REFERENCE

1. https://www.medline.com/product/TheraHoney-Gel/Honey-Dressings/Z05-PF13869

Transparent Films

ACTION

Transparent films are adhesive, semipermeable, polyurethane membrane dressings that vary in thickness and size. They are waterproof and impermeable to bacteria and contaminants, yet they permit water vapor to cross the barrier. These dressings maintain a moist healing environment, promoting formation of granulation tissue and autolysis of necrotic tissue.

INDICATIONS

Transparent films may be used as a primary or secondary dressing to prevent and manage stage 1 pressure ulcers, partial-thickness wounds with little or no exudate, and wounds with necrotic tissue or slough.

ADVANTAGES

- Retain moisture.
- Are impermeable to bacteria and other contaminants.
- Facilitate autolytic debridement.
- Allow wound observation.
- Do not require a secondary dressing.

DISADVANTAGES

- May not be recommended for infected wounds.
- Not recommended for wounds with moderate to heavy drainage because they don't absorb.
- Not recommended for use on fragile skin.
- Require a border of intact skin for adhesive edge of dressing.
- May be difficult to apply and handle.
- May dislodge in high-friction areas.

HCPCS CODE OVERVIEW

The HCPCS codes normally assigned to transparent film dressings are:
A6257—pad size <16 in^2.
A6258—pad size >16 in^2 but ≤48 in^2.
A6259—pad size >48 in^2.

New Product: BIOCLUSIVE™ Plus Transparent Film Dressing

Systagenix, An ACELITY™ Company

HOW SUPPLIED

BIOCLUSIVE™ Plus Transparent Film Dressing	2 3/8″ × 2 3/4″	A6257
BIOCLUSIVE™ Plus Transparent Film Dressing	4″ × 4 3/4″	A6258
BIOCLUSIVE™ Plus Transparent Film Dressing	5 7/8″ × 7 7/8″	A6258
BIOCLUSIVE™ Plus Transparent Film Dressing	7 3/8″ × 11 3/4″	A6259

ACTION

BIOCLUSIVE™ Plus Transparent Film Dressing is a self-adhesive dressing consisting of a transparent semi-permeable polyurethane film coating with an acrylic adhesive. BIOCLUSIVE™ Plus Dressing provides a bacterial barrier while also allowing the transmission of moisture vapor and oxygen, and facilitates a moist wound-healing environment. BIOCLUSIVE™ Plus Dressing allows visual inspection of the wound site and is flexible and conformable for use on difficult contours.

INDICATIONS

BIOCLUSIVE™ Plus Dressing is indicated for the management of wounds where there is no exudate, or light levels of exudate.
- BIOCLUSIVE™ Plus Dressings should be used under health care professional direction for the following indications:
  - Minor burns.
  - Donor sites.
  - Superficial pressure areas and leg ulcers.
  - Clean, closed, postoperative wounds.
  - Cuts and abrasions.
- BIOCLUSIVE™ Plus Dressing is also suitable for:
  - Securing of catheters.
  - Use as a secondary, cover dressing.
  - Reducing shear and friction.

CONTRAINDICATIONS

- BIOCLUSIVE™ Plus Dressing should not be used on patients with a known sensitivity to any of its components.
- BIOCLUSIVE™ Plus Dressing is not indicated for use on the following:
  - Full-thickness burns.
  - Deep cavity wounds.
  - Wound or catheter sites which are clinically infected.
  - Wounds treated with topical medicinal preparations.

APPLICATIONS

- If clinical infection is observed during the use of BIOCLUSIVE™ Plus Dressing, discontinue use and refer to local protocol for managing the infection.

TRANSPARENT FILMS

- The bacterial barrier of the dressing can be compromised if the dressing is damaged or punctured. Leakage of loss of adhesion to the skin will also compromise the bacterial barrier.
  - Prepare the wound according to the local wound management protocol.
  - Ensure that the skin surrounding the wound is clean, dry and free from grease, soaps, or detergents.
  - Choose an appropriate-size dressing to allow at least a 2-cm border to overlap the wound edge.
  - Peel open the package and remove the dressing.
  - Remove the larger, central release liner from the adhesive underside of the dressing (marked A).
  - Position the dressing centrally over the wound, adhesive side down.
  - Press the exposed adhesive side of the dressing onto the skin surrounding the wound.
  - Grasp the outer release liner tabs from the underside of the dressings (marked B).
  - Peel away the tabs and press the remaining edges of the dressing onto the skin using a rolling motion.
  - Ensure the dressing adheres well to the skin.
  - Once the dressing is secure, grasp the upper release liner tabs (marked C) and peel away from the center of the dressing outward.

REMOVAL

- Dressing change frequency is dictated by good wound care practice and will depend on the condition of the wound.
- BIOCLUSIVE™ Plus Dressing may be left in place for several days depending upon the amount of exudate.
- Gently peel and lift one corner of the dressing from the skin. Support the skin whilst peeling the dressing off by stretching horizontally (not vertically) and in the direction of hair growth.
- Care should be taken to avoid skin damage with repeated applications or on patients with fragile skin.
- Care should also be taken not to dislodge catheters or other devices.
- Use existing clinical protocols to clean the wound in order to remove any remaining exudate residue before wound assessment or the application of further dressings.
- Do not use if the package is damaged.
- Do not reuse.
- Do not resterilize.
- The use by date of this product is printed on the packaging.

TRANSPARENT FILMS

DermaView

DermaRite Industries, LLC

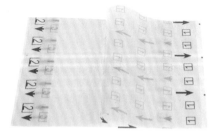

HOW SUPPLIED

Transparent Film Wound Dressing with Label and Grid	2" × 3"	A6257
Transparent Film Wound Dressing with Label and Grid	4" × 5"	A6258
Transparent Film Wound Dressing with Label and Grid	6" × 11"	A6259
Transparent Film Wound Dressing with Label and Grid, I.V.	2.375" × 2.75"	A6257
Transparent Film Wound Dressing with Label and Grid	2" × 11" yds	
Transparent Film Wound Dressing with Label and Grid	4" × 11" yds	

ACTION

DermaView™ is a nonabsorbent, moisture-vapor--permeable, self-adhesive transparent film wound dressing for noninfected wounds with minimal drainage. Allows visualization of wound, maintains a moist wound bed, and helps prevent bacterial contamination of wound.

INDICATIONS

May be used as a primary or secondary dressing. For the management of dry to lightly exuding wounds including noninfected wounds, partial-thickness ulcers, shallow full-thickness ulcers.

CONTRAINDICATIONS

- DermaView should not be used on people who are sensitive or allergic to the dressing and its components.

APPLICATION

- Cleanse the wound with the advised liquid to remove the residue according to the local infection control protocol. Deep wounds should be well irrigated.
- The skin around the wound should be clean and dry. Use skin barrier prep as needed.
- Remove the dressing from the package.
- If applicable, remove the middle paper panel from the front (nonsticky) side of the dressing.
- Remove the backing paper from the dressing.
- Apply the sticky side of the dressing to the moist wound bed overlapping 1 to 2 inches of dry skin; gently smooth into place.
- If applicable, remove the paper frame from the front (nonsticky) side of the dressing.

REMOVAL

- The dressing may be moistened to ease removal.
- Carefully remove adhesive dressings by holding the edge of the dressing and slowly pulling it parallel to the skin.
- Dispose of in accordance with local guidance.

REFERENCE

1. http://dermarite.com/product/dermaview/

TRANSPARENT FILMS

DermaView II

DermaRite Industries, LLC

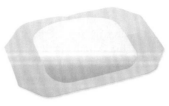

HOW SUPPLIED

Transparent Film Wound Dressing with Label	2.375" × 2.75"	A6257
Transparent Film Wound Dressing with Label	4" × 4.5"	A6257
Transparent Film Wound Dressing with Label	4" × 10"	A6258
Transparent Film Wound Dressing with Label	6" × 8"	A6259
Transparent Film Wound Dressing with Label	8" × 12"	A6259

ACTION

DermaView™ II is a nonabsorbent, moisture-vapor–permeable transparent film dressing with a picture-frame border for easy application. DermaView II is suitable for noninfected wounds with minimal drainage or as a secondary dressing. DermaView II maintains a moist wound bed and helps prevent bacterial contamination of the wound.

INDICATIONS

May be used as a primary or secondary dressing. For the management of minimally exuding wounds including noninfected wounds, partial-thickness ulcers, shallow full-thickness ulcers.

CONTRAINDICATIONS

- DermaView II should not be used on people who are sensitive or allergic to the dressing and its components.

APPLICATION

- Cleanse the wound with the advised liquid to remove the residue according to the local infection control protocol. Deep wounds should be well irrigated.
- The skin around the wound should be clean and dry. Use skin barrier prep as needed.
- Remove the dressing from the package.
- If applicable, remove the middle paper panel from the front (nonsticky) side of the dressing.
- Remove the backing paper from the dressing.
- Apply the sticky side of the dressing to the moist wound bed overlapping 1 to 2 inches of dry skin; gently smooth into place.
- Remove the paper frame from the front (nonsticky) side of the dressing.

REMOVAL

- Dressing may be moistened to ease removal.
- Carefully remove adhesive dressings by holding the edge of the dressing and slowly pulling it parallel to the skin.
- Dispose of in accordance with local guidance.

REFERENCE

1. http://dermarite.com/product/dermaview-ii/

Mepore® Film Transparent Film Dressing

Mölnlycke Health Care

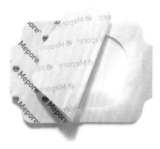

Mepore® Film

HOW SUPPLIED

Dressing	2.4″ × 2.6″	A6257
Dressing	4″ × 5″	A6258
Dressing	4″ × 10″	A6258
Dressing	6″ × 8.5″	A6259

ACTION

Mepore® Film is a breathable, transparent self-adhesive film dressing that conforms easily to body contours, helps protect the wound surface, and provides a barrier to leakage and bacterial contamination. Mepore® Film helps maintain a moist wound environment and the adhesive is gentle to the skin and wound site.

INDICATIONS

Designed for a wide range of clean wounds in the granulation phase, such as superficial burns, IV sites, abrasions, lacerations, superficial pressure ulcers, closed surgical wounds, and donor sites with low exudate levels, as well as for the prevention of skin breakdown.

CONTRAINDICATIONS

- Not for use on full-thickness wounds involving muscle, tendon, or bone.
- Not for use on third-degree burns.
- Mepore Film should not be applied on patients who are sensitive to acrylic adhesive.

APPLICATION

- Clean the wound area. Make sure that the surrounding skin is dry.
- Choose the correct dressing size to overlap the dry skin by at least 3/8″ (1 cm).
- For sizes 4″ × 10″ and 6″ × 8.5″ only: Remove center cutout paper and discard.
- Remove the protective backing to expose the adhesive.
- Position the dressing and smooth it onto the skin.
- Remove the paper frame and the two white paper side tabs.

REMOVAL

- The dressing may be left in place for several days, depending on the condition of the wound and surrounding skin.
- Lift a corner of the dressing and gently pull the film along the skin (in the direction of hair growth).

TRANSPARENT FILMS

MVP Transparent

Gentell

REORDER
GEN-16450
NDC 61554-164-04

Gentell®

MVP Dressing
Transparent Film 4" x 4.75" (10x12cm)

*Non-absorptive Moisture Vapor Permeable Dressing
with hypoallergenic adhesive to cover
and monitor low exudating wounds*

Directions
1. Flush the wound with Gentell Wound Cleanser and gently dry the skin surrounding the wound site.
2. As a primary dressing, apply directly to the wound surface.
3. As a secondary dressing, apply directly over primary treatment.
4. Change dressing daily or as order by a physician.

Gentell®
2701 Bartram Road
Bristol, PA 19007
215-788-2700 Fax 215-788-2713
www.gentell.com

HOW SUPPLIED

Film	4" × 4.75"	A6258

ACTION

Gentell MVP Transparent Film Dressing is a moisture vapor permeable transparent membrane coated with a layer of acrylic, hypoallergenic adhesive that can be used to cover low exuding wounds. Gentell MVP is a non-absorptive sterile dressing that is permeable to moisture vapor and oxygen, but impermeable to bacteria.

INDICATIONS

- Gentell MVP Transparent Film Dressing can be used as a primary treatment by applying as a breathable bacterial barrier to block outside contaminants.
- MVP can also be used as a secondary dressing for Stage II pressure ulcers, abrasions, skin tears, blisters, skin graft donor sites, superficial partial-thickness burns, autolytic debridement, skin protection against moisture as well as friction and clean, closed surgical incisions. MVP transparent dressings may also be used to cover and secure IV devices.

CONTRAINDICATIONS

- Do not use on infected wounds.

APPLICATION

- Flush the wound with Gentell Wound Cleanser and gently dry the skin surrounding the wound site.
- As a primary dressing, apply directly to the wound surface.
- As a secondary dressing, apply directly over primary treatment.

REMOVAL

- Change daily or as ordered by a physician.

Transeal Transparent Wound Dressing

DeRoyal

HOW SUPPLIED

Film	1 3/4" × 1 3/4"	A6257
Film	2 1/2" × 2 3/4"	A6257
Film	4" × 4 3/4"	A6258
Film	4" × 10"	A6258
Film	6" × 8"	A6258
Film	8" × 12"	A6259

ACTION

Transeal is a transparent, breathable polyurethane wound dressing coated with an acrylic, pressure-sensitive adhesive that acts as a second skin. Transeal has the highest vapor transmission rate available, yet it is impermeable to external contaminants, such as water, dirt, debris, and bacteria.

INDICATIONS

To prevent skin breakdown and to manage pressure ulcers (stages 1 to 4), partial- and full-thickness wounds, tunneling wounds, donor sites, IV sites, first- and second-degree burns, acute wounds, infected and noninfected wounds, draining wounds, and red, yellow, or black wounds; may be used as a primary or secondary dressing depending on wound type.

CONTRAINDICATIONS

- Contraindicated as a primary dressing for heavily draining wounds.

APPLICATION

- Clean and thoroughly dry the wound and surrounding skin.
- Peel off the backing layer of the dressing to expose the adhesive side of the dressing.
- Position the dressing over the wound and press it gently into place.
- Peel off the clear carrier film to leave the dressing in place.

REMOVAL

- Remove the dressing by gently peeling away in the direction of hair growth.

TRANSPARENT FILMS

3M™ Tegaderm™ HP Transparent Film Dressing

3M™ Tegaderm™ Transparent Film Dressing

3M™ Health Care

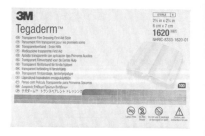

HOW SUPPLIED

3M™ Tegaderm™ HP Transparent Film Dressing

Film Sheet	2 3/8″ × 2 3/4″	A6257
Film Sheet	4″ × 4 3/4″	A6258
Film Sheet (Sacral)	4 1/2″ × 4 3/4″	A6258
Oval	2 1/8″ × 2 1/2″	A6257
Oval	5 1/2″ × 6 1/2″	A6258
Oval	4″ × 4 1/2″	A6257

3M™ Tegaderm™ Transparent Film Dressing

Frame Style	1 3/4″ × 1 3/4″	A6257
Frame Style	2 3/8″ × 2 3/4″	A6257
Frame Style	4″ × 4 3/4″	A6258
Frame Style	4″ × 10″	A6258
Frame Style	6″ × 8″	A6258
Frame Style	8″ × 12″	A6259
Frame Style with Border	2 3/8″ × 2 3/4″	A6257
Frame Style with Border	4″ × 4 3/4″	A6258
Frame Style (Oval)	4″ × 4 1/2″	A6258
First Aid Style	2 3/8″ × 2 3/4″	A6257
First Aid Style	4″ × 4 3/4″	A6258
Frame Style	2 3/8″ × 2 3/4″	A6257
Frame Style	4″ × 4 3/4″	A6258
Frame Style	4″ × 4 1/2″	A6258
Frame Style	2 3/8″ × 2 3/4″	A6257
Frame Style	4 × 4 3/4″	A6258

3M™ Tegaderm™ Transparent Film Roll

Film Roll	2″ × 11 yd	A6257-A6259
Film Roll	4″ × 11 yd	A6257-A6259
Film Roll	6″ × 11 yd	A6257-A6259

DESCRIPTION

3M™ Tegaderm™ Transparent Film Dressing consists of a thin film backing with a non-latex, hypo-allergenic adhesive. The dressing is breathable, allowing good oxygen and moisture vapor exchange. It is waterproof and impermeable to liquids, bacteria, and viruses. An intact dressing protects the site from outside contamination.

INDICATIONS

To cover and protect catheter sites and wounds, to maintain a moist environment for wound healing, or to facilitate autolytic debridement, as a secondary dressing, as a protective cover over at-risk skin, to secure devices to the skin, to cover first and second-degree burns, and as a protective eye covering up to 7 days wear time.

CONTRAINDICATIONS

- May be used on infected site only when under the care of a health care professional.
- Not intended to replace sutures or other primary wound closure methods.
- Antimicrobial ointments containing polyethylene glycols may compromise the strength of Tegaderm™ HP Transparent Film dressing.

APPLICATION

- Stop any bleeding at the site before applying dressing.
- Do not stretch dressing during application as tension can cause skin trauma.
- Make sure the skin is clean, free of soap residue and lotion and allowed to dry thoroughly before applying the dressing to prevent skin irritation, and to ensure good adhesion.
- Peel the liner from the dressing, exposing the adhesive surface.
- Center the dressing over the catheter site or wound.
- Apply firm pressure over entire transparent portion.
- While slowly peeling off the paper frame, smooth down the dressing edges with fingertips.

REMOVAL

Low and slow

- Gently grasp an edge, and slowly peel the dressing from the skin in the direction of hair growth. Avoid skin trauma by peeling the dressing back, rather than pulling it up from the skin.
  OR

Stretch and release

- Grasp one edge of the dressing and gently pull it straight out to stretch it and release the adhesion.

TRANSPARENT FILMS

Wound Fillers

ACTION

Wound fillers are available as pastes, granules, powders, beads, and gels that provide a moist healing environment, absorb exudate, and help debride the wound bed by softening the necrotic tissue.

INDICATIONS

Wound fillers may be used as primary dressings to manage partial- and full-thickness wounds, minimally to moderately exuding wounds, infected and noninfected wounds, and wounds requiring packing to fill dead space.

ADVANTAGES

- May be absorbent.
- Promote autolytic debridement.
- Are easy to apply and remove.
- May be used with other products.
- Fill dead space.

DISADVANTAGES

- Most not recommended for use in wounds with little or no exudate.
- Require secondary dressing.

HCPCS CODE OVERVIEW

The HCPCS codes normally assigned to wound fillers not elsewhere classified are:
A6261—gel/paste, per fluid ounce.
A6262—dry form, per gram.

Multidex Maltodextrin Wound

DeRoyal

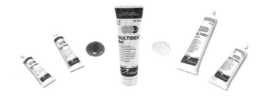

HOW SUPPLIED

Powder Tube	6-g	A6262
Powder Tube	12-g	A6262
Powder Tube	25-g	A6262
Powder Tube	45-g	A6262
Gel Tube	1/4 fl oz	A6248
Gel Tube	1/2 fl oz	A6248
Gel Tube	3 fl oz	A6248

ACTION

Multidex Maltodextrin Wound Dressing establishes and maintains a moist environment for tissue granulation by mixing with wound exudate, thus controlling dehydration, drainage, and odor.

INDICATIONS

To be used as a primary or secondary dressing to manage pressure ulcers (stages 2 to 4), venous stasis ulcers, diabetic ulcers, neuropathic ulcers, and poorly healing wounds; may also be used on tunneling wounds, partial- and full-thickness wounds, infected and noninfected wounds, wounds with heavy or purulent drainage, and red, yellow, or black wounds.

CONTRAINDICATIONS

- None provided by the manufacturer.

APPLICATION

- Irrigate the wound with normal saline solution.
- Apply the dressing over the entire wound to a minimum thickness of 1 1/8″ to 1 1/4″ (0.3 to 0.5 cm). For deep wounds, fill to the skin surface.
- Cover with a nonadherent dressing.

REMOVAL

- Remove the secondary dressing.
- Irrigate the wound with normal saline solution. Any remaining dressing may be left in the wound.

WOUND FILLERS

OTHER PRODUCTS

Other Products

This category comprises a wide variety of products used to facilitate skin and wound management. Each entry details the products:

- Action.
- Indications.
- Contraindications.
- Application.
- Removal.

Please refer to each product listing for further information about these products.

In this section, the manufacturer has either received an HCPCS code or hasn't yet received or applied for a code. It is the clinician's responsibility to verify coding of each product with the product's manufacturer.

New Product: Activon®
Manuka Honey Tube

Advancis Medical/DUKAL Corporation

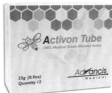

HOW SUPPLIED

Activon® Manuka Honey Tube	0.9 oz	A9270

ACTION

- Contains 100% pure Manuka honey with no additives.
- A wound filler ideal for debriding necrotic tissue.
- Eliminates odors.
- Maintains a moist wound-healing environment, facilitating faster healing of chronic wounds.
- Does not absorb into the blood stream, meaning it can be safely used on diabetic patients.

INDICATIONS

- Any wound.
- Slough, necrotic, and malodorous wounds.
- Pressure ulcers.
- Leg ulcers.
- Diabetic ulcers.
- Surgical wounds.
- Burns.
- Graft sites.
- Infected wounds.
- Cavity wounds.
- Sinuses.

CONTRAINDICATIONS

- Although the honey is not absorbed into the blood stream, we advise monitoring the levels of patients with diabetes.
- Do not use if allergic to bee venom.
- Discomfort can occasionally be experienced when honey is initially applied, it may be necessary to consider an appropriate level of analgesia. If discomfort continues, discontinue use and irrigate the wound with saline solution.

APPLICATION

- Twist off cap, apply liberally to the wound bed to a minimum depth of 5 mm.
- Cover with an appropriate secondary dressing.
- Activon® Tube is a single patient use only product, once opened use within 90 days.

REFERENCE

1. http://www.advancis.co.uk/products

New Product: Activon® Manuka Honey Tulle

Advancis Medical/DUKAL Corporation

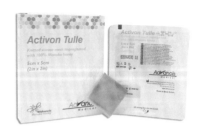

HOW SUPPLIED

| Activon® Manuka Honey Tulle | 2″ × 2″ | A9270 |
| Activon® Manuka Honey Tulle | 4″ × 4″ | A9270 |

ACTION

- A knitted viscose mesh primary dressing impregnated with 100% medical grade. Manuka honey
- Creates a moist healing environment and effectively eliminates wound odor.
- Allows exudate to pass through the dressing on wounds with low to moderate levels of exudate.
- Ideal to debride and deslough shallow wounds or where the exudate levels have started to decrease.
- Can be cut to size, increasing patient comfort and resulting in better periwound skin condition.
- Can be placed on the wound either side up, eliminating incorrect dressing application.

INDICATIONS

- Any wound.
- Sloughy, necrotic, and malodorous wounds.
- Dry wounds.
- Leg ulcers.
- Diabetic ulcers.
- Pressure sores.
- Infected wounds.

CONTRAINDICATIONS

- Although the honey is not absorbed into the blood stream, we advise monitoring the levels of patients with diabetes.
- Do not use if allergic to bee venom.
- Discomfort can occasionally be experienced when honey is initially applied, it may be necessary to consider an appropriate level of analgesia. If discomfort continues, discontinue use and irrigate the wound with saline solution.

APPLICATION

- Dressing is placed (either side down) onto the wound surface.
- Can be placed side by side to cover large wound areas or cut to size.
- Can be unfolded to cover larger areas, this reduces the concentration of honey at the wound site.

- Depending on the tissue type within the wound bed and level of exudate, your secondary dressing of choice could be a film dressing and/or bandage.
- In wounds with a high level of exudate an additional highly absorbent dressing, such as the Eclypse® super absorbent dressing, can be introduced to help manage exudate.

REMOVAL

- Up to 7 days.

New Product: DxWound

Millennium Health, LLC

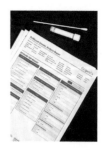

HOW SUPPLIED

DNA-Based Tests	Codes associated with Infectious Disease Molecular Diagnostic Testing

ACTION

DxWound is a DNA-based diagnostic tool that provides a rapid and comprehensive assessment of the microbial environment of a wound. The tests identify aerobic and anaerobic bacteria, fungi, and antibiotic resistance genes plus a virulence gene specific to *Staphylococcus aureus*, and compile the information into a single report delivered, generally, one business day after receipt of the specimen.

INDICATIONS

DxWound can be used for any patient suspected of having an skin and soft tissue infection or with clinical signs of an skin and soft tissue infection.

CONTRAINDICATIONS

- N/A.

APPLICATION

- DxWound utilizes a swab for sample collection. The Levine technique is suggested for collection of the sample: the swab is rotated over a 1-cm^2 area with sufficient pressure to express the liquid from within the wound tissue. The swab is then placed in a transport tube containing an inactivating solution that kills microorganisms at the same time as protecting the microbial DNA, thus preserving the wound microbiome in time at the point of specimen collection.

REMOVAL

- N/A.

REFERENCE

1. www.cogendx.com/resources/

Electrode Gel Pads and Connection Wires

Senergy Medical Group

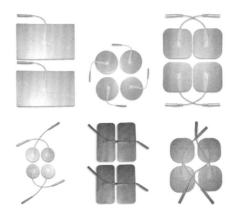

HOW SUPPLIED

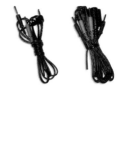

Electrode Gel, Pads	3" × 5" rectangle	A4556
Electrode Gel, Pads	3" round	A4556
Electrode Gel, Pads	2" × 2" square	A4556
Electrode Gel, Pads	1.375" round	A4556
Electrode Gel, Pads	1.75" × 3.75" rectangle for sensitive skin	A4556
Electrode Gel, Pads	1.75" × 1.75" square for sensitive skin	A4556
Connection Wires (2 lead and 4 lead)	42" long	A4557

Electrode gel pads and connection wires are available for purchase from Senergy Medical Group.

ACTION

Self-stick, reusable/disposable conductive pads can be used to stimulate specific areas with concentrated voltage and intensify the treatment on specific muscle or tissue for extended pain relief.

INDICATIONS

Refer to Tennant Biomodulator® indications.

CONTRAINDICATIONS

- Refer to Tennant Biomodulator contraindications.

APPLICATION

- Use directly on clean, dry, unbroken skin and place on either side of a wound for pain management. Conductive pads provide for extended, hands-free treatment.

REMOVAL

- Gently remove from the skin and return to the plastic sheet. Replace conductive pads when they no longer stick to the skin. Unplug connection wires from the Biomodulator.

REFERENCES

1. http://senergy.us/pads.html
2. www.senergy.us

Flexi-Seal™ PROTECT Fecal Management System*

ConvaTec

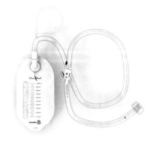

HOW SUPPLIED

Flexi-Seal PROTECT FMS Kit	1 kit or box
Flexi-Seal PROTECT FMS Replacement Collection Bags	10/box

ACTION

The Flexi-Seal™ PROTECT Fecal Management System contains, 1 soft catheter tube assembly, 1 Luer-Lock syringe, 1 Privacy bag with filter and 1 cinch clamp. The soft catheter is inserted into the rectum for fecal management to contain and divert fecal waste in order to protect the patient's skin and keep the bedding clean. There is a low-pressure retention balloon at the distal end and a connector for attaching the collection bag at the other end. There is a recess under the balloon for the clinician's finger allowing the device to be positioned digitally.

INDICATIONS

For use to manage fecal incontinence through the collection of liquid to semi-liquid stool and to provide access to administer medications.

CONTRAINDICATIONS

- This product is not intended for use:
  - for more than 29 consecutive days.
  - for pediatric patients (patients under 18 years of age) as its use has not been tested in this population.
- The Flexi-Seal™ PROTECT Fecal Management System should not be used on individuals who:
  - have suspected or confirmed rectal mucosal impairment, i.e. severe proctitis, ischemic proctitis, mucosal ulcerations.
  - have had rectal surgery within the last year.
  - have any rectal or anal injury.
  - have hemorrhoids of significant size and/or symptoms.
  - have a rectal or anal stricture or stenosis.
  - have a suspected or confirmed rectal/anal tumor.
  - have any in-dwelling rectal or anal device (e.g. thermometer) or delivery mechanism (e.g. suppositories or enemas) in place.
  - are sensitive to or who have had an allergic reaction to any component within the system.

APPLICATION

Preparation of device

- In addition to the device system, gloves and lubricant will be required.
- Unfold the length of the catheter to lay it flat on the bed, extending the collection bag toward the foot of the bed.
- Securely attach the collection bag to the connector at the end of the catheter.

Preparation of patient

- Position the patient in left side lying position; if unable to tolerate, position the patient so access to the rectum is possible.
- Remove any in-dwelling or anal device prior to insertion of the Flexi-Seal™ PROTECT device.
- Perform a digital rectal exam to evaluate suitability for insertion of device.

Insertion of device

- Remove the white cap from the inflation port. Using the syringe provided, remove the air that is in the balloon by attaching the syringe to the white inflation port (marked "≤45 mL") and withdrawing the plunger.

    Remove the supplied syringe and fill it with 45 mL of water or saline and connect the syringe to the white inflation port of the catheter.

    Insert a lubricated gloved finger into the blue finger pocket for digital guidance during device insertion (the finger pocket is located above the position indicator line).

    Coat the balloon end of the catheter with lubricant. Grasp the catheter and gently insert the balloon end through the anal sphincter until the balloon is beyond the external orifice and well inside the rectal vault. The finger may be removed or remain in place in the rectum during initial balloon inflation.

- Inflate the balloon with up to 45 ml of fluid by slowly depressing the syringe plunger. With the insertion finger removed, the green PROTECT indication dome will indicate once the balloon has reached the optimal fill level for the anatomy. Stop inflation once the green dome has signaled optimal fill. Under no circumstances should the balloon be inflated with more than 45 mL of fluid.

    If the green PROTECT indication dome indicates at less than 30 mL of fluid, withdraw the fluid and reposition the balloon in the rectal vault. After repositioning, fill the balloon as described above. Do not fill with more than 45 mL of fluid. The red PROTECT indication dome will start to indicate if the balloon is overfilled beyond the maximum 45 mL of fluid. If the red PROTECT indication dome is fully inflated, assess patient's position, fully deflate the balloon and repeat the balloon inflation process. Stop inflation once the green dome has signaled optimal fill.

- Remove the syringe from the inflation port, and gently pull on the soft catheter to check that the balloon is securely in the rectum and that it is positioned against the rectal floor. (Figure 6). Close the cap on the white inflation port to avoid misconnection issues such as inserting medication or irrigating through the wrong port.

- Position the length of the flexible catheter along patient's leg avoiding kinks and obstruction. Take note of the position indicator line relative to the patient's anus. Regularly observe changes in the location of the position indicator line as a means to determine movement of the retention balloon in the patient's rectum. This may indicate the need for the balloon or device to be re-positioned. In the event of expulsion of the device, deflate the balloon fully; rinse the balloon end of the catheter and reinsert following the instructions for 'Insertion of Device'. A rectal exam should be conducted prior to re-insertion to verify that no stool is present. If expulsion continues for more than three episodes discontinuation of the device should be considered.

- Hang the bag by the bead strap on the bedside at a position lower than that of the patient.

Irrigation of the device

- Port (marked "irriG./rx") and slowly depress the plunger. Clinicians should take extra care to use the blue irrigation/medication port only when irrigating. Do not irrigate through the white inflation port (marked "≤45 mL") as this would lead to over inflation of the retention balloon and the device would not be irrigated as intended.

- Repeat the irrigation procedure as often as necessary to maintain proper functioning of the device. Flushing the device as described above is an optional procedure for use only when needed to maintain the unobstructed flow of stool into the collection bag.
- If repeated flushing with water does not return the flow of stool through the catheter, the device should be inspected to ascertain that there is no external obstruction (i.e. pressure from a body part, piece of equipment, or resolution of diarrhea). If no source of obstruction of the device is detected, use of the device should be discontinued.

Maintenance of device

- Change the collection bag as needed. Discard used bags according to institutional protocol for disposal of medical waste. Observe the device frequently for obstructions from kinks, solid fecal particles or external pressure.

REMOVAL

- To remove the catheter from the rectum, the retention balloon must first be deflated. Remove the white cap from the inflation port. Attach the syringe to the white inflation port (marked "≤45 mL") and slowly withdraw all fluid from the retention balloon.
- Disconnect the syringe and discard. Grasp the catheter as close to the patient as possible and slowly remove from the anus. Dispose of the device in accordance with institutional protocol for disposal of medical waste. In the event that the balloon is difficult or impossible to deflate, cut the inflation lumen and drain out the water in the balloon. On no account should the device be removed from a patient with the balloon still inflated.

*See package insert for complete instructions for use.

Flexi-Seal™ SIGNAL Fecal Management System*

ConvaTec

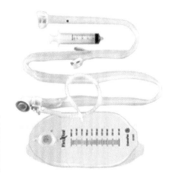

HOW SUPPLIED

Flexi-Seal SIGNAL FMS Kit	1 kit or box
Flexi-Seal SIGNAL FMS Replacement Collection Bags	10/box

ACTION

The Flexi-Seal™ SIGNAL Fecal Management System contains one soft silicone catheter tube assembly, one Luer-lock syringe, and three collection bags with filter. The soft silicone catheter is inserted into the rectum for fecal management to contain and divert fecal waste in order to protect the patient's skin and keep the bedding clean. There is a low-pressure retention balloon at one end and a connector for attaching the collection bag at the other end.

INDICATIONS

For the fecal management of patients with little or no bowel control and liquid or semi-liquid stool.

CONTRAINDICATIONS

- This product is not intended for use:
  - for more than 29 consecutive days.
  - for pediatric patients.
- The Flexi-Seal™ SIGNAL Fecal Management System should not be used on individuals who:
  - have suspected or confirmed rectal mucosal impairment, that is, severe proctitis, ischemic proctitis.
  - mucosal ulcerations.
  - have had rectal surgery within the last year.
  - have any rectal or anal injury.
  - have hemorrhoids of significant size and/or symptoms.
  - have a rectal or anal stricture or stenosis.
  - have a suspected or confirmed rectal/anal tumor.
  - have any indwelling rectal or anal device (e.g., thermometer) or delivery mechanism (e.g., suppositories or enemas) in place.
  - are sensitive to or who have had an allergic reaction to any component within the kit.

APPLICATION

Preparation of device

- In addition to the device kit, gloves and lubricant will be required.
- Using the syringe provided, remove any residual air that may be in the balloon by attaching the syringe to the inflation port and withdrawing the plunger. Ensure that the syringe is empty by expelling any air. Then fill this empty syringe with 45 mL tap water or saline. Do not overfill beyond 45 mL.
- Attach the syringe to the 45-mL inflation port with fill indicator (marked 45 mL).
- Securely snap the collection bag to the connector at the end of the catheter.

Preparation of patient

- Position the patient in the left-side–lying position; if unable to tolerate, position the patient so that access to the rectum is possible.
- Perform a digital rectal examination to evaluate suitability for insertion of the device.

Insertion of device

- Remove any indwelling or anal device prior to insertion of the Flexi-Seal™ SIGNAL FMS device.
  - Unfold the length of the catheter to lay it flat on the bed, extending the collection bag toward the foot of the bed. Insert a lubricated gloved index finger into the blue retention balloon cuff finger pocket for digital guidance during device insertion.

    The blue finger pocket is located above the position indicator line. Coat the balloon end of the catheter with lubricating jelly. Grasp the catheter and gently insert the balloon end through the anal sphincter until the balloon is beyond the external orifice and well inside the rectal vault. The finger may be removed or remain in place in the rectum during balloon inflation.
  - Inflate the balloon with 45 mL of water or saline by slowly depressing the syringe plunger. Under no circumstance should the balloon be inflated with more than 45 mL. The inflation port will expand as fluid is injected. Once the balloon has reached the optimal fill level or 45 mL has been injected, the indicator bubble will pop. The indicator bubble will remain popped while the balloon is at its optimal fill level.

    If the indicator bubble pops, or expands significantly, at less than 30 mL, withdraw the liquid and reposition the balloon in the rectal vault. After repositioning, fill the balloon as described above. If the fill indicator bubble does not pop, the balloon is underfilled. Use the syringe to withdraw fluid from the retention balloon and reinject until the indicator bubble pops, or 45 mL has been injected.

    Should the indicator bubble deflate or appear excessively inflated, this is an indication that the retention balloon is no longer at the optimal fill level. In this case, use the syringe to withdraw the fluid from the retention balloon and reinject until the indicator bubble pops, or 45 mL has been injected.
- Remove the syringe from the inflation port, and gently pull on the soft silicone catheter to check that the balloon is securely in the rectum and that it is positioned against the rectal floor.
- Position the length of the flexible silicone catheter along the patient's leg avoiding kinks and obstructions.
  - Take note of the position indicator line relative to the patient's anus. Regularly observe changes in the location of the position indicator line as a means to determine the movement of the retention balloon in the patient's rectum. This may indicate the need for the balloon or device to be repositioned.
- Hang the bag by the bead strap on the bedside at a position lower than that of the patient.

Irrigation of the device

- The silicone catheter can be rinsed by filling the syringe with tap water at room temperature and attaching the syringe to the blue irrigation port (marked IRRIG.) and depressing the plunger. Ensure the syringe is not inadvertently attached to the balloon inflation port (marked 45 mL).
- Repeat the irrigation procedure as often as necessary to maintain proper functioning of the device. Flushing the device as described above is an optional procedure for use only when needed to maintain the unobstructed flow of stool into the collection bag. If repeated flushing with water does not return the flow of stool through the catheter,

the device should be inspected to ascertain that there is no external obstruction (e.g., pressure from a body part, piece of equipment, or resolution of diarrhea). If no source of obstruction of the device is detected, use of the device should be discontinued.

Maintenance of device

- Change the collection bag as needed. Snap the cap onto each used bag and discard according to institutional protocol for disposal of medical waste. Observe the device frequently for obstructions from kinks, solid fecal particles, or external pressure.

REMOVAL

- To remove the catheter from the rectum, the retention balloon must first be deflated. Attach the syringe to the inflation port, and slowly withdraw all water from the retention balloon.
- Disconnect the syringe and discard.
- Grasp the catheter as close to the patient as possible, and slowly slide it out of the anus. Dispose of the device in accordance with institutional protocol for disposal of medical waste.

*See package insert for complete instructions for use.

OTHER PRODUCTS

New Product: Heelmedix Advanced Heel Protector

Medline Industries, Inc.

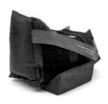

HOW SUPPLIED

Heelmedix Advanced Heel Protector	Petite
Heelmedix Advanced Heel Protector	Standard
Heelmedix Advanced Heel Protector	X-Large

ACTION

Heelmedix Advanced completely offloads the heel and helps to redistribute pressure.

INDICATIONS

Used for prevention through treatment of Stage IV pressure ulcers.

APPLICATION

- Open all of the straps.
- Flip the boot inside out. Place the lower leg on the long side of the boot, with the heel in the hole.
- Once the heel is properly placed in the hole, flip the sides of the boot up. Make sure the heel is elevated.
- Cross the two straps furthest from the foot across the leg. Make sure the straps are not touching the leg.
- Secure the two additional straps alongside the leg at a slight downward angle.
- Make sure the heel is elevated.
- Apply one or two optional wedges to outside/inside of boot for extra stabilization.

REMOVAL

- Remove the boot during skin checks.
- Do not walk in the Heelmedix heel protector.

InterDry®

Coloplast

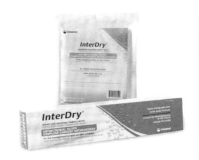

HOW SUPPLIED

Wicking Fabric	10 × 144″	none
Wicking Fabric	10 × 36″	none
Wicking Fabric	10 × 18″	none

ACTION

InterDry® is a nonsterile skin protectant comprised of polyurethane-coated polyester fabric impregnated with an antimicrobial silver complex as the active component. The fabric provides moisture transportation to keep the skin dry while the antimicrobial in the fabric reduces odor. The fabric's low-friction surface acts as a lubrication aid thereby reducing skin-to-skin friction. Provides a protective environment for the skin and an effective protection against microbial contamination in the fabric. The product reduces colonization of bacteria and yeast such as *Staphylococcus aureus, Staphylococcus epidermidis, Pseudomonas aeruginosa,* and *Candida albicans.* InterDry fabric contains 0.019% silver.

INDICATIONS

InterDry is a skin protectant indicated for management of skin folds and other skin-to-skin contact areas. Reduces microbial colonization in the fabric.

PRECAUTIONS

- InterDry fabric is not a wound dressing and should not be placed directly onto an open wound.
- Should not be used on patients with a known sensitivity to silver.

WARNINGS

- May cause transient skin staining. Excessive absorption of silver into the body may cause the skin to obtain a blue-grey appearance (Argyria).
- The safe use of InterDry fabric during pregnancy, lactation, and on children has not been demonstrated.
- May not be used to protect against urine and feces. If such soiling occurs, the fabric must be changed immediately.
- Creams or ointments used in conjunction with InterDry fabric may reduce the efficacy of the product.
- In vitro studies with this product have been shown to cause mild biological reactivity.

APPLICATION

- Wash the skin gently. Pat dry, do not rub.
- Cut the appropriate size of the fabric with clean scissors, allowing a minimum 2 in of the fabric exposed outside the skin fold for moisture evaporation.
- Lay a single layer of fabric in the skin fold, placing one edge of the fabric into the base of the skin fold. Gently smooth the rest of the fabric over the skin, keeping it flat. Leave at least 2 in of the fabric exposed outside of the skin fold.
- Secure the fabric in one of several ways; with the skin fold, with a small amount of tape, or tucked under clothing.

REMOVAL

- Each piece of InterDry may be used up to 5 days, depending on fabric soiling, odor, amount of moisture, and general skin condition.
- Remove the fabric before bathing and reuse when finished. When removing the fabric from skin folds, gently separate the skin fold and lift away the fabric.
- If you notice persistent symptoms of skin irritation or breakdown, talk with your doctor.

REFERENCE

1. https://www.interdry.com/

Large Body Tissue (Y) Electrode and Connection Wire

Senergy Medical Group

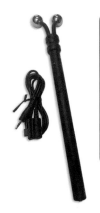

HOW SUPPLIED

Accessory	11″ long	A4556
Connection Wire	42″ long	A4557

For use with the Tennant Biomodulator, the stainless steel Large Body Tissue (Y) Electrode includes a connection wire.

ACTION

For use as an accessory with the Tennant Biomodulator to treat large areas such as the back, arms, and legs.

INDICATIONS

Refer to Tennant Biomodulator indications.

CONTRAINDICATIONS

- Refer to Tennant Biomodulator contraindications.

APPLICATION

- Use directly on dry, unbroken skin for extended treatment.

REMOVAL

- When treatment is complete, unplug the connection wire from the accessory and the Biomodulator accessory port. Clean the electrode with a sterilizing wipe.

REFERENCES

1. http://senergy.us/large-body-tissue-electrode.html
2. www.senergy.us

OWLS® Custom Orthoses

Orthomerica Products, Inc.

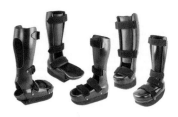

HOW SUPPLIED

OWLS Custom Orthoses	L1940
OWLS Custom Orthoses	L1960
OWLS Custom Orthoses	L1970
OWLS Custom Orthoses	L4631
	Additional add-on codes relative to custom design

ACTION

OWLS is a line of custom orthotic solutions designed to positively influence the disrupted biomechanics of walking for people with diabetic peripheral neuropathy and/or foot ulcerations. Specifically, OWLS positively impacts walking characteristics such as: (1) deceleration of the foot as it contacts the ground, (2) the timing and translation of the center of pressure, (3) offloading of the affected limb, and (4) immobilization of specific joints as needed.

INDICATIONS

Most diabetic ulcers are secondary to orthopedic anomalies and peripheral neuropathies. In these cases, maximal correction and offloading of the affected limb is imperative for the fastest and most effective outcome. The OWLS system promotes continued ambulation while stabilizing the foot and ankle during Charcot joint activity and/or wound-healing efforts. Unique orthotic designs are available for the treatment of Charcot foot syndrome, as well as heel, midfoot, and forefoot ulcerations.

CONTRAINDICATIONS

- Patients not participating in a wound care program or being treated for Charcot foot syndrome are not appropriate candidates.

APPLICATION

- The OWLS program is an interdisciplinary effort between the wound team, orthotist, and patient. An OWLS-trained orthotist will provide a thorough orthotic evaluation, casting or scanning session, and develop the most appropriate orthotic design to treat each patient's unique situation. Each OWLS custom orthosis begins with a cast or scan of the affected limb and is manufactured by Orthomerica. After delivery and fitting of the orthosis, the patient is seen for ongoing follow-up by the orthotic clinician as part of the comprehensive medical care program.

REMOVAL

- The OWLS program is delivered by the orthotist and overseen by the referring physician. Discharge from the orthotic treatment program is at the discretion of the referring physician and is usually continued for 1 to 3 months after initial healing has been determined.

REFERENCES

1. Hanft JR, Hall DT, Kapila A. A guide to preventative offloading of diabetic foot ulcers. *Podiatry Today.* 2011;24(12):60–67.
2. Galhoum AE, Abd-Ella MM. Charcot ankle neuroarthropathy pathology, diagnosis and management: A review of literature. *Orth & Rheum.* 2016;6(2):00218.
3. Armstrong DG, Issac AL, Bevilacqua NJ, et al. Offloading foot wounds in people with diabetes. *Wounds.* 2014;26(1):13–20.
4. Milne, TE, Rogers JR, Kinnear EM, et al. Developing an evidence-based clinical pathway for the assessment, diagnosis and management of acute Charcot neuro-arthropathy: A systematic review. *J Foot Ankle Research.* 2013;6:30.

OTHER PRODUCTS

New Product: PLUROGEL® Burn and Wound Dressing

Medline Industries, Inc.

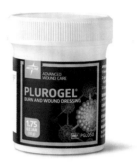

HOW SUPPLIED

PluroGel, Tube	20-g (35 ea/cs)
PluroGel, Tube	50-g (12 ea/cs)
PluroGel, Jar	50-g (24 ea/cs)
PluroGel, Jar	400-g (6 ea/cs)

NO HCPCS/CPT/APC codes available for Concentrated Surfactant Technology.

ACTION

PluroGel® Burn and Wound Dressing is a translucent, water soluble dressing. By design, PluroGel maintains moisture in the wound and protects the wound from dessication. PluroGel contains a noncytotoxic surfactant which helps promote autolytic debridement. As a concentrated surfactant gel, PluroGel softens, loosens, and traps necrotic tissue and debris, promoting a favorable healing environment. PluroGel is provided nonsterile for single-patient use. PluroGel is shown to disrupt and prevent biofilm (in vitro).

INDICATIONS

PluroGel® Burn and Wound Dressing is indicated for use on partial- and full-thickness, lightly to moderately draining wounds, first- and second-degree burns.

APPLICATION

- Cleanse the burn or wound in accordance with normal procedures.
- Apply directly to the burn or wound or onto sterile dressing. When using the jar format, apply PluroGel using a sterile applicator or sterile gloves.
- For lightly draining wounds, a thickness of 3 mm is recommended. For moderately draining wounds, a thickness of 5 mm (1/2 cm) is recommended.
- Secure with an appropriate absorbent secondary dressing.
- Maximum wear time up to 3 days.
  Note: PluroGel is biocompatible and can be used with any type of cleansers and any type of secondary dressing including antimicrobial silver, etc.

REMOVAL

- PluroGel® Burn and Wound Dressing can be removed with saline, sterile water, or wound cleanser depending on normal procedures.

OTHER PRODUCTS

REFERENCES

1. International Wound Infection Institute (IWII). Wound infection in clinical practice: Principles of best practice. *Wounds International.* 2016. http://www.woundinfection-institute.com/wp-content/uploads/2014/04/IWII-Consensus_Final-web.pdf

2. Jeong S, Schultz GS, Gibson DJ. Testing the influence of surfactant-based wound dressings on proteinase activity. *Int Wound J.* 2017;14(5):786–790.

3. Yang Q, Larose C, Porta AD, et al. A surfactant-based wound dressing can reduce bacterial biofilms in a porcine skin explant model. *Int Wound J.* 2017;14(2):408–413.

SensiLase PAD-IQ® System

Väsamed, Inc.

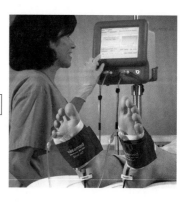

HOW SUPPLIED

| Ischemic Vascular Disease | G8547 | 93923 |

Diagnostic Test Equipment Peripheral Artery Disease/ Wound Healing and Health Information Technology— web-based data communication and management services.

ACTION

The SensiLase PAD-IQ® System ("SensiLase PAD-IQ") generates two noninvasive vascular tests: Skin Perfusion Pressure (SPP) and Pulse Volume Recording (PVR). SPP, a quantitative evaluation of microcirculatory perfusion in the skin, is measured using a laser Doppler sensor and an occlusive pressure cuff to evaluate reactive hyperemia. All measurements are completed automatically, bilaterally, and simultaneously in order to save time. A graph displays pressure and perfusion during cuff deflation and indicates the pressure at which skin perfusion is found to return. Other information observable from the graph includes percentage perfusion increase above baseline, total response time, perfusion reappearance time, and perfusion contour. PVR uses air plethysmography to evaluate variations in the volume of blood passing through a limb during each cardiac cycle. In combination, these tests help determine the severity and level of disease in the extremities. SensiLase PAD-IQ has a DICOM interface for Worklist and Storage servers. SensiLase PAD-IQ features customized Studycast software and services which provide web-accessible SensiLase PAD-IQ data. Studycast System studies are uploaded in 2 minutes or less and feature two-way physician test data interpretation and optimal treatment path decisions.

INDICATIONS

SensiLase PAD-IQ is used in the Wound Care Center to:
- Perform peripheral vascular assessments on all patients with lower-extremity ulcers to rule out arterial ischemia. SPP is clinically demonstrated to accurately predict the wound-healing outcome.
- Assess the degree of arterial perfusion at the site of the wound in advance of HBO therapy to meet the pretherapy vascular assessment requirement.
- Determine the optimal level of amputation by measuring the site where there is adequate perfusion for healing to occur.
- Plan compression wrap therapy in patients with edema to rule out arterial ischemia both pre- and post-compression wrap.
  SensiLase PAD-IQ Studycast Data Communication Networking is used in the Wound Care Center to:
- Send completed SensiLase tests via a HIPAA-compliant secure internet server to a physician for rapid test interpretation from any internet-connected device, allowing streamlined patient care.
- Facilitate a collaborative-care multidisciplinary team to treat these complex patients.
- Integrate with electronic medical records to streamline patient care and support an optimal care treatment pathway.

CONTRAINDICATIONS
- None known.

APPLICATION

- SPP is performed in the angiosome (distal arterial anatomy) where the ulcer is present.
- Bilateral SPP measurements can be obtained in less than 10 minutes.
- Similar to a regular blood pressure test, SensiLase SPP is reported in mm Hg.
- Utilizing a laser Doppler to detect capillary perfusion, the SensiLase measures the first return of perfusion following controlled release of cuff occlusion. The SPP value is the cuff pressure at the point of reperfusion and is a measurement with reactive hyperemia.
- PVR is measured following SPP assessment; it is performed at different limb levels to assess changes in limb volume with each cardiac cycle.
- SensiLase PAD-IQ SPP tests will determine if there is adequate perfusion in the region of the ulcer for a likely healing outcome.
- SensiLase PAD-IQ tests should be performed following revascularization therapy (bypass surgery or endovascular) to measure changes in perfusion.

REMOVAL

- SPP/PVR tests require patient contact for only a brief testing period. Disposable accessories are provided that support institutional cross-contamination initiatives.

REFERENCE

1. http://www.vasamed.com/index.php/clinicians/clinical-references

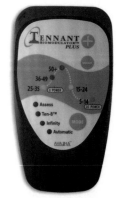

Tennant Biomodulator® *PLUS*

Senergy Medical Group

HOW SUPPLIED

TENS Unit	4.5″ × 2.5″ × 1.25″	E0720
		DME 1399

Handheld, battery-operated, class-2 prescription medical device FDA-cleared for pain relief (FDA classification 882.5890 neurology transcutaneous electrical nerve stimulator for pain relief). Health Canada License and CE Mark 2460. GSA Contract Holder Contract V797D-50488. Manufactured with both foreign and domestic components and serviced in the U.S.

ACTION

Tennant Biomodulator Technology

The Tennant Biomodulator *PLUS* is **no ordinary** TENS or biofeedback unit. The microcurrent technology is unique in the way it engages the body's natural resources to assist the processes of pain management and rehabilitation. Standard TENS units temporarily mask pain, inhibiting the healing process. The Tennant *PLUS* is designed to break the *pain cycle.*

The interactive technology offers a simplified, user-friendly interface that provides immediate access to four preset stimulation patterns to treat a full range of pain caused by injuries and other conditions.

Microcurrent technology works with tiny currents, closer to the type and amount that naturally occur in the body. By comparison, the current used by typical TENS devices is thousands of times greater than the natural body current. Although, patients sometimes may feel a slight tingling sensation under the electrodes, it is not necessary to feel this to achieve results.

The Biomodulator uses neuromodulation technology designed to stimulate the body's natural release of endorphins and neuropeptides into the blood stream. The Biomodulator works by giving the cells the energy they are lacking. When the cells are restored to their optimal level of energy, it supports the healing process.

- Nitric oxide causes vascular dilation and thereby increases blood circulation. This is critical to wound healing, reduction of edema, and treatment of diabetic neuropathy.
- Endorphins are the body's natural pain-management chemicals.
- Neuropeptides are the body's regulatory elements that promote accelerated healing.
- ATP is responsible for the energy level of the cell.

The Tennant Biomodulator *PLUS* uses a unique technology and patent-pending frequency sets, not available with any other brand or company. This technology may be used as an alternative therapy and in conjunction with conventional medical treatments provided by healthcare practitioners.

Technical Specifications	
Pulse duration	<2 ms
Pulse frequency	25 to 150 Hz
Output voltage	Up to 650 V
Output current	Up to 2300 µA
Timeout	60 mins
Waveform	HVPC, pulsed, damped, biphasic, asymmetrical, sinusoidal

Technical Comparison	
Tennant Biomodulator *PLUS*	**Conventional TENS**
21st century technology	1970s technology
Voltage range: Up to 650 V	Voltage range: 0 to 40 V
Amperage range: Microamps $(10^{-6}$ A)	Amperage range: Milliamps $(10^{-3}$ A)
Signals in the frequency range of 25 to 150 Hz	Signals in the frequency range of 15 to 351 Hz
Damped, asymmetrical, biphasic, sinusoidal, waveform	Square waveform, monophasic or biphasic symmetrical or asymmetrical
Signaling varies based upon changes in impedance of the tissue (cybernetic loop technology)	Signaling is typically the same continuous pattern (no cybernetic loop technology)
Cybernetic look technology prevents neurological habituation and accommodation for more effective pain management	Repetitive signals often cause neurological habituation and accommodation, which severely limits effectiveness of pain management
Reaction Feedback Technology; device indicates changes in relative impedance	No feedback

INDICATIONS

Symptomatic relief and management of chronic, intractable pain.
Adjunctive treatment in the management of postsurgical and posttraumatic pain.

CONTRAINDICATIONS

- Do not use on persons with a demand-type cardiac pacemaker, implanted defibrillator, or other implanted electronic device. Such use could cuase electric shock, burns, electrical interference, or death.
- Do not use if pregnant or nursing.

CAUTION

Do not use on a stroke patient until a possible blood clot has had time to resolve.
Do not rub the device over a vessel that might contain a blood clot, for example, a tender varicose vein or the carotid arteries.
Do not use when someone is under the influence of alcohol or other drugs.

Do not use the electrode directly on the eyeball.

Do not use on a patient who is very sensitive to electromagnetic frequencies, for example, someone who can't be around a computer.

Do not use on a patient who doesn't want you to use it.

APPLICATION

- This battery-operated, handheld device has a built-in electrode that can be applied directly on unbroken skin on or near areas of pain. The device also has an accessory port for use with the large body tissue (Y) electrode, the Tennant Biotransducer®, self-stick reusable/disposable conductive pads and other accessories available from Senergy Medical Group.

REMOVAL

- When the treatment is complete, remove the device electrode from the skin and clean with a sterilizing wipe.

REFERENCES

1. http://senergy.us/biomodulator-plus.html
2. http://senergy.us/

Tennant Biomodulator® PRO

Senergy Medical Group

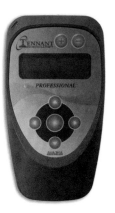

HOW SUPPLIED

TENS	4.5″ × 2.5″ × 1.25″	E0720
		DME 1399

Handheld, battery-operated class-2 prescription medical device, FDA-cleared for pain relief (FDA classification 882.5890 neurology transcutaneous electrical nerve stimulator for pain relief). Health Canada License and CE Mark 2460. GSA Contract Holder Contract V797D-50488. Manufactured with both foreign and domestic components and serviced in the U.S.

ACTION

Tennant Biomodulator Technology

The Tennant Biomodulator PRO is **no ordinary** TENS unit. The microcurrent technology is unique in the way it engages the body's natural resources to assist the processes of pain management and rehabilitation. Standard TENS units temporarily mask pain, inhibiting the healing process. The PRO is designed to break the *pain cycle*.

Microcurrent technology works with tiny currents, closer to the type and amount that naturally occur in the body. By comparison, the current used by typical TENS devices is thousands of times greater than the natural body current. Although, patients sometimes may feel a slight tingling sensation under the electrodes, it is not necessary to feel this to achieve results.

The Biomodulator uses neuromodulation technology designed to stimulate the body's natural release of endorphins and neuropeptides into the blood stream. The Biomodulator works by giving the cells the energy they are lacking. When the cells are restored to their optimal level of energy, it supports the healing process.

- Nitric oxide causes vascular dilation and thereby increases blood circulation. This is critical to wound healing, reduction of edema, and treatment of diabetic neuropathy.
- Endorphins are the body's natural pain management chemicals.
- Neuropeptides are the body's regulatory elements that promote accelerated healing.
- ATP is responsible for the energy level of the cell.

The Tennant Biomodulator PRO uses a unique technology and patent-pending frequency sets, not available with any other brand or company. This technology may be used as an alternative therapy and in conjunction with conventional medical treatments provided by healthcare practitioners. In addition to the 50 preset advanced frequency sets, the PRO has four programmable modes.

Technical Specifications	
Pulse duration	<2 ms
Pulse frequency	0.5 to 2500 Hz
Output voltage	Up to 650 V
Output current	Up to 4400 µA
Timeout	60 minutes
Waveform	HVPC, pulsed, damped, biphasic, asymmetrical, sinusoidal

Technical Comparison	
Tennant Biomodulator PRO	**Conventional TENS**
21st century technology	1970s technology
Voltage range: Up to 650 V	Voltage range: 0 to 40 V
Amperage range: Microamps (10^{-6} A)	Amperage range: Milliamps (10^{-3} A)
Signals in the frequency range of 0.5 to 2500 Hz	Signals in the frequency range of 15 to 351 Hz
Damped, asymmetrical, biphasic, sinusoidal, waveform	Square waveform, monophasic or biphasic symmetrical or asymmetrical
Signaling varies based upon changes in impedance of the tissue (cybernetic loop technology)	Signaling is typically the same continuous pattern (no cybernetic loop technology)
Cybernetic look technology prevents neurological habituation and accommodation for more effective pain management	Repetitive signals often cause neurological habituation and accommodation, which severely limits effectiveness of pain management
Reaction Feedback Technology; device indicates changes in relative impedance	No feedback

INDICATIONS

Symptomatic relief and management of chronic, intractable pain.

Adjunctive treatment in the management of postsurgical and posttraumatic pain.

CONTRAINDICATIONS

- Do not use on persons with a demand-type cardiac pacemaker, implanted defibrillator, or other implanted electronic device. Such use could cuase electric shock, burns, electrical interference, or death.
- Do not use if pregnant or nursing.

CAUTION

Do not use on a stroke patient until a possible blood clot has had time to resolve.

Do not rub the device over a vessel that might contain a blood clot, for example, a tender varicose vein or the carotid arteries.

Do not use when someone is under the influence of alcohol or other drugs.

Do not use the electrode directly on the eyeball.

Do not use on a patient who is very sensitive to electromagnetic frequencies, for example, someone who can't be around a computer.

Do not use on a patient who doesn't want you to use it.

APPLICATION

- This handheld, battery-operated device has built-in electrodes that can be applied directly on clean, dry, unbroken skin on or near areas of pain. The device also has an accessory port for use with the large body tissue (Y) electrode, the Tennant Biotransducer®, self-stick reusable/disposable conductive pads, and other accessories available from Senergy Medical Group.

REMOVAL

- When the treatment is complete, remove the device electrode from the skin and clean the electrode with a sterilizing wipe.

REFERENCES

1. http://senergy.us/biomodulator-pro.html
2. http://senergy.us/

Tennant Biotransducer® CrystalWave and Connection Wire

Senergy Medical Group

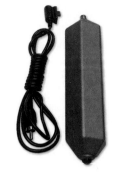

HOW SUPPLIED

Accessory	6.75″ × 1.5″	A4556
		DME 1399
Connection Wire	42″ long	A4557

The Tennant Biotransducer is sold as an accessory to the Tennant Biomodulator®.

ACTION

The Tennant Biotransducer provides no-touch, painless therapy into the tissue, through bandages, casts, or fabric. It uses a combination of technologies including actuation, piezoelectricity, semiconduction, and modulation to create a field that will transmit the frequencies of the Tennant Biomodulator into the tissue more efficiently.

INDICATIONS

Refer to Tennant Biomodulator indications.

CONTRAINDICATIONS

• Refer to Tennant Biomodulator contraindications.

APPLICATION

• Tennant Biotransducer may be used for pain management over the injured tissue, including wounds. No skin contact is necessary and it can transmit voltage and frequency through bandages, casts, or fabric.

REMOVAL

• Unplug the connection wire from the Biomodulator and the Biotransducer for storage.

REFERENCE

1. http://senergy.us/

UltraMIST® Ultrasound Healing Therapy

Celularity, Inc.

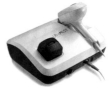

HOW SUPPLIED

UltraMIST Therapy System incl. Treatment Wand	12" × 10" × 7.5"
UltraMIST Disposable Applicator	5" × 5" × 2.5"
CPT Code: 97610	

ACTION

UltraMIST® delivers low frequency (40 kHz), nonthermal ultrasonic energy without surface contact through a fluid (e.g., saline) mist to the wound bed and the energy continues to travel below the wound surface. The ultrasound energy creates a pressure wave "pushing" the cells on and below the wound surface. These mechanical forces cause microstrains that deform the flexible cell membranes. Cells have a physiologic response to membrane deformation that results in the promotion of healing.

INDICATIONS

May be used on all types of wounds (chronic, acute, and/or surgical) to promote wound healing. May be used by itself or in conjunction with other wound therapies and/or procedures.

CONTRAINDICATIONS

- Not for use near electronic implants/prosthesis (e.g., near or over the heart or over the thoracic area if the patient is using a cardiac pacemaker).
- Not for use on the lower back during pregnancy or over the pregnant uterus.
- Not for use over areas of malignancies.

APPLICATION

- Clean the entire system using a disinfectant wipe.
- Ensure the treatment wand cable is attached and fully seated to the front of the generator.
- With the power switch off, plug the system power cord into an electrical outlet. Turn the power switch located on the back of the generator to the "on" position.
- Use the keypad on the treatment wand to enter the size of each wound to be treated per the screen prompts. The total fluid (e.g., saline) requirement for the combined treatment area is displayed (approximately 100 mL for every 25 cm^2). Select the appropriate fluid (e.g., saline) bag size.
- Remove the applicator from the packaging. Press the applicator onto the treatment wand.
- Insert the applicator tubing into the treatment wand tubing channel and attach the tubing clip to the treatment wand cable. Place the treatment wand in the cradle once completed.
- Insert the spike from the tubing fully into the fluid (e.g., saline) bag.
- Allow the fluid (e.g., saline) to run through the applicator tubing until it is noted at the distal tip. Close the tubing clamp. Loop the applicator tubing from the fluid (e.g., saline) bag through the pump from the left to the right, center on tubing guides, and close the pump door.
- Administer UltraMIST treatment by slowly moving the treatment wand in a horizontal and vertical pattern over the wound, keeping the ultrasound tip at a distance of 1 to 1.5 cm from the wound bed. UltraMIST ultrasound is delivered via a gentle fluid (e.g., saline) mist and penetrates in and below the wound bed.
- The ultrasound and fluid (e.g., saline) will automatically turn off after the allotted treatment time.

REMOVAL

- Turn power switch to off. Clamp the tubing with the pinch clamp.
- Remove the tubing from the treatment wand channel and pump, remove the applicator from the treatment wand and fluid (e.g., saline) bag from the adjustable hook and discard.
- Clean the entire system using a disinfectant wipe.
- For complete product information, please consult UltraMIST Instructions for Use.

REFERENCES

1. Driver VR, Yao M, Miller CJ. Noncontact low-frequency ultrasound therapy in the treatment of chronic wounds: A meta-analysis. *Wound Rep Reg.* 2011;19:475–480.
2. Gibbons GW, Orgill DP, Serena TE, et al. A prospective, randomized, controlled trial comparing the effects of noncontact, low-frequency ultrasound to standard care in healing venous leg ulcers. *Ostomy Wound Manage.* 2015;61(1):16–29.
3. Prather JH, Tummel EK, Patel AB, et al. A prospective, randomized controlled trial comparing the effects of noncontact low-frequency ultrasound with standard care in healing split-thickness donor sites. *J Am Coll Surg.* 2015;221(2):309–318.
4. Honaker JS, Forston MR, Davis EA, et al. The effect of adjunctive noncontact low frequency ultrasound on deep tissue pressure injury. *Wound Rep Reg.* 2016;24(6):1081–1088.

Skin Care Products and Additional Dressings and Products

Overview

Part II provides a comprehensive listing of skin care products as well as additional dressing and products. When reviewing the skin care products, it is paramount that providers take these proactive steps in clinical practice to develop sound skin care prevention and intervention pathways. To that end, the clinician must understand the anatomy and physiology of the skin, current practice guidelines, and indications and contraindications of skin care products used in clinical practice.

Use the skin care products within this section to help you develop a skin care formulary for your facility to include products under categories such as:

- Antifungals and antimicrobials (topical): products that inhibit the growth of organisms that cause superficial skin infections, such as yeast.
- Liquid skin protectants (also called skin sealants): products that protect the skin by forming a transparent protective barrier.
- Moisture barriers (also called skin protectants): ointments, creams, or pastes that protect the skin from urinary and fecal incontinence by shielding the skin from irritants or moisture (e.g., dimethicone, petrolatum, and zinc oxide).
- Skin cleansers: pH-balanced products used to provide moisture and to effectively remove urine, feces, or both without patient discomfort.
- Therapeutic moisturizing products: lotions and creams used to replace lost lipids in skin.

Part II also provides a comprehensive listing of additional products: Tapes and closures, wound pouches, wound cleansers, gauzes, elastic bandages, and compression bandage systems.

Because of the high volume of general products that are manufactured, the section groups similar products into tables. Each table may include more than one category. In that case, as appropriate, each representative category and its respective Healthcare Common Procedure Coding System (HCPCS) code are identified above the table. It is the clinician's responsibility to understand the actions, indications, advantages, disadvantages, and reimbursement information for each product prior to its use.

Inclusion in these tables does not mean that the manufacturers have applied for or received the HCPCS code identified above the tables. The provider and supplier are responsible for verifying the correct HCPCS codes before submitting claims to any payer. Please refer to individual product listings for further information about each product and verify coding of each product with the product's manufacturer.

ANTIFUNGALS AND ANTIMICROBIALS

The pH of the skin is in the acidic range but varies in different areas of the body. The pH is important because it regulates some of the functions of the stratum corneum, including its permeability function; the integrity and cohesion of skin cells, or what holds the cells together; and the defense against bacteria and fungi. Skin flora, or the microorganisms that live on or infect the skin, grow differently based on the skin pH. Antifungal and antimicrobial products inhibit the growth of organisms that cause superficial skin infections, such as yeast. These products are formulated as creams, ointments, lotions, or powders and may be found in select moisture barriers.

Because of the variation in coding for antifungals and antimicrobials, it is the clinician's responsibility to verify coding and payment of each product with the manufacturer.

Product Name	Manufacturer/Distributor
Aloe Vesta® Clear Antifungal Ointment	ConvaTec
Baza® Antifungal Cream	Coloplast
Critic-Aid® Clear Antifungal	Coloplast
DermaFungal Antifungal Cream	DermaRite Industries, LLC
Micro-Guard® Powder	Coloplast
Remedy Olivamine Antifungal Cream	Medline Industries, Inc.
Remedy Phytoplex Antifungal Powder	Medline Industries, Inc.
Remedy Phytoplex Antifungal Ointment	Medline Industries, Inc.
SECURA Antifungal Extra Thick	Smith & Nephew, Inc. Wound Management
SECURA Antifungal Greaseless	Smith & Nephew, Inc. Wound Management
Soothe & Cool INZO Antifungal Cream	Medline Industries, Inc.
3M™ Cavilon™ Antifungal Cream	3M Health Care

COMPRESSION BANDAGE SYSTEMS

Compression therapy products are used to manage edema and promote the return of venous blood flow to the heart. Conventional management with zinc oxide–impregnated bandaging systems, such as an Unna boot, provides inelastic compression. Multilayered, sustained, graduated, high-compression bandages aid in the management of wounds caused by venous insufficiency.

Each component used in the compression therapy system is billed using a specific code for the component, if available. It is the clinician's responsibility to verify coding and payment of each product with the manufacturer.

The HCPCS codes normally assigned to compression bandage systems are:

Light compression bandage

A6448: Width < 3″ per yard.
A6449: Width ≥ 3″ and < 5″ per yard.
A6450: Width ≥ 5″ per yard.

Moderate-high compression bandage

A6451: Moderate-compression bandage, load resistance of 1.25 to 1.34 ft lb at 50% maximum stretch, width >3″ and < 5″ per yard.
A6452: High-compression bandage, load resistance ≥ 1.35 ft lb at 50% maximum stretch, width ≥3″ and < 5″ per yard.

Gradient compression wrap

A6545: Gradient compression wrap, non-elastic, below knee, 30–50 mm hg, each.

Self-adherent bandage

A6453: Width <3″ per yard.
A6454: Width ≥3″ and <5″ per yard.
A6455: Width ≥5″ per yard.

Conforming bandage

A6442: Width <3″ per yard.
A6443: Width ≥3″ and <5″ per yard.
A6444: Width >5″ per yard.

A6445: Width <3″ per yard.
A6446: Width ≥3″ and <5″ per yard.
A6447: Width ≥5″ per yard.

Padding bandage

A6441: Width ≥ 3″ and < 5″ per yard.

Zinc paste–impregnated bandage

A6456: Width ≥3″ and <5″ per yard.

Name of Product	Manufacturer/ Distributor	Type of Compression	Subcategory
• = New Product			
3M™ Coban™ 2 Two-Layer Light Compression System	3M Health Care	Inelastic	2 layer cohesive compression system
DeWrap	DeRoyal	Elastic	Multilayer compression system
Fourflex	Medline Industries, Inc.	Elastic	Multilayer compression system
circaid® juxtacures®	medi USA	Inelastic	Compression garments for lower leg
circaid® juxtafit®	medi USA	Inelastic	Compression garments for lower leg
COMPRECARES®	Medline Industries, Inc.	Inelastic	Compression garments for lower leg
circaid® juxtalite®	medi USA	Inelastic	Compression garments for lower leg
• circaid juxtalite hd	• medi USA	• Inelastic	Gradient compression for lower leg
mediven® dual layer	medi USA	Inelastic	Two layer compression stocking system
mediven® plus	medi USA	Elastic	Compression stockings
PROFORE LF (Latex-Free) Lite Multi-Layer Reduced Compression Bandage System	Smith & Nephew, Inc. Wound Management	Elastic	Multilayer compression system
PROFORE LF (Latex-Free) Multi-Layer High Compression Bandage System	Smith & Nephew, Inc. Wound Management	Elastic	Multilayer compression system
PROFORE Multi-Layer High Compression Bandage System	Smith & Nephew, Inc. Wound Management	Elastic	Multilayer compression system
Threeflex	Medline Industries, Inc.	Elastic	Multilayer compression system

Name of Product	Manufacturer/ Distributor	Type of Compression	Subcategory
3M™ Coban™ 2 Two-Layer Compression System	3M Health Care	Inelastic	2 layer cohesive compression system
UNNA-FLEX Plus Venous Ulcer	ConvaTec	Elastic	Unna boot
UNNA-FLEX Plus Venous Ulcer Convenience Pack	ConvaTec	Inelastic	Unna boot/paste bandage
Unna-Z	Medline Industries, Inc.	Inelastic	Unna boots
Unna-Z Stretch and Unna-Z Stretch with Calamine	Medline Industries, Inc.	Inelastic	
Unna-Z with Calamine	Medline Industries, Inc.	Inelastic	Unna boots
VISCOPASTE PB7	Smith & Nephew, Inc., Wound Management	Inelastic	Paste bandage
• CoFlex TLC	• Medline Industries, Inc.	• Inelastic	• CoFlex TLC
• CoFlex TLC Lite	• Medline Industries, Inc.	• Inelastic	• CoFlex TLC Lite
• FlexPress 4	• DermaRite Industries, LLC	• Elastic	• Multilayer compression system
• UnnaRite	• DermaRite Industries, LLC	• Inelastic	• Unna boots
• UnnaRite C	• DermaRite Industries, LLC	• Inelastic	• Unna boots
• EXTREMIT-EASE® Compression Garment	• AMERX Health Care Corporation	• Inelastic	• Gradient compression wrap, below knee

CONFORMING BANDAGES

It is the clinician's responsibility to verify the coding and payment of each product with the manufacturer. The HCPCS codes normally assigned to conforming bandages are:

Conforming bandage, nonsterile

A6442: Width <3″ per yard.
A6443: Width ≥3″ and <5″ per yard.
A6444: Width ≥5″ per yard.

Conforming bandage, sterile

A6445: Width <3″ per yard.
A6446: Width ≥3″ and <5″ per yard.
A6447: Width ≥5″ per yard.

Packing strips, nonimpregnated

A6407: Up to 2″ wide, per linear yard.

Product Name	Manufacturer/Distributor
Bulkee Lite 100% Cotton Bandage—Nonsterile	Medline Industries, Inc.
Albahealth® Packing Strips	DUKAL Corporation
Bulkee Lite 100% Cotton Bandage—Sterile	Medline Industries, Inc.
Bulkee II® 100% Cotton Gauze Bandage—Sterile	Medline Industries, Inc.
Conforming Stretch Gauze	DUKAL Corporation
Fluftex Rolls	DeRoyal
Medline Packing Strips—Plain	Medline Industries, Inc.
Medline Packing Strips—with Iodoform	Medline Industries, Inc.
Medline Conforming Bandages—Sterile	Medline Industries, Inc.
Medline Conforming Bandages—Nonsterile	Medline Industries, Inc.
Bulkee II® 100% Cotton Gauze Bandage—Nonsterile	Medline Industries, Inc.

ELASTIC BANDAGE ROLLS

It is the clinician's responsibility to verify the coding and payment of each product with the manufacturer. The HCPCS codes normally assigned to elastic bandage rolls are:

Light compression bandage

A6448: Width <3″ per yard.
A6449: Width ≥3″ and <5″ per yard.
A6450: Width ≥5″ per yard.

Moderate-high compression bandage

A6451: Moderate compression bandage, load resistance of 1.25 to 1.34 ft lb at 50% maximum stretch, width ≥3″ and <5″ per yard.
A6452: High compression bandage, load resistance greater than or equal to 1.35 ft lb at 50% maximum stretch, width ≥3″ and <5″ per yard.

Self-adherent bandage

A6453: Width <3″ per yard.
A6454: Width ≥3″ and <5″ per yard.
A6455: Width ≥5″ per yard.
A6457: Tubular dressing with or without elastic, any width, per linear yard.

Product Name	Manufacturer/Distributor
• = New Product	
Matrix Elastic Bandage—Latex Free, Hook and Loop on Both Ends	Medline Industries, Inc.
Medigrip Elastic Tubular Bandage	Medline Industries, Inc.
Premium Elastic Bandages	DUKAL Corporation
Setopress® High Compression Bandage	Mölnlycke Health Care

Product Name	Manufacturer/Distributor
Soft-Wrap Elastic Bandage—Latex Free, with clips	Medline Industries, Inc.
SurePress High Compression Bandage	ConvaTec
• SurePress® Absorbent Padding	ConvaTec
Swift-Wrap Elastic Bandage—Latex Free, Hook and Loop on One End	Medline Industries, Inc.
3M™ Coban™ Self-Adherent Wrap	3M Health Care
Tubifast Garments	Mölnlycke Health Care
Tubifast 2-Way Stretch Tubular Retention Dressing	Mölnlycke Health Care
Tubigrip Arthro-pad Support bandage	Mölnlycke Health Care
Tubigrip Shaped Support Bandage	Mölnlycke Health Care
Tubigrip Tubular Support Bandage	Mölnlycke Health Care
• 3M™ Coban™ LF Latex Free Self-Adherent Wrap with Hand Tear	3M Health Care

GAUZE, IMPREGNATED WITH OTHER THAN WATER, NORMAL SALINE, OR HYDROGEL, WITHOUT ADHESIVE BORDER

Impregnated gauze dressings are woven or nonwoven materials in which substances such as iodinated agents, petrolatum, zinc compounds, crystalline sodium chloride, chlorhexidine gluconate, bismuth tribromophenate, aqueous saline, or other agents have been incorporated into the dressing material by the manufacturer.

It is the clinician's responsibility to verify the coding and payment of each product with the manufacturer. The HCPCS codes normally assigned to gauze, impregnated with other than water, normal saline, or hydrogel, without adhesive border are:

A6222: Pad size $\leq$16 in^2.

A6223: Pad size >16 in^2 but $\leq$48 in^2.

A6224: Pad size >48 in^2.

The HCPCS codes normally assigned to gauze, impregnated, other than water, normal saline, or zinc paste, sterile, any width, per linear yard.

A6266: Any width, per linear yard.

Product Name	Manufacturer/Distributor
• = New Product	
• Albahealth® Oil Emulsion Dressings	DUKAL Corporation
• Albahealth® Petrolatum Gauze Dressings	DUKAL Corporation
• Albahealth® Xeroform Petrolatum Gauze Dressing	DUKAL Corporation
Curad Oil Emulsion Dressing	Medline Industries, Inc.
Curad Petrolatum Gauze Dressing	Medline Industries, Inc.
Curad Xeroform Gauze Dressing	Medline Industries, Inc.
CUTICERIN Low Adherent Dressing	Smith & Nephew, Inc. Wound Management
Honey Gauze	Gentell

Product Name	Manufacturer/Distributor
• Medline Packing Strips with Iodoform	Medline Industries, Inc.
Mesalt® Sodium Chloride Wound Cleansing Dressing	Mölnlycke Health Care
Mesalt® Sodium Chloride Ribbon	Mölnlycke Health Care
Oil Emulsion	DeRoyal
Oil Emulsion	Gentell
Xeroform	DeRoyal
Xeroform	Gentell
• Oil Emulsion Dressing	• DermaRite Industries, LLC
• Petrolatum Gauze	• DermaRite Industries, LLC
• Xeroform	• DermaRite Industries, LLC

GAUZE, IMPREGNATED WITH WATER OR NORMAL SALINE, WITHOUT ADHESIVE BORDER

It is the clinician's responsibility to verify the coding and payment of each product with the manufacturer. The HCPCS codes normally assigned to gauze, impregnated with water or normal saline, without an adhesive border are:

A6228: Pad size ≤16 in².
A6229: Pad size >16 in² but ≤48 in².
A6230: Pad size >48 in².

Product Name	Manufacturer/Distributor
CUTICERIN Low Adherent Dressing	Smith & Nephew, Inc. Wound Management

GAUZE, NONIMPREGNATED, WITH ADHESIVE BORDER

It is the clinician's responsibility to verify the coding and payment of each product with the manufacturer. The HCPCS codes normally assigned to gauze, nonimpregnated, with an adhesive border are:

A6219: Pad size ≤16 in².
A6220: Pad size >16 in² but ≤48 in².
A6221: Pad size >48 in².

Product Name	Manufacturer/Distributor
AMERX® Bordered Gauze Dressing	AMERX Health Care Corporation
Sterile Bordered Gauze	DermaRite Industries, LLC
Bordered Gauze	Gentell
COVRSITE	Smith & Nephew, Inc., Wound Management Division
DeRoyal Covaderm Thin	DeRoyal
Medline Bordered Gauze	Medline Industries, Inc.
Mepore Self-Adhesive Absorbent Dressing	Mölnlycke Health Care
Mepore Pro	Mölnlycke Health Care
3M™ Medipore™ +Pad Soft Cloth Adhesive Wound Dressing	3M™ Health Care

GAUZE, NONIMPREGNATED, WITHOUT ADHESIVE BORDER

It is the clinician's responsibility to verify the coding and payment of each product with the manufacturer. The HCPCS codes normally assigned to gauze, nonimpregnated, without an adhesive border are:

Gauze, nonimpregnated, sterile

A6402: Pad size ≤16 in^2.
A6403: Pad size >16 in^2 but ≤48 in^2.
A6404: Pad size >48 in^2.

Gauze, nonimpregnated, nonsterile

A6216: Pad size ≤16 in^2.
A6217: Pad size >16 in^2 but ≤48 in^2.
A6218: Pad size >48 in^2.

Product Name	Manufacturer/Distributor
Avant Gauze Drain Sponge	Medline Industries, Inc.
Avant Gauze—Nonsterile	Medline Industries, Inc.
Bulkee Super Fluff Sponges	Medline Industries, Inc.
FLUFTEX Sponges	DeRoyal
Medline Gauze Pads—Bulk, Nonsterile	Medline Industries, Inc.
Medline Gauze Pads—Sterile	Medline Industries, Inc.
Sof-Form	Medline Industries, Inc.
Combine ABD Pads	DUKAL Corporation
Caliber™ Type VII Gauze Sponge	DUKAL Corporation

LIQUID SKIN PROTECTANTS

Liquid skin protectants, or skin sealants, are formulated with a polymer and solvent. When the product is applied to the skin, the solvent evaporates, and the polymer dries to form a transparent, protective barrier. Select liquid skin protectants may irritate denuded or compromised skin. The clinician should be aware that liquid skin protectants can be formulated with or without alcohol. Liquid skin protectants are manufactured in wipes, swabs, sprays, and foam applicators.

Because of the variation in coding for liquid skin protectants, it is the clinician's responsibility to verify the coding and payment of each product with the manufacturer.

Product Name	Manufacturer/Distributor
Prep™ Protective Skin Barrier	Coloplast
DermaPrep (pads)	DermaRite Industries, LLC
No-Sting Skin-Prep Spray	Smith & Nephew, Inc. Wound Management
No-Sting Skin-Prep Swabs	Smith & Nephew, Inc. Wound Management
No-Sting Skin-Prep Wipes	Smith & Nephew, Inc. Wound Management
Sensi-Care® Sting Free Skin Barrier	ConvaTec

Product Name	Manufacturer/Distributor
StingFree (pads & spray)	DermaRite Industries, LLC
SurePrep® RapidDry Wipes	Medline Industries, Inc.
SurePrep® RapidDry Wands	Medline Industries, Inc.
3M™ Cavilon™ No Sting Barrier Film	3M Health Care
3M™ Cavilon™ Advanced Skin Protectant	3M Health Care
SurePrep® Protective Wipes	Medline Industries, Inc.
SurePrep® No-Sting Wipes	Medline Industries, Inc.
SurePrep® No-Sting Wands	Medline Industries, Inc.
Marathon® Cyanoacrylate (solvent-free)	Medline Industries, Inc.

MOISTURE BARRIERS

Moisture barriers, sometimes called skin protectants, are ointments, creams, or pastes that shield the skin from exposure to irritants or moisture from sources such as incontinence, perspiration, and enzymatic and wound drainage. Three common ingredients found in moisture barriers include dimethicone, petrolatum, and zinc oxide or a combination thereof. Some products are formulated with additional properties such as antibacterial, antiyeast, or antifungal ingredients. A moisture barrier may be formulated with a skin cleanser or as a standalone paste, cream, powder, or ointment. Once the moisture barrier is applied to the skin, it may appear clear, translucent, or opaque depending on the formulation.

Because of the variation in coding for moisture barriers, it is the clinician's responsibility to verify coding and payment of each product with the manufacturer.

Product Name	Manufacturer/Distributor
A&D+E Ointment	Gentell
Aloe Vesta® Clear Barrier Spray	ConvaTec
Aloe Vesta® Protective Ointment	ConvaTec
AMERIGEL® Barrier Lotion	AMERX Health Care Corporation
Baza® Clear Ointment	Coloplast
Baza® Protect Ointment	Coloplast
Critic-Aid® Clear	Coloplast
Critic-Aid® Skin Paste	Coloplast
DermaMed Ointment	DermaRite Industries, LLC
DermaSeptin Ointment	DermaRite Industries, LLC
Essentials INZO Barrier Cream	Medline Industries, Inc.
LanoDerm	DermaRite Industries, LLC
PeriGuard Ointment	DermaRite Industries, LLC
Petroleum Jelly	Gentell
Remedy Essentials Barrier Skin Protectant Ointment	Medline Industries, Inc.

Product Name	Manufacturer/Distributor
Remedy Essentials Zinc Paste	Medline Industries, Inc.
Remedy Intensive Skin Therapy Calazime Protectant Paste	Medline Industries, Inc.
Remedy Intensive Skin Therapy Hydraguard-D Silicone Cream	Medline Industries, Inc.
Remedy Olivamine Calazime Protectant Paste	Medline Industries, Inc.
Remedy Olivamine Clear-Aid Skin Protectant	Medline Industries, Inc.
Remedy Olivamine Dimethicone Skin Protectant Cream	Medline Industries, Inc.
Remedy Olivamine Nutrashield Skin Protectant Cream	Medline Industries, Inc.
Remedy Phytoplex Clear-Aid Ointment	Medline Industries, Inc.
Remedy Phytoplex Hydraguard Silicone Cream	Medline Industries, Inc.
Remedy Phytoplex Z-Guard Paste	Medline Industries, Inc.
Renew Dimethicone	DermaRite Industries, LLC
Renew Lotion Body Cleanser	DermaRite Industries, LLC
Renew PeriProtect	DermaRite Industries, LLC
SECURA Dimethicone Protectant	Smith & Nephew, Inc. Wound Management
SECURA Extra Protective Cream	Smith & Nephew, Inc. Wound Management
SECURA Protective Cream	Smith & Nephew, Inc. Wound Management
SECURA Protective Ointment	Smith & Nephew, Inc. Wound Management
Sensi-Care® Clear Zinc	ConvaTec
Sensi-Care® Protective Barrier	ConvaTec
Shield & Protect™ Anti-Fungal Barrier Cream	Gentell
Shield & Protect™ Barrier Cream	Gentell
Soothe & Cool Cornstarch Body Powder	Medline Industries, Inc.
Soothe & Cool Moisture Guard Skin Protectant	Medline Industries, Inc.
Super Max Barrier Cream	Gentell
Zinc Oxide Ointment	Gentell
3M™ Cavilon™ Durable Barrier Cream	3M Health Care
3M™ Cavilon™ 3-in-1 Incontinence Care Lotion	3M Health Care
4-N-1	DermaRite Industries, LLC

SKIN CLEANSERS

Skin cleansing removes unwanted microorganisms while maintaining the skin's barrier function. The characteristics of skin cleansers vary according to the needs of those using the product. For example, skin cleansers are available as a rinse or no-rinse formulation, an all-in-one product that cleanses, moisturizes, and protects or a variation thereof. In addition, some products are manufactured for cleansing the entire body or only the perineal area. Therefore, when choosing a skin cleanser, it is important to understand the ingredients and total formulation and match the product to the patient's clinical goals.

Because of the variation in coding for skin cleansers, it is the clinician's responsibility to verify coding and payment of each product with the manufacturer.

Product Name	Manufacturer/Distributor
Aloe Vesta Bathing Cloths	ConvaTec
Aloe Vesta Body Wash & Shampoo	ConvaTec
Aloe Vesta Cleansing Foam	ConvaTec
Added: Aloe Vesta Perineal/Skin Cleanser	ConvaTec
AlphaBath Body Oil	DermaRite Industries, LLC
Baza Cleanse & Protect® Lotion	Coloplast
Bedside-Care® EasiCleanse®	Coloplast
Bedside-Care® Foam	Coloplast
Bedside-Care® Sensitive Skin Foam	Coloplast
Bedside-Care® Spray	Coloplast
Bedside-Care® Perineal Wash	Coloplast
Bedside-Care® Sensitive Skin Spray	Coloplast
Clean & Free Rinse-Free Full-Body Wash & Peri-Cleanser	DermaRite Industries, LLC
DermaRain Extra Mild Body Wash & Shampoo	DermaRite Industries, LLC
DermaVera Skin & Hair Cleanser	DermaRite Industries, LLC
Gentle Rain® Extra Mild	Coloplast
Liquid Clean Skin Cleanser	Gentell
PeriFresh Rinse-Free Perineal Cleanser	DermaRite Industries, LLC
PeriGiene	DermaRite Industries, LLC
Perineal Spray	Gentell
Remedy Olivamine Cleansing Body Lotion	Medline Industries, Inc.
Remedy Olivamine Foaming Body Cleanser	Medline Industries, Inc.
Remedy Phytoplex Hydrating No-Rinse Cleansing Foam	Medline Industries, Inc.
Remedy Phytoplex Hydrating Shampoo & Body Wash	Medline Industries, Inc.

Product Name	Manufacturer/Distributor
Remedy Phytoplex Hydrating Spray Cleanser	Medline Industries, Inc.
Remedy Phytoplex Cleansing Body Lotion	Medline Industries, Inc.
Remedy Essentials Shampoo & Body Wash Gel	Medline Industries, Inc.
Remedy Essentials No-Rinse Cleansing Spray	Medline Industries, Inc.
Remedy No-Rinse Cleansing Foam	Medline Industries, Inc.
Soothe & Cool Foaming Body Cleanser No-Rinse	Medline Industries, Inc.
Soothe & Cool Shampoo & Body Wash	Medline Industries, Inc.
Soothe & Cool Total Body Cleanser, No Rinse	Medline Industries, Inc.
SECURA Moisturizing Cleanser	Smith & Nephew, Inc. Wound Management
SECURA Personal Cleanser	Smith & Nephew, Inc. Wound Management
SECURA Total Body Foam Cleanser	Smith & Nephew, Inc. Wound Management
Sensi-Care® Body Wash & Shampoo	ConvaTec
Sensi-Care® Perineal/Skin Cleanser	ConvaTec
Sensi-Care® Skin Protectant Incontinence Wipes	ConvaTec
Soothe & Cool Shampoo & Body Wash	Medline Industries, Inc.
3-N-1 Cleansing Foam	DermaRite Industries, LLC
3M™ Cavilon™ No-Rinse Skin Cleanser	3M Health Care
3M™ Cavilon™ 3-in-1 Incontinence Care Lotion	3M Health Care
TotalBath Skin & Hair Cleanser	DermaRite Industries, LLC
TotalFoam Foam Body Wash & Shampoo with Aloe Vera	DermaRite Industries, LLC
Renew Full-Body Foaming Cleanser	DermaRite Industries, LLC
Renew Hair & Body Wash	DermaRite Industries, LLC

SURGICAL DRESSING HOLDER, NON-REUSABLE, EACH

Surgical dressing holders are nonreusable, hypoallergenic products used in place of standard surgical tapes to avoid removing and reapplying tape during dressing changes.

The HCPCS code normally assigned to abdominal dressing holders or binders is A4461. It is the clinician's responsibility to verify the coding and payment of each product with the manufacturer.

Product Name	Manufacturer/Distributor
Medfix Montgomery Straps	Medline Industries, Inc.

TAPES

Securing a wound cover is an essential step in the management process. One way to secure a wound cover is with the use of tapes. Each product is manufactured using various materials, widths, adhesives, and hypoallergenic properties.

It is the clinician's responsibility to verify the coding and payment of each product with the manufacturer. The HCPCS codes normally assigned tapes and closures are:

A4450: Nonwaterproof, per 18 in^2.

A4452: Waterproof, per 18 in^2.

Product Name	Manufacturer/Distributor
• = New Product	
Medfix Dressing Retention Tape	Medline Industries, Inc.
Medfix EZ Dressing Retention Tape	Medline Industries, Inc.
Mefix® Self-Adhesive Fabric Tape	Mölnlycke Health Care
• Mepitac® Self Adherent Comfortable Fixation Tape	Mölnlycke Health Care
3M™ Blenderm™ Surgical Tape	3M Health Care
3M™ Durapore™ Surgical Tape	3M Health Care
3M™ Kind Removal Silicone Tape	3M Health Care
3M™ Medipore™ H Solf Cloth Surgical Tape	3M Health Care
3M™ Medipore™ Dress-It Pre-cut Dressing Covers	3M Health Care
3M™ Medipore™ Soft Cloth Surgical Tape	3M Health Care
3M™ Microfoam™ Surgical Tape	3M Health Care
3M™ Micropore™ Tan Surgical Tape	3M Health Care
3M™ Micropore™ Surgical Tape	3M Health Care
3M™ Transpore™ Surgical Tape	3M Health Care
3M™ Transpore™ White Surgical Tape	3M Health Care
3M™ Multipore™ Dry Surgical Tape	3M Health Care
• Cloth Tape	DUKAL Corporation
• Paper Tape	DUKAL Corporation
• Retention Tape	DUKAL Corporation
• Transparent Tape	DUKAL Corporation
• FixTape™	Gentell
• Gentac Silicone Tape	Medline Industries, Inc.
• Pinc Tape	Medline Industries, Inc.
• PRIMAFIX Plus Retention Tape	Smith & Nephew
• RiteFix Non-woven Dressing Retention Tape	• DermaRite Industries, LLC
• ComfiTape Silicone Adhesive Tape	• DermaRite Industries, LLC

THERAPEUTIC MOISTURIZERS

One of the main functions of the skin is to hold in moisture. The epidermis produces lipids, oily substances that limit the passage of water into or out of the skin. If the skin is deficient in lipids, moisture can escape. The loss of moisture causes dry, flaky, itchy skin. Therapeutic moisturizers replace skin lipids and maintain skin hydration. These products can be found as creams, lotions, or ointments with or without an antimicrobial ingredient. Common ingredients found in therapeutic moisturizers include emollients and humectants. Some products are applied daily while other products are indicated to be applied more frequently.

Because of the variation in coding for therapeutic moisturizers, it is the clinician's responsibility to verify the coding and payment of each product with the manufacturer.

Product Name	Manufacturer/Distributor
Aloe Vesta® Daily Moisturizer	ConvaTec
AMERIGEL® Care Lotion	AMERX Health Care Corporation
Atrac-Tain® Cream	Coloplast
DermaCerin Moisturizing Cream	DermaRite Industries, LLC
DermaDaily Moisturizing Lotion	DermaRite Industries, LLC
DermaPhor Moisturizing Ointment	DermaRite Industries, LLC
DermaSarra Anti-Itch Lotion	DermaRite Industries, LLC
DermaVantage Moisturizing Lotion	DermaRite Industries, LLC
LubriSilk Dry Skin Care Lotion	DermaRite Industries, LLC
Remedy Olivamine Skin Repair Cream	Medline Industries, Inc.
Remedy Phytoplex Nourishing Skin Cream	Medline Industries, Inc.
Renew Skin Repair Cream	DermaRite Industries, LLC
Restore Cleanser & Moisturizer	Hollister Wound Care
SECURA Moisturizing Cream	Smith & Nephew, Inc. Wound Management
SECURA Moisturizing Lotion	Smith & Nephew, Inc. Wound Management
Sensi-Care® Body Cream	ConvaTec
Remedy Essentials Moisturizing Body Lotion	Medline Industries, Inc.
Soothe & Cool Herbal Moisturizing Body Lotion	Medline Industries, Inc.
Soothe & Cool Moisturizing Body Lotion	Medline Industries, Inc.
Soothe & Cool Skin Cream	Medline Industries, Inc.
Sween Cream®	Coloplast
Sween® 24 Cream	Coloplast
Sween® Lotion	Coloplast
3M™ Cavilon™ Extra Dry Skin Cream	3M Health Care
3M™ Cavilon™ Moisturizing Hand Lotion	3M Health Care
3M™ Cavilon™ 3-in-1 Incontinence Care Lotion	3M Health Care
Remedy Intensive Skin Therapy Skin Repair Cream	Medline Industries, Inc.

WOUND CLEANSERS

Wound cleansers are an essential step in wound management. These solutions are used to remove debris or foreign materials from the wound. Each cleanser listed provides the health care professional with proactive products for positive outcomes.

It is the clinician's responsibility to verify the coding and payment of each product with the manufacturer. The HCPCS code normally assigned wound cleansers is: A6260—any type, any size.

Product Name	Manufacturer/Distributor
• = New Product	
AMERIGEL® Saline Wound Wash	AMERX Health Care Corporation
• Anasept® Antimicrobial Skin and Wound Cleanser	Anacapa Technologies, Inc.
• Anasept® Antimicrobial Wound Irrigation Solution	Anacapa Technologies, Inc.
CarraKlenz Wound and Skin Cleanser	Medline Industries, Inc.
DermaKlenz Wound Cleanser	DermaRite Industries
DERMAL WOUND CLEANSER	Smith & Nephew, Wound Management Division
• Vashe® Wound Solution	SteadMed Medical
MicroKlenz Antimicrobial First Aid Antiseptic	Medline Industries, Inc.
• Prontosan® Wound Irrigation Solution 40 mL	• B. Braun Medical Inc.
• Prontosan® Wound Irrigation Solution, 350 mL	• B. Braun Medical Inc.
• Prontosan® Wound Gel	• B. Braun Medical Inc.
• Prontosan® Wound Gel X	• B. Braun Medical Inc.
• Prophase Wound Cleanser	• Medline Industries, Inc
Restore Wound Cleanser	Hollister Wound Care
SAF-Clens AF Dermal Wound Cleanser	ConvaTec
SafeWash Saline	DermaRite Industries, LLC
Sea-Clens® Wound Cleanser	Coloplast
Skintegrity Wound Cleanser	Medline Industries, Inc.
3M™ Tegaderm™ Wound Cleanser	3M™ Health Care
UltraKlenz Wound and Skin Cleanser	Medline Industries, Inc.
Wound Cleanser	Gentell

Manufacturer Resource Guide

3M
www.3m.com/medical

Acelity
www.acelity.com

Allosource
www.allosource.org

AMERX Health Care Corp.
www.amerxhc.com

Amniox Medical
www.amnioxmedical.com

Anacapa Technologies, Inc.
www.anacapa-tech.net

Aroa Biosurgery Limited
Marketed in the US by Appulse
www.aroabio.com

B. Braun Medical Inc.
www.BBraunUSA.com

Celularity Inc.
www.ultramist.com
www.celularity.com

Coloplast
www.coloplast.us

ConvaTec
www.convatec.com

DermaRite Industries, LLC
www.dermarite.com

DeRoyal
www.deroyal.com

DUKAL Corporation
www.dukal.com

ETS Wound Care LLC
www.etswoundcare.com

Ferris Mfg. Corp.
www.PolyMem.com

Gentell
www.gentell.com

Hollister Incorporated
www.hollister.com

Kerecis
www.kerecis.com

medi USA
www.mediusa.com

Medline Industries, Inc.
www.medline.com

Millennium Health, LLC
www.cogendx.com

MiMedx Group, Inc.
www.mimedx.com

Molnlycke
www.molnlycke.us

Orthomerica Products, Inc.
www.orthomerica.com

Osiris Therapeutics, Inc.
www.osiris.com/

OSNovative Systems, Inc.
www.enluxtrawoundcare.com

Senergy Medical Group
www.senergy.us

Smith & Nephew, Inc.
www.smith-nephew.com

Southwest Technologies, Inc.
www.elastogel.com

TRX BioSurgery
www.tissueregenixus.com

Urgo Medical
www.urgomedical.us

Vasamed Inc.
www.vasamed.com

Wound Care Innovations, LLC
www.sanaramedtech.com

Index

---

t refers to a table.

t refers to a table.